NEPHROLOGY RESEARCH AND CLINICAL DEVELOPMENTS

ESSENTIALS AND UPDATES IN UROLOGIC ONCOLOGY (2 VOLUME SET)

VOLUME 2

PHILIPPE E. SPIESS
EDITOR-IN-CHIEF

MATHEW BIAGIOLI
MAYER FISHMAN
JORGE LOCKHART
JULIO M. POW-SANG
WADE J. SEXTON
ASSOCIATE EDITORS

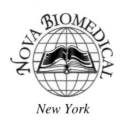

New York

NOTICE TO THE READER

The Publisher has taken reasonable care in the preparation of this book, but makes no expressed or implied warranty of any kind and assumes no responsibility for any errors or omissions. No liability is assumed for incidental or consequential damages in connection with or arising out of information contained in this book. The Publisher shall not be liable for any special, consequential, or exemplary damages resulting, in whole or in part, from the readers' use of, or reliance upon, this material. Any parts of this book based on government reports are so indicated and copyright is claimed for those parts to the extent applicable to compilations of such works.

Independent verification should be sought for any data, advice or recommendations contained in this book. In addition, no responsibility is assumed by the publisher for any injury and/or damage to persons or property arising from any methods, products, instructions, ideas or otherwise contained in this publication.

This publication is designed to provide accurate and authoritative information with regard to the subject matter covered herein. It is sold with the clear understanding that the Publisher is not engaged in rendering legal or any other professional services. If legal or any other expert assistance is required, the services of a competent person should be sought. FROM A DECLARATION OF PARTICIPANTS JOINTLY ADOPTED BY A COMMITTEE OF THE AMERICAN BAR ASSOCIATION AND A COMMITTEE OF PUBLISHERS.

Additional color graphics may be available in the e-book version of this book.

Library of Congress Cataloging-in-Publication Data

ISBN: 978-1-62081-494-9

Library of Congress Control Number: 2012936705

Published by Nova Science Publishers, Inc. † New York

Contents

Volume 2

Section 5. Kidney Cancer

Toni K. Choueiri and Philippe E. Spiess
Section Editors

In: Essentials and Updates in Urologic Oncology
Editor: Philippe E. Spiess

ISBN: 978-1-62081-494-9
© 2013 Nova Science Publishers, Inc.

Chapter XXII

Epidemiology and Risk Factors for Renal Cell Carcinoma

Sandhya R. Rao and Philippe E. Spiess
Department of Genitourinary Oncology,
Moffitt Cancer Center, Tampa, Florida, US

Abstract

Renal cell carcinoma (RCC) which accounts for nearly 90% of all renal malignancies has been steadily rising in incidence in both the United States and most European countries over the last several decades. In the United States, this increase has been noted across all racial and age groups. Smoking, obesity, hypertension, the rising incidence of medical renal disease, and germline mutations may account for these increasing rates of RCC. This chapter will give some insight into the epidemiology, clinical presentation, staging, and proposed risk factors for RCC.

Introduction

Kidney cancer consists of malignant tumors arising from the renal parenchyma. Kidney cancer is the ninth most common cancer in developed countries accounting for approximately 2% of all malignancies worldwide. In 2011, 60,920 new cases and 13,120 deaths are expected from kidney cancer within the U.S. [1] RCC accounts for approximately 90% of all renal malignancies. Approximately 80% of renal cell cancers are clear cell adenocarcinomas, the remainder being papillary (15%), chromophobe (5%), and collecting duct carcinomas or other rare variant histologies (<1%).

Descriptive Epidemiology

Incidence

Globally, the incidence of kidney cancer varies more than 10-fold between populations and geographic areas suggesting a strong role of lifestyle factors as well as genetic predisposition. [2] The highest rates of RCC are found in North America, Europe, and Australia, with the lowest incidences in Asia and Africa. In Europe, there have been regional differences in rates and trends over time, with the higher rates remaining in several countries across central and eastern Europe, whereas rates have been declining in Sweden, Poland, Finland and the Netherlands. [3] In the United States, the incidence rates for RCC have been rising steadily for more than 3 decades and the annual incidence rose by 2.6% per year from 1997 to 2007. [4] RCC is more common in men than in women regardless of racial/ethnic origins, with a male to female ratio of 2:1. In the United States, increases in incidence have been more rapid however in females than in males and in African Americans than in Caucasians. [5, 6]

Both the increasing incidence observed over the past decades in almost all areas and the geographic and racial differences could be in large part be due to better imaging modalities which has led to an increase in incidentally detected RCCs, which tend to be at a lower stage and more likely localized and asymptomatic. An increasing incidence has however been noted in large and advanced stage renal cell tumors accounting in good part for the overall increase in incidence. [6-8]

Mortality

The worldwide mortality rates of kidney cancer were estimated to be 116,000 in 2008 constituting 1.5% of all cancer deaths. Similarly the incidence and mortality rates vary considerably among various geographical regions. In the United States, it was estimated that 13,000 deaths from kidney cancer occurred in 2010, making it the tenth most common cause of cancer deaths among men. [9] Death rates were highest among American Indians and Alaska Natives. Among women, mortality rates were in general about half of those of men.

In Europe, death rates increased until the early 1990s and thereafter declined or stabilized. [10] Nevertheless, at the turn of the century, there was a greater than threefold difference in kidney cancer mortality rates within Europe, with high rates remaining in the Czech Republic and Baltic countries and the lowest rates in Greece, Spain, Portugal, and Romania. [10, 11]

The diagnosis of RCC presenting as smaller tumors and at an earlier clinical stage may also be responsible for the recent plateauing in mortality rates within the United States and many European nations. The decreased mortality rates among patients presenting with advanced stage RCC could have also resulted from improved systemic therapies and multimodal treatment approaches to advanced disease.

Survival

Relative survival rates for kidney cancer are higher in the United States than in Europe. [13] From 2000 to 2002, data using 47 European cancer registries (EUROCARE-4), reported a mean 5-year relative survival for kidney cancer of 55.7% compared to 62.6% reported from 13 U.S. SEER registries. [12] In the United States, the 5-year survival rates for RCC increased from 1983 to 2002 across all clinical stages. The improvement in survival was most prominent for patients with small tumors less than 2 cm. [13] For localized disease, survival rates increased from 91.7% in 1988 to 92.8% in 2002 with no change in rates for regional (63.7% to 64.2%) and distant metastatic disease (12.1% to 11.9%) respectively. [14] Across all tumor stages and genders, African Americans generally had lower 5-year relative survival rates than Caucasians.

Clinical Presentation

The three classic diagnostic features of RCC are abdominal pain, a palpable mass, and hematuria, but these signs and symptoms are rarely seen and typically denote advanced disease. [15] The most reliable of the three is hematuria, but it is usually intermittent and may be microscopic; thus, the tumor may remain silent until it attains a large size and clinical stage. Spontaneous perirenal hemorrhage is a less common but important presentation of RCC. The widespread use of ultrasonography and CT has led to an increase in incidentally detected RCCs which tend to be of a lower clinical stage and more likely localized and asymptomatic at diagnosis. [16] Other indicators of advanced disease include generalized constitutional symptoms, such as fever, malaise, weakness, weight loss and night sweats, and the physical examination findings of palpable cervical lymphadenopathy, nonreducing varicocele (typically right sided) , and bilateral lower extremity edema due to venous involvement. Symptoms can also be directly related to metastatic disease, such as bone pain, new onset seizures or sensory/motor deficits, and persistent cough or hemoptysis.

RCC is sometimes termed the "internist's tumor", because it tends to produce a diversity of systemic symptoms not related to the kidney itself. In addition to fever and constitutional symptoms as mentioned earlier, RCC can present as a number of paraneoplastic syndromes, ascribed to abnormal hormone production. [17-19]

Hypercalcemia has been reported in up to 13% of patients with RCC and can be due to either a paraneoplastic syndrome or metastatic bone lesions. The etiology of hypercalcemia resulting from a paraneoplastic syndrome most commonly results from parathormone related peptide secretion. [20] The signs and symptoms of hypercalcemia are often nonspecific and include nausea, anorexia, fatigue, and decreased deep tendon reflexes. Other paraneoplastic syndromes include hypertension and polycythemia. Hypertension is related to increased production of renin directly by the tumor; compression or encasement of the renal artery or an arteriovenous fistula within the tumor. [17, 21] Polycythemia is attributed to increased production of erythropoietin. [22, 23] Stauffer syndrome also termed non-metastatic hepatic dysfunction has been reported in between 3% to 20% of RCC cases. [24-26] It is characterized by elevation of alkaline phosphatase, erythrocyte sedimentation rate, alpha-2 globulin, and gamma-glutamyl transferase, thrombocytopenia, prolongation of prothrombin time, and hepatosplenomegaly, in the absence of hepatic metastasis. Elevated serum levels of IL-6 have been found in patients with Stauffer syndrome, and it is believed that this and other cytokines may play a role in the pathogenesis of this disorder. Hepatic function typically normalizes after nephrectomy in 60% to 70% of cases. Persistence or recurrence of hepatic dysfunction is almost always indicative of the presence of viable tumor and thus represents a poor prognostic finding.[17]

Tumor Histology and Grading and Clinical Staging

Tumor Histology

An updated classification of malignant epithelial tumors of the kidney was presented by the World Health Organization in 2004 based on pathology and genetic abnormalities. RCC was recognized as comprising several different tumor subtypes each having a distinct genetic basis and unique clinical features. The classification of RCC is based on correlative cytogenetic, genetic, and histologic studies of both familial and sporadic tumors. [26, 27] It is now clear that all these tumors arise from the renal tubular epithelium. The major tumour histological types are as follows:

Clear cell carcinoma. This is the most common histology, accounting for 70% to 80% of RCC. [27] The tumors are made up of cells with clear or granular cytoplasm and are nonpapillary. The majority (95%) are sporadic though they can be familial. In 98% of these tumors, whether familial, sporadic, or associated with VHL, there is loss of genetic sequences on the short arm of chromosome 3. Grossly, these tumors are typically yellow /tanned with hemorrhagic areas when they are bivalved. On microscopic examination, clear cell RCC can include clear cell, granular cell, or mixed types. Clear cell RCC has a worse prognosis when compared with chromophobe or papillary histologic subtypes. [28, 29]

Papillary RCC is the second most common histologic subtype, accounting for 10% to 15% of renal cancers and is frequently multicentric in origin. It is characterized by a papillary growth pattern and also occurs in both familial and sporadic forms. The most common cytogenetic abnormalities are trisomies 7, 16, 17, and loss of chromosome Y in male patients in the sporadic form, and trisomy 7 in the familial form. Two variants have been described: Type 1 papillary RCC, the more common form, consisting of basophilic cells with scant cytoplasm and type 2 papillary RCC include potentially more aggressive variants with eosinophilic cells and an abundant granular cytoplasm [30, 31] These two subtypes correspond with two familial RCC syndromes: hereditary papillary RCC syndrome (type 1) and hereditary leiomyomatosis and RCC syndrome (type 2). [32]

Chromophobe RCC represents 3% to 5% of RCC and is composed of cells with prominent cell membranes and pale eosinophilic cytoplasm with a fine reticular pattern that has been described as a "plant cell" appearance, usually with a halo formation around the nucleus. Eosinophilic variants of chromophobic RCC have also been described and constitute about 30% of cases. Electron microscopy reveals numerous 150- to 300-nm microvesicles which stain positive for Hale colloidal iron and are the defining feature of chromophobe RCC. [33] On cytogenetic examination these tumors show multiple chromosome losses and extreme hypodiploidy i.e. chromosome number less than diploid number. Chromophobe RCC is thought to be derived from the intercalated cells of the collecting duct, exhibiting alterations of mitochondria that are frequently observed in the oncocytosis, (a spectrum of changes in the kidneys harboring oncocytomas. It includes multifocal oncocytic transformation of renal tubules, which may undergo cystic transformation, and infiltration of neoplastic oncocytes among tubules) with or without Birt-Hogg-Dubé (BHD) syndrome. A histologic distinction from renal oncocytoma can be difficult and requires careful histological evaluation and use of immunostains. Chromophobe RCC has a better prognosis compared to clear cell and papillary histological subtypes with more than 90% of patients remaining cancer-free 5 or more years following treatment. However, high-grade tumors, including those exhibiting sarcomatoid differentiation or metastatic spread have a poorer outcome.

Collecting duct (Bellini duct) carcinoma (CDC) represents approximately 1% or less of renal epithelial neoplasms arising from collecting duct cells within the renal medulla. They frequently occur in younger patients in the third, fourth, or fifth decades of life and the majority present with metastatic disease typically displaying Fuhrman grade 3 or 4 nuclear features. [34] CDC are usually centrally located in the kidney, ranging in size from 2.5 to 12 cm and exhibiting a firm grey-white gross appearance. Upper tract imaging often may suggest an urothelial carcinoma rather than RCC. Several chromosomal losses and deletions have been described with this tumor histology, but a distinguishing genetic pattern has not yet been characterized. Histologically these tumors are characterized by nests of malignant cells enmeshed within a prominent fibrotic stroma, typically located in the renal medulla.

Renal medullary carcinoma is a rapidly growing rare tumor within the renal medulla regarded as an aggressive variant of CDC. [27] It occurs almost exclusively in young black males with the sickle cell trait often presenting within the third decade of life. [35] Many cases are both locally-advanced and metastatic at the time of diagnosis portending a poor prognosis. [36]

Other RCC Histologies

Renal carcinoma associated with Xp11.2 translocations/TFE3 gene fusions, renal cell carcinoma associated with neuroblastoma, mucinous and tubular, spindle cell carcinoma, and renal cell carcinoma, unclassified RCC are other uncommon histologic subtypes which have been described as well.

Grading

Several grading systems for RCC have been proposed based on tumor cell cytoplasmic and/or architectural features. The four-tiered Fuhrman nuclear grading system has been most frequently utilized and is now recognized as an independent prognostic factor for clear cell RCC in particular (Table 1). [37] Tumor grade is assigned according to the highest grade present. Recent studies have indicated that grading of papillary RCC should be based on nucleolar prominence alone and that the components of the Fuhrman grading classification do not provide prognostic information for the chromophobe RCC histology. [38, 39]

Table 1. Fuhrman's Classification System for Nuclear Grading in RCC

GRADE	NUCLEAR SIZE	NUCLEAR OUTLINE	NUCLEOLI
1	10 mm	Round, uniform	Absent or inconspicuous
2	15 mm	Irregular	Small
3	20 mm	Irregular	Prominent
4	≥20 mm	Bizarre, often multilobed	Prominent, heavy chromatin clumps

Staging

Staging of RCC is assigned based on the Union Internationale Contre le Cancer/American Joint Committee on Cancer (UICC/AJCC) 2010 classification of primary RCC. The TNM classification for RCC has undergone several modifications in the past 3 decades (in 1987, 1993, 1997, 2002, and most recently in 2010) in an effort to more accurately reflect tumor biology, prognosis, and guide treatment recommendations.

T stage: In 1987, the size cut-off between T1 and T2 was established at 2.5 cm, but was later demonstrated to have little prognostic value. [40] In 1997, this cut off of 2.5 cm between T1 and T2 was increased to 7 cm whereby improving the prognostic validity of this staging system. Analysis of the Surveillance, Epidemiology, and End Results (SEER) program database demonstrated survival differences between 5, 7.5, and 10 cm tumor diameter cut points, and the 7 cm cut point between stages T1 and T2 was adopted because it reflected the mean tumor size in the database thus nicely stratifying RCC patients and their outcomes. [41, 42] In 2002, the T1 clinical stage was subdivided into T1a and T1b substages, separated by a size cut-off of 4 cm reflecting excellent treatment outcomes for patients with small (≤4 cm), unilateral, renal tumors managed by either partial or radical nephrectomy.[43, 44[

The most recent change in 2010 was a subdivision of T2 tumors: T2a tumors between 7 and 10 cm, and T2b representing tumors greater than 10 cm, but confined to the renal parenchyma, supported by a number of studies demonstrating prognostic relevance of this size cut off. [45-48]

This change was validated in a multicentric study by Novara et al. who concluded that the latest changes in the clinical staging system for RCC are a powerful predictor of cancer specific survival (CSS). [49]

Other major revisions were as well made to the staging system. Contiguous extension of tumor into the ipsilateral adrenal gland is now classified as T4 and metastatic involvement of either adrenal gland as M1, reflecting likely patterns of tumor dissemination. The decision to classify direct adrenal invasion as stage T4 was driven by several studies, all of which demonstrated that tumors with adrenal invasion had the same aggressive clinical behavior of those extending beyond Gerota's fascia. [50, 51]

Moreover, tumors with renal vein involvement or perinephric fat involvement were downstaged from stage T3b to stage T3a because of the more favorable prognosis of isolated renal venous tumor thrombus. Any nodal involvement is now classified as N1 regardless of the number of nodes involved because the prognostic relevance of the previous version was not observed.

Risk Factors

Cigarette Smoking

Cigarette smoking is considered to be a causal risk factor for RCC by both the International Agency for Research on Cancer (IARC) and the U.S. Surgeon General. [52, 53] Approximately 20% to 30% of renal cell cancers among men and 10% to 20% among women are estimated to be attributable to cigarette smoking. A meta-analysis of 24 studies (19 case controlled and 5 cohort) studies demonstrated a relative risk of developing RCC of 1.38 for smokers compared to non-smokers. [54] Compared to non-smokers, smoking increased the risk of RCC by 54% among men and 22% among women. [55] The association between smoking and RCC is however relatively weak, but a clear dose–response relationship is evident with the risk doubling among men and increasing 58% among women who smoked more than a pack of cigarettes per day. Smoking fewer cigarettes per day for a longer number of years posted a greater RCC risk than smoking at a higher frequency for a shorter duration of time. Smoking cessation encouragingly reduces the risk, but only among long-term quitters of 10 years or more. [56]

Cigarette smoke has a wide range of carcinogenic compounds including polycyclic aromatic hydrocarbons, aromatic amines, heterocyclic amines, and N-nitrosamines which can both initiate and promote tumor development in animals. Cigarette smoking is hypothesized to increase RCC risk through chronic tissue hypoxia due to carbon monoxide exposure and smoking-related conditions such as chronic obstructive pulmonary disease. [57] In addition, RCC patients were shown to have a higher level of DNA damage in their peripheral blood lymphocytes induced by a tobacco-specific N-nitrosamine compared to control subjects. Deletions in chromosome 3p, a frequent site of genetic alterations in RCC, were also shown to be more common in cultured peripheral blood lymphocyte cells from RCC patients than in control subjects after being exposed to benzol-pyrene diol epoxide, a major constituent of cigarette smoke. [58]

Hypertension

Hypertension has been associated with the risk of RCC in several large prospective cohort studies. [59-62] One case–control and three cohort studies observed an increased risk of RCC with elevated blood pressure, with a clear dose–response relationship reported in two of the studies. [59, 61-63] Individuals with systolic blood pressures $\geq$ 160 mm Hg or diastolic pressures $\geq$ 100 mm Hg were found to have a two-fold or higher risk compared to individuals with a systolic blood pressure below 120 mmHg and a diastolic blood pressure below 80 mmHg, respectively. The contributions of blood pressure level and antihypertensive medication use independent of each other have been difficult to decipher since most studies are based on a diagnosis of hypertension that is inevitably linked to treatment with antihypertensive medication. However, the current evidence suggests that it is hypertension in and of itself and not the medication that is the main determinant of RCC risk.

Although there is a high correlation between obesity and hypertension, their associations with RCC risk have been shown to be independent of each other. The risk among individuals who are both obese and hypertensive is higher than those who have only one of these conditions. The mechanism by which high blood pressure may affect RCC risk remains unclear. It has been hypothesized that hypertension-induced renal injury and metabolic or functional changes within the renal tubule induced by hypertension increases its susceptibility to carcinogens. Chronic renal hypoxia and lipid peroxidation with formation of reactive oxygen species has also been implicated. [64]

Obesity

RCC has been consistently associated with obesity in most case-control test and cohort studies that have evaluated this relationship including recent large prospective studies in the Netherlands, Norway, and the United States. Although early studies showed the association primarily in women, most studies have demonstrated a dose-response relationship with increasing body mass index (BMI) that is equally strong in men and women. [65,66] A meta-analysis of 17 epidemiologic studies showed that every 5 kg/m^2 increase in BMI increases the risk of RCC by 24% in men and 34% in women. Studies investigating body fat distribution also suggest an increased risk of RCC with increasing waist circumference or waist-to-hip ratio but evidence is insufficient to conclude that abdominal obesity is a risk factor for RCC independently of BMI or total body weight. [67-69] Limited data suggest an increased risk of RCC with weight gain or weight fluctuations. Most studies found a dose-response relationship with increasing BMI. Waist circumference and waist-to-hip ratio provide an estimate of abdominal or centripetal obesity, a powerful contributor to metabolic abnormalities such as insulin resistance and hyperinsulinemia.

The increasing prevalence of obesity may partly explain the overall increased incidence of RCC but does not explain the recent plateauing of incidence RCC noted in some countries. The proportion of RCC cases directly attributable to obesity and overweight has been estimated to be about 40% in the US and Canada and up to about 30% in most European countries. [70-72]

The mechanisms by which obesity influences renal carcinogenesis is unclear, but several plausible hypotheses have been proposed. These include chronic tissue hypoxia, insulin resistance, increased levels of growth factors such as insulin-like growth factor 1 (IGF-I) and high circulating levels of leptin and a compensatory hyperinsulinemia, obesity-induced inflammatory response, lipid peroxidation, and oxidative stress. [73,74] Obesity may act by promoting hormonal changes, such as increased peptide levels, and steroid hormones and the production of adipokines which are cytokines (cell-to-cell signaling proteins) secreted by adipose tissue. Sex steroid hormones may affect renal cell proliferation and growth by direct endocrine receptor-mediated effects, by the regulation of receptor concentrations, or through paracrine growth factors such as epidermal growth factor. Further, obesity is related to several endocrine disorders such as decreased levels of sex hormone-binding globulin and progesterone, anovulation, and insulin resistance. Lower adiponectin levels have also been observed among RCC patients as compared to healthy controls. Obesity may also predispose to a higher glomerular filtration rate and renal plasma flow independent of hypertension as well as to nephrosclerosis, which may in turn render the kidney more susceptible to carcinogenesis. Other conjectured mechanisms for this association include elevated cholesterol levels and down-regulation of the low-density lipoprotein receptor, lower levels of vitamin D, and increases in adipose tissue-derived hormones and cytokines such as leptin and adiponectin. [70,75]

Physical Activity

Data examining the relationship between physical activity and RCC risk are still limited, but most studies suggest an inverse association between the risk of RCC and leisure time and/or occupational activity levels. The inverse trend was observed for current exercise, routine physical activity, recreational activity, or a composite of energy expenditure within a typical day. [74,75] Physical activity may decrease RCC risk through a number of related pathways including lowering body weight and blood pressure, improving insulin sensitivity, and reducing chronic inflammation and oxidative stress. [65,76-78]

Diet and Nutrition

Fruits and Vegetables

Diets rich in fruits and vegetables contain putative anticarcinogenic and antimutagenic substances and have been proposed to potentially prevent cancer. However, convincing evidence for a protective role of these dietary components in cancer development is currently lacking for most malignancies, including RCC. Although high fruit and vegetable consumption was associated with a decreased risk of RCC in a pooled analysis of several cohort studies other large prospective studies have failed to validate such an association. [79]

Alcohol and Other Beverages

Recent studies suggest that alcohol consumption is inversely associated with RCC risk in a dose- dependent manner although the association is not statistically significant. [80, 81]

There was an estimated 28% reduction in risk among those who drank ≥15 gram/day, equivalent to slightly more than one alcoholic drink per day. [82] The inverse association was observed for all types of alcoholic drinks, including beer, wine, and liquor. A potential mechanism by which moderate consumption of alcohol may decrease RCC cancer risk is proposed through an improvement in insulin sensitivity whereby lowering the risk of type 2 diabetes, production of insulin-like growth factor-I, and the subsequent risk of RCC. [83] In contrast, total fluid intake from all beverages, including coffee, tea, milk, juice, soda, and water, has not been consistently linked to the risk of RCC. Data on other beverages including coffee, tea, soft drinks or juices are therefore inconclusive at this time.

Meat and Fish

Meat intake has been hypothesized to elevate the risk of RCC, presumably because of its content of fat and protein. Constituents of cooked meat such as heterocyclic amines, polycyclic aromatic hydrocarbons, and amongst cured meat, nitrites and nitrates may mediate renal carcinogenesis. [84, 85] Although many case-controlled studies found a positive association between the consumption of poultry, processed meat, red meat, and all meat products with RCC, prospective studies from both North America and Europe were not corroborative. In addition, a prospective Swedish cohort study reported a lower risk of RCC among women with high consumption of fatty fish products. [86]

Other Medical Conditions and Medications

End-Stage Renal Disease

The incidence of RCC in patients with end-stage renal disease (ESRD) developing acquired renal cystic disease (ARCD) is reported to be 3 to 6 times higher than in the general population. [87] The age at RCC development in such patients is younger and the ratio of male to female is higher amongst patients with ESRD. An increased risk of RCC has also been seen in the native kidney among renal transplant patients which is presumed to be a result of the immunosuppressing medications such patients are placed on. [88-90] Proliferation of proximal tubular epithelial cells is the chief pathogenic mechanism of cyst formation but hormones, growth factors, and their receptors may stimulate cell proliferation and promote subsequent carcinogenesis. Type 2 diabetes mellitus has as well been linked to RCC risk in several studies, but whether its role is independent of those of obesity and hypertension is controversial. Survivors of certain childhood cancers and other malignancies such as esophageal adenocarcinoma have as well been shown to have an increased risk of subsequent RCC development.[91] Similarly, patients with RCC have been shown to have an elevated risk of a second primary neoplasm including RCC of the contralateral kidney. [92, 93] Statins are widely used drugs for the treatment of lipid disorders and have been shown to inhibit renal cancer cell growth *in vitro* and decrease the amount of pulmonary metastasis in animals administered oral doses of statins. However, their potential effectiveness for the primary prevention of cancer is unclear. Although a retrospective study from the US Veteran Affair database reported a 50% reduced risk of RCC among statin users compared to non-users, the influence of dose, duration, and type of statin was not addressed. [94] Use of aspirin and other nonsteroidal anti-inflammatory drugs has as well not been consistently associated with RCC risk though this association has been hypothesized.

Reproductive Factors and Hormones

Some retrospective studies have shown that oral contraceptive use among nonsmokers was associated with a decreased risk of RCC. [95,96] Several case-controlled and prospective cohort studies have found a positive correlation between RCC and high parity. [95,97] Mechanisms underlying this observed association however remain unclear although pregnancy-induced hypertension, and renal stress, along with hormonal fluctuations of pregnancy may play a role. [98]

Genetic Factors

RCC occurs in both sporadic and hereditary forms. Having a first degree relative with kidney cancer has been associated with a two- to four-fold increased risk of RCC in most contemporary studies. [99] Approximately, 2–3% of RCC can be directly attributable to inherited genetic defects.

In this regard, four familial renal cell carcinoma syndromes have been described. The von Hippel–Lindau (VHL) syndrome is a dominantly inherited multi-organ disorder presenting with potential tumors in the kidneys, pancreas, adrenal glands, epididymis, eyes, spine, and cerebellum. [100] The cumulative risk of RCC in such patients is more than 70% by the age of 60 years, and RCC is the most common cause of death. [101] The VHL tumor-suppressor gene which is located on the short arm of chromosome 3p is inactivated by one of several mechanisms including mutation and silencing by DNA methylation.[102] This gene is exclusively involved in conventional (clear cell) RCC. Hereditary papillary RCC caused by mutations in the c-Met proto-oncogene has been associated with type 1 papillary RCC.[103]

Familial leiomyomatosis and RCC linked to mutations in the fumarate hydratase gene has been associated with type 2 papillary RCC with a propensity for aggressive tumor biology. Such patients can present with cutaneous leiomyomas, and women often have a history of hysterectomy for uterine bleeding. [104, 105]

BHD syndrome caused by mutations in the folliculin tumor suppressor gene and associated with a spectrum of RCC of varying histologic subtypes (chromophobe, clear cell, or papillary) has as well been described. [102, 106]

Conclusion

Much of the recent increases in incidence of RCC is attributable to the diagnosis of early stage tumors, suggesting that the increased use of abdominal imaging may explain such reported rising incidence rates. The vast majority of currently incidentally detected renal tumors are small, localized, and asymptomatic at the time of diagnosis. Cigarette smoking, obesity and hypertension are well-established risk factors for RCC. Genetic variations may explain current disparities in reported incidence rates of RCC across various patient populations and geographical areas. Continued efforts to decipher the underlying etiology of RCC are greatly needed to better delineate how this malignancy can be obviated in a significant proportion of patients.

References

[1]   Siegel, R., Ward, E., Brawley, O. et al.: Cancer statistics, 2011: the impact of eliminating socioeconomic and racial disparities on premature cancer deaths. *CA Cancer J Clin*, 61: 212, 2011

[2]   Curado,M.P.,et al.: Cancer Incidence in Five Continents,Vol IX. In: *IARC Scientific Publications* No. 160: Lyon:IARC, vol. Vol IX, 2007

[3]   Karim-Kos, H. E., de Vries, E., Soerjomataram, I. et al.: Recent trends of cancer in Europe: a combined approach of incidence, survival and mortality for 17 cancer sites since the 1990s. *Eur J Cancer,* 44: 1345, 2008

[4]   SEER cancer statistics review 1975-2007.national cancer institute.2010. Available at *http://seer.cancer.gov/csr/1975_2007.*

[5]   Chow, W. H., Devesa, S. S., Warren, J. L. et al.: Rising incidence of renal cell cancer in the United States. *JAMA,* 281: 1628, 1999

[6]   Kosary C L, M. J. K.: Kideny and Renal Pelvis. In: *Cancer Statistics Review* 1973-1990. Edited by R. L. Miller B A, Hankey B E National Cancer Institute.: NIH Pub.No 93-2789;, vol. XI-X22, 1993

[7]   Mathew, A., Devesa, S. S., Fraumeni, J. F., Jr. et al.: Global increases in kidney cancer incidence, 1973-1992. *Eur J Cancer Prev,* 11: 171, 2002

[8]   Hollingsworth, J. M., Miller, D. C., Daignault, S. et al.: Rising incidence of small renal masses: a need to reassess treatment effect. *J Natl Cancer Inst,* 98: 1331, 2006

[9]   Jemal, A., Siegel, R., Xu, J. et al.: Cancer statistics, 2010. *CA Cancer J Clin,* 60: 277, 2010

[10] Levi, F., Ferlay, J., Galeone, C. et al.: The changing pattern of kidney cancer incidence and mortality in Europe. *BJU Int,* 101: 949, 2008

[11] Levi, F., Lucchini, F., Negri, E. et al.: Declining mortality from kidney cancer in Europe. *Ann Oncol,* 15: 1130, 2004

[12] Verdecchia, A., Francisci, S., Brenner, H. et al.: Recent cancer survival in Europe: a 2000-02 period analysis of EUROCARE-4 data. *Lancet Oncol,* 8: 784, 2007

[13] Chow, W. H., Linehan, W. M., Devesa, S. S.: Re: Rising incidence of small renal masses: a need to reassess treatment effect. *J Natl Cancer Inst,* 99: 569, 2007

[14] Sun, M., Thuret, R., Abdollah, F. et al.: Age-adjusted incidence, mortality, and survival rates of stage-specific renal cell carcinoma in North America: a trend analysis. *Eur Urol,* 59: 135, 2011

[15] Jayson, M., Sanders, H.: Increased incidence of serendipitously discovered renal cell carcinoma. *Urology,* 51: 203, 1998

[16] Decastro, G. J., McKiernan, J. M.: Epidemiology, clinical staging, and presentation of renal cell carcinoma. *Urol Clin North Am,* 35: 581, 2008

[17] Sufrin, G., Chasan, S., Golio, A. et al.: Paraneoplastic and serologic syndromes of renal adenocarcinoma. *Semin Urol,* 7: 158, 1989

[18] Gold, P. J., Fefer, A., Thompson, J. A.: Paraneoplastic manifestations of renal cell carcinoma. *Semin Urol Oncol,* 14: 216, 1996

[19] Hagel, C., Stavrou, D., Hansen, H. C.: Paraneoplastic frontal lobe disorder and ataxia in renal cell carcinoma. *Neuropathol Appl Neurobiol,* 31: 97, 2005

[20] Mundy, G. R.: Pathophysiology of cancer-associated hypercalcemia. *Semin Oncol,* 17: 10, 1990

[21] Robertson, F. M., Cendron, M., Klauber, G. T. et al.: Renal cell carcinoma in association with tuberous sclerosis in children. *J Pediatr Surg,* 31: 729, 1996

[22] Gross, A. J., Wolff, M., Fandrey, J. et al.: Prevalence of paraneoplastic erythropoietin production by renal cell carcinomas. *Clin Investig,* 72: 337, 1994

[23] Wiesener, M. S., Munchenhagen, P., Glaser, M. et al.: Erythropoietin gene expression in renal carcinoma is considerably more frequent than paraneoplastic polycythemia. *Int J Cancer,* 121: 2434, 2007

[24] H, S. M.: Nephrogenic Hepatosplenomegaly. *Gastroenterology*, 40: 694, 1961

[25] Rosenblum, S. L.: Paraneoplastic syndromes associated with renal cell carcinoma. *J S C Med Assoc,* 83: 375, 1987

[26] Young, A. N., Master, V. A., Paner, G. P. et al.: Renal epithelial neoplasms: diagnostic applications of gene expression profiling. *Adv Anat Pathol*, 15: 28, 2008

[27] Eble, J. N., Sauter,G., et al: WHO Classification of Tumours: Pathology and Genetics of Tumours of the Urinary System and Male Genital Organs,. Lyon. France: *IARC Press*, 2004

[28] Cheville, J. C., Lohse, C. M., Zincke, H. et al.: Comparisons of outcome and prognostic features among histologic subtypes of renal cell carcinoma. *Am J Surg Pathol,* 27: 612, 2003

[29] Beck, S. D., Patel, M. I., Snyder, M. E. et al.: Effect of papillary and chromophobe cell type on disease-free survival after nephrectomy for renal cell carcinoma. *Ann Surg Oncol,* 11: 71, 2004

[30] Delahunt, B., Eble, J. N.: Papillary renal cell carcinoma: a clinicopathologic and immunohistochemical study of 105 tumors. *Mod Pathol,* 10: 537, 1997

[31] Pignot, G., Elie, C., Conquy, S. et al.: Survival analysis of 130 patients with papillary renal cell carcinoma: prognostic utility of type 1 and type 2 subclassification. *Urology,* 69: 230, 2007

[32] Rosner, I., Bratslavsky, G., Pinto, P. A. et al.: The clinical implications of the genetics of renal cell carcinoma. *Urol Oncol,* 27: 131, 2009

[33] Nagashima, Y.: Chromophobe renal cell carcinoma: clinical, pathological and molecular biological aspects. *Pathol Int*, 50: 872, 2000

[34] Tokuda, N., Naito, S., Matsuzaki, O. et al.: Collecting duct (Bellini duct) renal cell carcinoma: a nationwide survey in Japan. *J Urol,* 176: 40, 2006

[35] Davis, C. J., Jr., Mostofi, F. K., Sesterhenn, I. A.: Renal medullary carcinoma. The seventh sickle cell nephropathy. *Am J Surg Pathol,* 19: 1, 1995

[36] Zhou, M.: Pathology of Renal Cell Carcinoma. In: *Renal Cell Carcinoma.* Edited by B. I. Rini, Campbell, S.c.,. Shelton,CT: People's Medical Publishing House, pp. 1-14, 2009

[37] Fuhrman, S. A., Lasky, L. C., Limas, C.: Prognostic significance of morphologic parameters in renal cell carcinoma. *Am J Surg Pathol,* 6: 655, 1982

[38] Sika-Paotonu, D., Bethwaite, P. B., McCredie, M. R. et al.: Nucleolar grade but not Fuhrman grade is applicable to papillary renal cell carcinoma. *Am J Surg Pathol,* 30: 1091, 2006

[39] Delahunt, B., Sika-Paotonu, D., Bethwaite, P. B. et al.: Fuhrman grading is not appropriate for chromophobe renal cell carcinoma. *Am J Surg Pathol,* 31: 957, 2007

[40] Moch, H., Gasser, T., Amin, M. B. et al.: Prognostic utility of the recently recommended histologic classification and revised TNM staging system of renal cell carcinoma: a Swiss experience with 588 tumors. *Cancer,* 89: 604, 2000

[41] Guinan, P., Sobin, L. H., Algaba, F. et al.: TNM staging of renal cell carcinoma: Workgroup No. 3. Union International Contre le Cancer (UICC) and the American Joint Committee on Cancer (AJCC). *Cancer,* 80: 992, 1997

[42] Ficarra, V., Novara, G., Galfano, A. et al.: Neoplasm staging and organ-confined renal cell carcinoma: a systematic review. *Eur Urol,* 46: 559, 2004

[43] Gettman, M. T., Blute, M. L., Spotts, B. et al.: Pathologic staging of renal cell carcinoma: significance of tumor classification with the 1997 TNM staging system. *Cancer*, 91: 354, 2001

[44] Hafez, K. S., Fergany, A. F., Novick, A. C.: Nephron sparing surgery for localized renal cell carcinoma: impact of tumor size on patient survival, tumor recurrence and TNM staging. *J Urol,* 162: 1930, 1999

[45] Frank, I., Blute, M. L., Leibovich, B. C. et al.: Independent validation of the 2002 American Joint Committee on cancer primary tumor classification for renal cell carcinoma using a large, single institution cohort. *J Urol,* 173: 1889, 2005

[46] Edge,S.B., Byrd,D.R.,Comptom,C.C., (ed.): *AJCC cancer staging manual,7th ed.* New York: Springer, pp. 479-489, 2010

[47] Frank, I., Blute, M. L., Leibovich, B. C. et al.: pT2 classification for renal cell carcinoma. Can its accuracy be improved? *J Urol,* 173: 380, 2005

[48] Klatte, T., Patard, J. J., Goel, R. H. et al.: Prognostic impact of tumor size on pT2 renal cell carcinoma: an international multicenter experience. *J Urol,* 178: 35, 2007

[49] Novara, G., Ficarra, V., Antonelli, A. et al.: Validation of the 2009 TNM version in a large multi-institutional cohort of patients treated for renal cell carcinoma: are further improvements needed? *Eur Urol,* 58: 588, 2010

[50] Thompson, R. H., Cheville, J. C., Lohse, C. M. et al.: Reclassification of patients with pT3 and pT4 renal cell carcinoma improves prognostic accuracy. *Cancer*, 104: 53, 2005

[51] Ficarra, V., Galfano, A., Guille, F. et al.: A new staging system for locally advanced (pT3-4) renal cell carcinoma: a multicenter European study including 2,000 patients. *J Urol,* 178: 418, 2007

[52] Sasco, A. J., Secretan, M. B., Straif, K.: Tobacco smoking and cancer: a brief review of recent epidemiological evidence. *Lung Cancer*, 45 Suppl 2: S3, 2004

[53] *U.S. Department vof Health and Human Services.The Health Consequences of Smoking: A Report of the Surgeon General.* Atlanta,GA., : U.S. Department of Health and Human Services,Centers for Disease Control and Prevention, National Center for Chronic Disease Preventionand Health Promotion, Office on Smoking and Health, 2004

[54] Hunt, J. D., van der Hel, O. L., McMillan, G. P. et al.: Renal cell carcinoma in relation to cigarette smoking: meta-analysis of 24 studies. *Int J Cancer,* 114: 101, 2005

[55] Parker, A. S., Cerhan, J. R., Janney, C. A. et al.: Smoking cessation and renal cell carcinoma. *Ann Epidemiol*, 13: 245, 2003

[56] Sharifi, N., Farrar, W. L.: Perturbations in hypoxia detection: a shared link between hereditary and sporadic tumor formation? *Med Hypotheses*, 66: 732, 2006

[57] Zhu, Y., Horikawa, Y., Yang, H. et al.: BPDE induced lymphocytic chromosome 3p deletions may predict renal cell carcinoma risk. *J Urol,* 179: 2416, 2008

[58] Chow, W. H., Gridley, G., Fraumeni, J. F., Jr. et al.: Obesity, hypertension, and the risk of kidney cancer in men. *N Engl J Med,* 343: 1305, 2000

[59] Flaherty, K. T., Fuchs, C. S., Colditz, G. A. et al.: A prospective study of body mass index, hypertension, and smoking and the risk of renal cell carcinoma (United States). *Cancer Causes Control*, 16: 1099, 2005

[60] Fryzek, J. P., Poulsen, A. H., Johnsen, S. P. et al.: A cohort study of antihypertensive treatments and risk of renal cell cancer. *Br J Cancer*, 92: 1302, 2005

[61] Vatten, L. J., Trichopoulos, D., Holmen, J. et al.: Blood pressure and renal cancer risk: the HUNT Study in Norway. *Br J Cancer*, 97: 112, 2007

[62] Weikert, S., Boeing, H., Pischon, T. et al.: Blood pressure and risk of renal cell carcinoma in the European prospective investigation into cancer and nutrition. *Am J Epidemiol,* 167: 438, 2008

[63] Shapiro, J. A., Williams, M. A., Weiss, N. S. et al.: Hypertension, antihypertensive medication use, and risk of renal cell carcinoma. *Am J Epidemiol,* 149: 521, 1999

[64] Gago-Dominguez, M., Castelao, J. E., Yuan, J. M. et al.: Lipid peroxidation: a novel and unifying concept of the etiology of renal cell carcinoma (United States). *Cancer Causes Control,* 13: 287, 2002

[65] Renehan, A. G., Tyson, M., Egger, M. et al.: Body-mass index and incidence of cancer: a systematic review and meta-analysis of prospective observational studies. *Lancet,* 371: 569, 2008

[66] Adams, K. F., Leitzmann, M. F., Albanes, D. et al.: Body size and renal cell cancer incidence in a large US cohort study. *Am J Epidemiol,* 168: 268, 2008

[67] Luo, J., Margolis, K. L., Adami, H. O. et al.: Body size, weight cycling, and risk of renal cell carcinoma among postmenopausal women: the Women's Health Initiative (United States). *Am J Epidemiol,* 166: 752, 2007

[68] Pischon, T., Lahmann, P. H., Boeing, H. et al.: Body size and risk of renal cell carcinoma in the European Prospective Investigation into Cancer and Nutrition (EPIC). *Int J Cancer,* 118: 728, 2006

[69] Bergstrom, A., Hsieh, C. C., Lindblad, P. et al.: Obesity and renal cell cancer--a quantitative review. *Br J Cancer,* 85: 984, 2001

[70] Calle, E. E., Kaaks, R.: Overweight, obesity and cancer: epidemiological evidence and proposed mechanisms. *Nat Rev Cancer,* 4: 579, 2004

[71] Bergstrom, A., Pisani, P., Tenet, V. et al.: Overweight as an avoidable cause of cancer in Europe. *Int J Cancer,* 91: 421, 2001

[72] Klinghoffer, Z., Yang, B., Kapoor, A. et al.: Obesity and renal cell carcinoma: epidemiology, underlying mechanisms and management considerations. *Expert Rev Anticancer Ther,* 9: 975, 2009

[73] Moyad, M. A.: Obesity, interrelated mechanisms, and exposures and kidney cancer. *Semin Urol Oncol,* 19: 270, 2001

[74] Mahabir, S., Leitzmann, M. F., Pietinen, P. et al.: Physical activity and renal cell cancer risk in a cohort of male smokers. *Int J Cancer,* 108: 600, 2004

[75] Moore, S. C., Chow, W. H., Schatzkin, A. et al.: Physical activity during adulthood and adolescence in relation to renal cell cancer. *Am J Epidemiol,* 168: 149, 2008

[76] Jakicic, J. M., Marcus, B. H., Gallagher, K. I. et al.: Effect of exercise duration and intensity on weight loss in overweight, sedentary women: a randomized trial. *JAMA,* 290: 1323, 2003

[77] Stewart, K. J., Bacher, A. C., Turner, K. L. et al.: Effect of exercise on blood pressure in older persons: a randomized controlled trial. *Arch Intern Med,* 165: 756, 2005

[78] Mora, S., Cook, N., Buring, J. E. et al.: Physical activity and reduced risk of cardiovascular events: potential mediating mechanisms. *Circulation,* 116: 2110, 2007

[79] Ljungberg, B., Campbell, S. C., Cho, H. Y. et al.: The epidemiology of renal cell carcinoma. *Eur Urol,* 60: 615, 2011

[80] Rashidkhani, B., Akesson, A., Lindblad, P. et al.: Major dietary patterns and risk of renal cell carcinoma in a prospective cohort of Swedish women. *J Nutr,* 135: 1757, 2005

[81] Mahabir, S., Leitzmann, M. F., Virtanen, M. J. et al.: Prospective study of alcohol drinking and renal cell cancer risk in a cohort of finnish male smokers. *Cancer Epidemiol Biomarkers Prev*, 14: 170, 2005

[82] Lee, J. E., Hunter, D. J., Spiegelman, D. et al.: Alcohol intake and renal cell cancer in a pooled analysis of 12 prospective studies. *J Natl Cancer Inst,* 99: 801, 2007

[83] Lazarus, R., Sparrow, D., Weiss, S. T.: Alcohol intake and insulin levels. The Normative Aging Study. *Am J Epidemiol,* 145: 909, 1997

[84] Augustsson, K., Skog, K., Jagerstad, M. et al.: Dietary heterocyclic amines and cancer of the colon, rectum, bladder, and kidney: a population-based study. *Lancet*, 353: 703, 1999

[85] De Stefani, E., Fierro, L., Mendilaharsu, M. et al.: Meat intake, 'mate' drinking and renal cell cancer in Uruguay: a case-control study. *Br J Cancer*, 78: 1239, 1998

[86] Wolk, A., Larsson, S. C., Johansson, J. E. et al.: Long-term fatty fish consumption and renal cell carcinoma incidence in women. *JAMA*, 296: 1371, 2006

[87] Port, F. K., Nissenson, A. R.: Outcome of end-stage renal disease in patients with rare causes of renal failure. II. Renal or systemic neoplasms. *Q J Med,* 73: 1161, 1989

[88] Kliem, V., Kolditz, M., Behrend, M. et al.: Risk of renal cell carcinoma after kidney transplantation. *Clin Transplant*, 11: 255, 1997

[89] Neuzillet, Y., Lay, F., Luccioni, A. et al.: De novo renal cell carcinoma of native kidney in renal transplant recipients. *Cancer*, 103: 251, 2005

[90] Das, A., Thomas, S., Zablotska, L. B. et al.: Association of esophageal adenocarcinoma with other subsequent primary cancers. *J Clin Gastroenterol,* 40: 405, 2006

[91] Thompson, R. H., Leibovich, B. C., Cheville, J. C. et al.: Second primary malignancies associated with renal cell carcinoma histological subtypes. *J Urol*, 176: 900, 2006

[92] Beisland, C., Talleraas, O., Bakke, A. et al.: Multiple primary malignancies in patients with renal cell carcinoma: a national population-based cohort study. *BJU Int*, 97: 698, 2006

[93] Khurana, V., Caldito, G., Ankem, M.: Statins might reduce risk of renal cell carcinoma in humans: case-control study of 500,000 veterans. Urology, 71: 118, 2008

[94] Lindblad, P., Mellemgaard, A., Schlehofer, B. et al.: International renal-cell cancer study. V. Reproductive factors, gynecologic operations and exogenous hormones. *Int J Cancer,* 61: 192, 1995

[95] Kabat, G. C., Silvera, S. A., Miller, A. B. et al.: A cohort study of reproductive and hormonal factors and renal cell cancer risk in women. *Br J Cancer*, 96: 845, 2007

[96] Altman, D., Yin, L., Johansson, A. et al.: Risk of renal cell carcinoma after hysterectomy. *Arch Intern Med,* 170: 2011, 2010

[97] Langner, C., Ratschek, M., Rehak, P. et al.: Steroid hormone receptor expression in renal cell carcinoma: an immunohistochemical analysis of 182 tumors. *J Urol,* 171: 611, 2004

[98] Noordzij, M. A., Mickisch, G. H.: The genetic make-up of renal cell tumors. *Urol Res*, 32: 251, 2004

[99] Linehan, W. M., Vasselli, J., Srinivasan, R. et al.: Genetic basis of cancer of the kidney: disease-specific approaches to therapy. *Clin Cancer Res,* 10: 6282S, 2004

[100] Axwijk, P. H., Kluijt, I., de Jong, D. et al.: Hereditary causes of kidney tumours. *Eur J Clin Invest,* 40: 433, 2010

[101] Choyke, P. L., Glenn, G. M., Walther, M. M. et al.: von Hippel-Lindau disease: genetic, clinical, and imaging features. *Radiology*, 194: 629, 1995

[102] Maher, E. R.: Inherited renal cell carcinoma. Br J Urol, 78: 542, 1996

[103] Kim, W. Y., Kaelin, W. G.: Role of VHL gene mutation in human cancer. *J Clin Oncol*, 22: 4991, 2004

[104] Coleman, J. A.: Familial and hereditary renal cancer syndromes. *Urol Clin North Am*, 35: 563, 2008

[105] Pfaffenroth, E. C., Linehan, W. M.: Genetic basis for kidney cancer: opportunity for disease-specific approaches to therapy. *Expert Opin Biol Ther*, 8: 779, 2008

[106] Van Poppel, H., Nilsson, S., Algaba, F. et al.: Precancerous lesions in the kidney. *Scand J Urol Nephrol Suppl:* 136, 2000

In: Essentials and Updates in Urologic Oncology
Editor: Philippe E. Spiess

ISBN: 978-1-62081-494-9
© 2013 Nova Science Publishers, Inc.

Chapter XXIII

Surgical Management of Renal Cell Carcinoma

David D. Buethe and Philippe E. Spiess

Department of Genitourinary Oncology, Moffitt Cancer Center, Tampa, Florida, US

Abstract

The surgical management of renal cell carcinoma (RCC) has evolved dramatically over the past two decades. With a rising incidence and cancer-specific mortality, continued attention should be given to evolving treatment options for RCC. A surgically curable disease, RCC has been traditionally managed by open radical nephrectomy. However, laparoscopic techniques have quickly been adopted and the increasing awareness of the morbidities associated with chronic kidney disease (CKD) have necessitated the implementation and constant innovation of nephron-sparing surgical alternatives. As the population ages and body imaging has become more common place, proportionately more small renal masses (SRMs) of less than 4 cm are identified in often less than ideal surgical candidates. This has prompted the evolution of percutaneous thermal ablative techniques as well as the option of active surveillance in well selected cases. Despite the downward stage migration, up to 30% of primary renal lesions still initially present as metastatic disease with such patients often benefiting from upfront cytoreductive nephrectomy.

I. Introduction

RCC currently accounts for an estimated 3 to 4% of newly diagnosed adult malignancies in the U.S. [1] Despite recent reports of downward stage migration, smaller tumor size at time of diagnosis, and a rise in incidentally diagnosed tumors due to readily available imaging techniques, there remains an increasing incidence of RCC along with a rising cancer-specific death rate. [2-5] This is somewhat surprising in an era when the increased utilization of extirpative surgery has kept pace with this reported rise in incidence. [2] Further, it's startling that 25-30% of RCCs are diagnosed due to symptoms resulting from metastatic disease which is associated with a dismal 0-20% 5-year survival. [6,7]

II. Preoperative Evaluation

A. Imaging

Non-invasive imaging such as ultrasound (US), computerized tomography (CT), and magnetic resonance imaging (MRI) are integral in tumor characterization and clinical staging of RCC. In fact, greater than 70% of newly diagnosed RCCs are incidental findings on imaging studies obtained for unrelated reasons. [8]

Ultrasound

Renal US is inexpensive, readily available, and does not necessitate ionized radiation exposure nor iodinated contrast injection. However, US does not adequately provide information regarding the extent of potentially locally advanced disease, metastatic disease, or the renal vasculature vital in surgical planning. Further, RCC can present isoechoic to the adjacent normal renal parenchyma making it difficult to identify small lesions that do not significantly distort the renal architecture. Thus, CT and MRI are often subsequently necessary to evaluate renal lesions identified by renal US.

Transesophogeal echocardiography (TEE) can be utilized to preoperatively the evaluate the extent of tumor thrombus within the inferior vena cava (IVC) of patients with locally advanced RCC. In a 13 patient prospective study in 1997, the accuracy of TEE in identifying the presence and level of IVC tumor thrombus was found to be 85% as compared to 90% for MRI. [9] However, the benefits of real-time intraoperative TEE can be significant for the surgical team. [10-12]

Computerized Tomography

CT of the abdomen and pelvis without and with intravenous contrast has become the gold standard with respect to the evaluation and staging of renal masses. [6,13] Beyond the assessment of a suspected primary renal lesion, CT allows for detailed characterization of the tumors location within the renal unit, ipisilateral renal vasculature relevant to surgical planning, evaluation of the contralateral renal unit, as well as assessment of the potential presence of regional adenopathy and/or distant sites of metastasis. It's now common practice to utilize 4-phase imaging inclusive of a pre-contrast, an arterial, a venous, and a delayed contrasted phase with as well 3-dimensional reconstruction. However, only 2 sets of images are truly necessary; one before and one after the administration of intravenous contrast. This allows for assessment of potential enhancement by the lesion in question, generally defined as a change of $\geq$15-20 Houndsfield units (HUs) between the pre- and post-contrast series, which is a hallmark of renal tumors. [14-16] While most benign lesions cannot be distinguished from those which are malignant utilizing CT, lipid rich angiomyolipomas (AMLs) tend to declare themselves with the pathognomonic finding of a lesion comprised partly of fat as defined by the finding of regions displaying negative Hus readings. The optimal threshold for AMLs has recently been reported as a value less than -10 HU's on non-enhanced CT. [17]

The Bosniak classification system pertaining to the characterization of cystic renal lesions relies on CT to evaluate lesions for the presence of calcifications, degree of enhancement and assessment of septations. Notably, CT findings concerning for malignancy include calcifications within the wall or septa of a cyst, a lesion with a density $\geq$ 20 HU, irregular septations, or septations measuring > 1 mm in width. [18] Using the criteria outlined in Table 1, nine studies (521 patients) designed to assign a risk of malignancy to each specific Bosniak classification identified the risk of malignancy to be 1.7, 18.5, 33.0 and 92.5% for categories I, II, III, and IV; respectively. However, one of the studies combined categories I and II and another, which was the only one to differentiate the category of IIF, combined categories II, IIF, and III. [18] A later study by Graumann *et al.* evaluated the 6 available studies inclusive of >30 patients and found a positive correlation between the Bosniak classification and risk of malignancy with the following associations: category I, 0%; category II, 15.6%; category IIF, 0%; category III, 65.3%; and category IV, 91.7%. Only 3 of the studies allotted for a IIF classification. [19]

Table 1. The Bosniak Classification of Renal Cysts

Bosniak Category	Features
I	A simple benign cyst with a hairline thin wall that does not contain septa, calcification or solid components. It measures as water density and does not enhance with contrast Material
II	A benign cyst that might contain a few hairline thin septa. Fine calcification might be present in the wall or septa. Uniformly high-attenuation lesions of <3 cm that are sharply marginated and do not enhance.
IIF	These cysts might contain more hairline thin septa. Minimal enhancement of a hairline thin septum or wall can be seen and there might be minimal thickening of the septa or wall. The cyst might contain calcification that might be nodular and thick but there is no contrast enhancement. There are no enhancing soft-tissue elements. Totally intrarenal non-enhancing high-attenuation renal lesions of ≥3 cm are also included in this category. These lesions are generally well marginated.
III	These lesions are indeterminate cystic masses that have thickened irregular walls or septa in which enhancement can be seen.
IV	These lesions are clearly malignant cystic lesions that contain enhancing soft-tissue components.

Adapted with permission from Warren and McFarlane. BJU 2005.[18]

Contrast Induced Nephropathy (CIN)

As the literature would suggest, 26% of patients being considered for either radical or partial nephrectomy suffer from concomitant chronic kidney disease (CKD) as defined by a derived estimated glomerular filtration rate (eGFR) of <60 ml/min/1.73m^2 despite potentially exhibiting a serum creatinine within the accepted normal range. [20] One should be aware that this is the most prevalent risk factor for CIN associated with intravenous contrast enhanced CT. Although serum creatinine is often used as a surrogate measure of renal function, a more accurate means of calculating an eGFR is the use of a 24-hour creatinine clearance or utilizing a technetium-99 diethylentriaminepentaacetic acid (DTPA) nuclear renal scan. Otherwise, calculations taking into account a patient's serum creatinine, age, race, and gender, known as the Modification Diet in Renal Disease (MDRD) and Chronic Kidney Disease Epidemiology (CKD-EPI) equations are available and readily applied via available online calculators. (www.mdrd.com) [21,22]

For those at risk for CIN, hydration with 154 mEq/L of bicarbonate in 5% dextrose water (D5W) or 0.9% normal saline (NS) before and after the procedure is recommended. The optimal agent and dose is not defined but suggested administration of 154 mEq/L of bicarbonate in D5W at 3 ml/kg/hr for 1 hour prior and 1ml/kg/hr for 6 hours after the imaging procedure or 1.5 ml/kg/hr for 6 hours prior and 6 hours after the images are acquired. Despite the evaluation of prophylactic N-acetylcysteine administration in multiple publications, the evidence is conflicting and the administration N-acetylcysteine prior to intravenous contrast exposure is not currently a recommended protective measure. Lastly, if a patient is at risk for CIN and taking potentially nephrotoxic drugs, a discussion should be had about cessation of such medications 24 hours prior to intended imaging. Specifically, metformin should be discontinued 48 hours prior to and withheld 48 hours after the procedure among those with an eGFR <45 ml/min/1.73m^2.[23]

Contrast Allergy

Another barrier to obtaining contrast-enhanced CT is a patient's historic intolerance to fish/shellfish or a hypersensitivity to topical iodine containing solutions. One should be aware that such reactions are, in actuality, rarely an immune response directly related to iodine which is a naturally present essential trace mineral. While those patients relaying such prior sensitivities are 3 times more likely than individuals without documented allergies to experience a reaction to iodinated contrast media (ICM), this number is similar to those individuals with other food allergies or asthma. [24] However, true ICM-related reactions do occur in 0.7-3.1% patients receiving low-osmolar non-ionic contrast media; with severe reactions much less prevalent. The most significant prognosticator of having an adverse reaction is a prior episode of such a reaction; 21-60% of those with previous reactions will experience an adverse event when re-exposed. [25]

With regards to prophylaxis, fully assessing the severity of prior reactions and the use of clinical judgment is essential, as prophylaxis does not guarantee that an adverse reaction will not occur. [25] That said, premedication protocols exist for those patients deemed at high-risk for ICM adverse reactions should a contrasted study be necessary. In 1980, the Greenberger protocol was published and called for the oral administration of 50 mg of prednisone at 13, 7, and 1 hour prior to the intended scan as well as an intramuscular (IM) injection of 50 mg of diphenhydramine 1 hour prior to imaging. Using the above protocol, 147 contrast-enhanced studies were performed without a single severe reaction and only 6.8% of the patients experienced any type of reaction. [26]

Magnetic Resonance Imaging

MRI is similar to CT in that it provides a means of obtaining detailed characterization of renal masses but offers the advantages of no requirement for ionizing radiation or iodinated intravenous contrast. Instead, images are acquired before and after the intravenous administration of gadolinium-based contrast agent (GBCA). Thus, MRI is an attractive modality of renal assessment in those who describe prior adverse reactions related to iodinated substances. While the study numbers are small, two different prospective observational studies have compared the sensitivity, specificity, and diagnostic accuracy of both multidetector CT and MRI when evaluating for an IVC tumor thrombus. No statistical analysis was provided in either study but in each small series CT correctly indentified the presence of an IVC thrombus more often than did MRI. Grossly looking at the data, the two imaging modalities are equivalent with respect to identifying the presence of a tumor thrombus within the IVC with sensitivities ranging from 93 to 100%. [27,28]

Nephrogenic Systemic Fibrosis

Nephrogenic systemic fibrosis (NSF) is a rare entity reported in patients with significant renal impairment and exposure to GBCAs. However, the mechanistic relationship is not known. Clinical symptoms generally present as indurated skin associated with nodules and plaques associated with flexion contractures limiting the range of motion. It is important to remember that it has never been reported in those with an eGFR >30 mL/min/1.73m^2. In fact, those with an eGFR >30 mL/min/1..73m^2 are considered to be at extremely low to no risk of developing NSF as long as a dose of GBCA of 0.1mmol/kg or less is utilized. Further, there is no evidence to support that those with an eGFR >60 mL/min/m^2 are at an increased risk of developing NSF. Thus, the current recommendation of the United States Federal Drug Administration regarding the use of GBCA's is to screen patients at risk for renal insufficiency and avoid the administration of GBCA's in patients with an eGFR <30 mL/min/1.73m^2. [29]

Positron Emission Tomography/Computerized Tomography (PET/CT)

The role PET/CT for the characterization of localized RCC is minimal to none at the present time. Given that the fluorine-18 fluorodeoxyglucose (F-18 FDG) is excreted in the urine, it is difficult to discern background urine excretion from hypermetabolic tumors. The reported sensitivities of PET/CT for primary renal tumors are quite varied. In a very small prospective study involving only 18 patients for which PET/CT images were acquired prior to extirpative surgery, the sensitivity and specificity were found to be 46.6% and 66.6%, respectively. However, all IVC/renal tumor thrombi and distant sites of metastasis were identified. [30]

B. Staging

Currently, renal masses are characterized by their size, perinephric invasion, confinement to Gerota's fascia, presence and degree of venous invasion, regional lymph node involvement, and presence of distant sites of metastasis, all of which are conveyed utilizing the TNM staging system as outlined by the American Joint Committee on Cancer (AJCC) 2010 (see Chapter 22). [31] T1 lesions are those ≤ 7 cm in greatest diameter confined within Gerota's fascia; with T1a and T1b denoting ≤ 4cm and > 4 cm but ≤ 7cm, respectively. T2 lesions are those > 7cm in size yet still lying completely within Gerota's fascia; T2a lesions defined as those ≤ 10cm and T2b lesions appropriately >10cm. The T3 classification identifies a lesion as involving the venous system (renal vein or IVC) or the perinephric tissue within Gerota's fascia excepting the ipsilateral adrenal gland. A T3a tumor invades either the perinephric/renal sinus fat or extends into the renal vein or a segmental vein. Lesions categorized as T3b or T3c are delineated by level of IVC involvement by tumor thrombus. Tumor thrombus ceasing below the diaphragm and without invasion into the venous wall are categorized as T3b and those tumors associated with tumor thrombus extending above the level of the diaphragm or which are invasive into the venous wall are described as T3c. The classification of T4 tumors is reserved for those tumors extending into the ipsilateral adrenal gland or beyond Gerota's fascia. The presence of regional adenopathy or distant sites of metastasis is communicated by the notation N1 or M1 respectively while the absence of such features is conveyed using the annotations N0 and M0, respectively. [31] The premise of such a staging system is to provide a means of communication between healthcare workers to easily convey the extent of a renal malignancy in a given case as well as a prognostic tool to predict future outcomes with respect to risk of recurrence, progression, and survival. The validity of the current TNM staging system was provided by a 16 center study which retrospectively evaluated the cancer-specific survival of 5339 patients treated with either radical nephrectomy (RN) or partial nephrectomy. The 5-year cancer-specific survival ranged from 94.9% in those with pT1a disease to 27.1% in those with pT4 disease; with a significant cancer-specific survival difference noted in all stepped categories except for the pT2b-pT3a and the pT3c-pT4 discriminating steps. [32]

The Heidelberg classification system is utilitized to identify the histologic subtypes of renal malignancies [33] while the Fuhrman grading system is used to define the cellular morphology of individual cancer cells; with types I – IV applicable only to the most common clear cell subtype and the terminology high and low-grade applied to the remaining subtypes (See Chapter 22). [34]

C. Role of Percutaneous Biopsy

The role of percutaneous biopsy has long been debated due to concerns regarding non-diagnostic specimens and the accuracy of such biopsies. Particularly, the negative predictive value (NPV), as defined by dividing the truly negative biopsies by the sum of the truly negative biopsies and falsely negative biopsies, has been in question. Generally, negative diagnostic results, which are the premise for no further clinical evaluation, must have a low false-negative rate termed a high NPV) However, the rising incidence of SRMs and incidentally discovered renal lesions along with a rising interest in thermal ablative techniques or active surveillance as primary treatment options for such lesions has resurrected interest in the role of percutaneous renal biopsy. [2-5,35]

Recent efforts describing the histological findings on percutaneous biopsies of SRMs have reported the non-diagnostic rates to be 16-19%. Of the diagnostic specimens, approximately 80% were found to be malignant, RCC being the most common finding. Of the benign specimens, oncocytoma and angiomyolipoma (AML) were the most common histologic subtypes identified and accounting for 67-79% of the benign lesions. [36,37] Of note, the diagnostic rate dropped to 67% in cystic lesions. [30] On multivariate analysis, tumors of larger size and solid nature (as opposed to cystic) were more likely to be associated with this diagnostic finding.[36] This distribution is substantiated by Kutikov et al.'s single center study that evaluated the pathologic specimens of 143 patients undergoing partial nephrectomy for a sporadic solitary lesion ranging in size from 0.6 to 8cm. Twenty-three (16.1%) were found to be composed of a benign pathology; 7/44 (15.9%) < 2cm, 14/85 (16.5%) 2-4cm, and 2/14 (14.3%) > 4cm. Of the benign lesions, 10 of 23 (43.5%) were AMLs, 8/23 (34.8%) were oncocytomas, 3/23 (13%) were benign renal cysts. [38]

The gold-standard for evaluation of the accuracy of a percutaneous biopsy for SRMs is the subsequent surgical resection of the renal lesion in question. This protocol was reported by an Austrian group in 2008 who found the NPV to be 70% and 80%, respectively for FNA and core biopsies performed on solid renal lesions.[39] The positive predictive value (PPV), as defined by the truly positive biopsies divided by the sum of truly positive biopsies and the false positive biopsies, was 100% denoting that there were no false positive percutaneous renal biopsies. [37,40] These findings are supported by a small retrospective review of 23 renal lesions subjected to CT-guided percutaneous biopsy of renal masses which found the sensitivity and specificity to be 93% and 100%, respectively. This is a very small series but the NPV was 75% and the PPV 100%. [40] It should again be noted that the diagnostic rate dropped to 67% in those lesions described as cystic in nature. [37]

In a prospective study in which 44 patients were subjected to simultaneous FNA with cytology (FNAC) and core biopsies via the same 17-gauge coaxial needle, the theoretical benefits of FNAC with respect to fewer complications were not realized and the study was continued using only core biopsies. Again, the specificity and PPV were both 100%, NPV 81.3% and sensitivity 95.2%. [39]

In light of the aforementioned data along with the exceedingly rare incidence of biopsy tract seeding, low complication rate, and less than 2% complication rate which requires intervention, [39,41] the AUA only advocates obtaining a renal biopsy for clinically stage 1 renal masses in patients with a wide array of treatment options ranging form surgery to observation. However, a biopsy is not advocated in healthy patients unwilling to accept the uncertainty of a biopsy or patients who will only consider conservative treatment options regardless of potential biopsy results. [6] Further indications for renal mass biopsy include a clinical picture suggestive of a renal lesion concerning for a distant site of metastasis or in the clinical context of a prior malignancy, or a minimally enhancing < 3 cm renal lesion.

D. Metastatic Evaluation

After a suspicious renal mass is identified, it's imperative to complete a thorough evaluation of the patient's health history via a complete history and physical examination before engaging in a detailed conversation about potential treatment strategies. Blood and urine samples should be evaluated by means of a complete blood count, comprehensive metabolic panel, and urinalysis. If further imaging is necessary to better characterize the lesion(s), to aid surgical planning or to up-date outdated films, these should be ordered as appropriate (see Section IIIA). A chest x-ray or CT scan of the chest is used to screen for pulmonary lesions. Should imaging be concerning for a centrally located renal lesion or an upper tract urothelial carcinoma, urine cytology, and/or ureteroscopy +/- biopsy should be considered. Bone scans and/or an MRI of the brain should be obtained when clinically indicated. If relevant to choosing a management strategy, a needle biopsy of the lesion may be considered (see Section IIIC). [42]

Paraneoplastic Syndromes

Paraneoplastic syndromes (PNS) are the resultant systemic signs or symptoms attributed to proteins inappropriately released directly from or due to the presence of renal tumors. The proteins often serve in an endocrine fashion as hormones, such as parathyroid hormone-related peptide (PTH-rP), and are not a consequence of local disease. Further, the clinical evidence of a PNS often dissipates after extirpation of the primary lesion or management of metastatic disease. As of 1996, 20% of RCCs were associated with paraneoplastic syndromes as outlined in Table 2. [43] However, in 2003, Kim *et al.* questioned whether the downward stage migration and a rise in incidentally discovered renal masses had changed the frequency of PNS. [2-5,44] In this study, anemia (52%), cachexia related findings (35%), and reversible hepatic dysfunction (often referred to as Stauffer's Syndrome) were the most common findings associated with localized and metastatic RCC. [44]

Table 2. Incidence of Systemic Syndromes Associated with Renal Cell Carcinoma

Syndrome	%
Elevated erythrocte sedimentation rate	55.6
Hypertension	37.5
Anemia	36.3
Cachexia, weight loss	34.5
Pyrexia	17.2
Abnormal liver function	14.4
Hypercalcemia	4.9
Polycythemia	3.5
Neuromyopathy	3.2
Amyloidosis	2

Adapted with permission from Gold *et al. Semin Urol Oncol 1996.*[43]

With respect to clinical ramifications, Kim *et al.* demonstrated that the presence of just one cachexia-related finding such as hypoalbuminemia, weight loss, anorexia, and malaise, was a significant predictor of cancer-specific survival (CSS) on multivariate analysis inclusive of the TNM staging system, ECOG performance status, and Fuhrman grade in those with both localized and metastatic RCC. For those with localized RCC, the 2-year survival was 79% and 95%, respectively for those displaying a cachexia-related finding at time of diagnosis versus those that did not (p <0.0001). The median survival was 12 and 31 months, respectively for those with metastatic RCC with or without an associated cachexia-related finding at time of diagnosis (p <0.001).

Also clinically relevant is the presence of hypercalcemia resultant of either osteolytic bone metastasis or a PNS. In the scenario of a PNS, hypercalcemia is attributed to the effects of PTH-rP mimicking the effects of parathyroid hormone as well the cytokine IL-6 which acts synergistically when co-expressed with PTH-rP. [45-47] The clinical manifestations include nausea, anorexia, fatigue, decreased deep tendon reflexes, and even an altered mental status. However, hypercalcemia is the only PNS that can be managed medically using vigorous hydration followed by furosemide driven diuresis, steroids, I.V. bisphosphonates and calcitonin. [43,45] Further implications stem from the association of corrected hypercalcemia of >9.48-10mg/dL with poor outcomes pertaining to the progression-free survival (PFS) and overall survival (OS) in those with mRCC. Furthermore, corrected calcium levels have been incorporated into prognostic tools used for the stratification of survival in those with mRCC. [48-50].

E. Perioperative Considerations

Antibiotic Prophylaxis

Over the last decade, the recommendations regarding prophylactic antibiotic administration has changed with respect to those with valvular heart disease or the presence of implanted orthopedic hardware. It should be noted that the American Heart Association no longer recommends antimicrobial prophylaxis solely for the prevention of infectious endocarditis. [51] Further, antimicrobial prophylaxis is not indicated preoperatively for surgically treated urologic patients on the basis of present orthopedic pins, plates, or screws. Nor are antimicrobials routinely indicated for urologic patients who have had prior total joint replacements, excepting for those patients who area at increased risk for bacteremia and hematogenous seeding of the total joint implant due to the nature of the urologic procedure. The presence of malignancy entering the collecting system during a partial nephrectomy would meet such criteria and would warrant prophylaxis with either a single dose of an oral fluoroquinolone 1-2 hours prior to surgery or a combination of intravenous ampicillin and gentamicin 30-60 minutes prior to surgery using vancomycin as a substitute among those who are penicillin allergic. [52]

Table 3. Recommended Antimicrobial Prophylaxis per AUA Best Practice Guidelines

Procedure	Organisms	Prophylaxis Indicated	Antimicrobials (s) of Choice	Alternative Antimicrobials(s)	Duration of Therapy*
		Lower Tract Instrumentation			
Removal of external urinary catheter	GU tract†	If risk factors‡§	-Fluoroquinolone¶	-Aminoglycoside ± Ampicillin¶ -1st/2nd gen.	≤24 hours¶
			-TMP-SMX¶	Cephalosporin¶	
		Upper Tract Instrumentation			
Percutaneous renal surgery	GU tract and skin‡‡	All	-1st/2nd gen. Cephalosporin	-Ampicillin/Sulbactam	≤24 hours
			-Aminoglycoside + Metronidazole or Clindamycin	-Fluoroquinolone	
		Open or Laparoscopic Surgery			
Without entering the urinary tract	Skin	If risk factors	-1st gen. Cephalosporin	-Clindamycin	Single Dose
Involving entry into the urinary tract	GU tract and skin	All	-1st/2nd gen. Cephalosporin -Aminoglycoside + Metronidazole or Clindamycin	-Ampicillin/Sulbactam -Fluoroquinolone	≤24 hours

* Additional antimicrobial therapy may be recommended at time of removal of an externalized urinary catheter.

† GU tract: Common urinary organisms are: *E. coli, Proteus sp., Klebsiella sp., Enterococcus.*

‡ Patient-related factors affecting host response to surgical infections may alter antimicrobial prophylaxis strategy.

§ If urine culture shows no growth prior to the procedure, antimicrobial phrophylaxis is not necessary.

¶ Or full course of culture-directed antimicrobials for documented infection (which is treatment, not prophylaxis)

‡‡ Skin: Common skin organisms are *S. aureus,* coagulase negative *Staph. Sp.,* Group A *Strep. sp.*

Adapted with permission from Wolf *et al. J Urol* 2008.53

Outside of the special considerations commented on above, the American Urology Association (AUA) currently recommends a single dose of a 1st generation cephalosporin for instances, such as a radical nephrectomy, in which the urinary tract will not be entered, using a single dose of clindamycin as a substitute in those reporting a penicillin allergy. For those renal procedures that include entry into the urinary tract (including percutaneous procedures), a 1st or 2nd generation cephalosporin or a combination of an aminoglycoside and either metronidazole or clindamycin is recommended. Alternatively, ampicillin/sulbactam or a fluoroquinolone would be appropriate. All antimicrobials should be instituted prior to surgery and be administered for less than 24 hours (Table 3). [53]

All patients found to have an active infection of colonization should be treated with a culture-specific antibiotic to sterilize the urine or reduce the bacterial colony counts prior to surgery. [53]

Table 4. Sumary of recommendations for DVT Prophylaxis per AUA Best Practice Statement

Level of Risk	Prophylactic Treatment
Low Risk	● No prophylaxis other than early ambulation
Moderate Risk	● Heparin 5000 units every 12 hours subcutaneous starting after surgery
	● OR *Enoxaparin 40 mg (Cr Cl < 30 mL/min = 30 mg) subcutaneous daily
	● OR Pneumatic compression device if risk of bleeding is high
High Risk	● Heparin 5000 units every 8 hours subcutaneous starting after surgery and adjuvant pneumatic compression device
	● OR *Enoxaparin 40 mg (Cr Cl < 30 mL/min = 30 mg) subcutaneous daily
	● OR Pneumatic compression device if risk of bleeding is high
Very High Risk	●*Enoxaparin 40 mg (Cr Cl < 30 mL/min = 30mg) subcutaneous daily **and** adjuvant pneumatic compression device,
	● OR Heparin 5000 units every 8 hours subcutaneous starting after surgery **and** adjuvant pneumatic compression device

*Guidelines and Cautions for Enoxaparin Use

● In patients with a body weight > 150 Kg, consider increasing prophylaxis dose of Enoxaparin to 40 mg subcutaneous every 12 hours.

● Withhold Enoxaparin generally fro at least 2 to 3 days after major trauma, and then only consider use after review of current patient condition and risk benefit ratio

● For planned manipulation of an epidural or spinal catheter (insertion, removal), Enoxaparin should be avoided/held for 24 hours BEFORE planned manipulation and should be resumbed no earlier than 2 hours FOLLOWING manipulation.

● Special testing may be indicated for Enoxaparin in a patient with a history of heparin-induced thrombocytopenia

● **The risks of bleeding must be weighed against the benefits of prophylaxis in determining the timing of initiation of DVT pharmacologic prophylaxis in combination with mechanical prophylaxis.**

Adapted with permission from Forrest *et al. J Urol* 2009.[55]

Deep Venous Thrombosis Prophylaxis

Efforts to prevent the development of deep venous thrombosis (DVT) and thromboembolic events such as pulmonary emboli are a necessity for the urologic oncologist. Using the risk factors and risk stratification system outlined by the American College of Chest Physicians (ACCP) in 2004, those with renal malignancies often exhibit multiple risk factors of DVT such as: increasing age, obesity, smoking, need for surgery, need for central venous catheterization, and the intrinsic presence of malignancy in such patients. Thus, these patients could be easily be deemed high or highest risk for development of DVT.[54] Adopting the recommendations of the ACCP, in 2009 the American Urologic Association (AUA) issued a best practice guideline specifically outlining the recommended DVT prophylaxis and these can be seen in Tables 4. [55] The tenants of DVT prophylaxis include preoperative placement of graduated compression stockings and/or intermittent pneumatic compression devices, early ambulation, and early institution of risk-specific pharmacologic prophylaxis when not contraindicated. With regards to special considerations, unfractionated heparin should be substituted for low-molecular weight heparins, such as enoxeparin or dalteparin, in those with a creatinine clearance of <30 ml/min.

IV. Surgical Management of Localized Renal Cell Carcinoma

Surgical extirpation remains the gold-standard for management of localized RCC due to the derived benefits of histological confirmation of diagnosis, accurate staging, and likely ability to achieve cure. However, it's important to understand the rapidly evolving nature and applicability of the array of therapeutic procedures from open radical nephrectomy to robot-assisted laparoscopic partial nephrectomy that are currently available to patients.

A. Radical Nephrectomy

Open radical nephrectomy (ORN), consisting of the removal of the kidney, the ipsilateral adrenal gland still encompassed by Gerota's fascia, and regional lymph nodes as described by Robson in 1969, [56] remained the modality of choice for the management of all renal masses for years due to the high achievement of cancer control as measured by local tumor control, progression-free survival (PFS), recurrence-free survival (RFS), and cancer-specific survival (CSS) whereby serving as the gold standard to which all other treatments are compared.

Ipsilateral Adrenalectomy

With downward stage migration of renal lesions and the increasing utilization of nephron-sparing surgery (NSS) for T1 renal masses, the necessity for ipsilateral adrenalectomy has became scrutinized in recent years. Lane *et al.* reported on 2,065 laparoscopic partial nephrectomies of which 48 underwent a concomitant ipsilateral adrenalectomy for either preoperative or intraoperative concerns for ipsilateral adrenal involvement. Of the 48 adrenal glands resected, only 1 was involved by direct extension of the renal tumor, 2 exhibited metastatic RCC, and 3 were found to constitute other adrenal neoplasms. Of the 2,017 patients with an intact ipsilateral adrenal gland, only 11 were later identified to have developed metachronous adrenal metastasis. [57] These findings are echoed by recently published data by Kutikov *et al.* who examined 179 patients undergoing radical or partial nephrectomy for lesions ≥7 cm, of which 91 underwent concurrent total ipsilateral adrenalectomy. Of the 91 adrenals examined, only 4 (4.4%) of the adrenal specimens were histologically involved by RCC. In that same cohort of patients, preoperative imaging had suggested abnormal adrenal findings in 12 (including all 4 positive specimens), thus the sensitivity was 100% (4 of 4), the specificity 90.1% (79 of 87), PPV 33% (4 of 12), and more importantly, the NPV was 100% (79 of 79). Further, of the 4 involved adrenal glands, only 1 (1.8%) of 57 patients with clinically N0 and M0 status were among these 4 cases.[58] This is consistent with O'Malley *et al.'s* systemic review of the role of ipsilateral adrenalectomy in which they found that the incidence of synchronous ipsilateral adrenal involvement ranged from 1 to 5%. [59] Despite a documented significant direct correlation between tumor size, renal vein involvement, regional, and distant metastasis, no benefit in overall-survival was garnered from performing a concomitant ipsilateral adrenalectomy in those without clinical or radiologic suspicion of adrenal involvement. [57-59]

Further, the historic notion that an upper pole location precludes an adrenal sparing procedure has not withstood the test of time. [58] Thus, ipsilateral adrenalectomy at time of extirpative surgery for renal cell carcinoma is not advocated in those without radiologic and operative findings suggestive of adrenal involvement. [13]

Regional Lymphadenectomy

The argument over the necessity for performing a regional lymph node dissection at the time of radical or partial nephrectomy has recently gained a bit of clarity although still debated among some within the urologic oncology community. In 2009, Blom *et al.* first published results regarding a prospective, randomized EORTC intergroup phase 3 study comparing the outcomes of those managed with radical nephrectomy versus radical nephrectomy and regional lymphadenectomy (LND). Seven-hundred and thirty-two lesions amenable to inclusion as defined as clinical stage T1 to T3 tumors (using the 1978 TNM staging system) without radiologic or clinical findings of regional or distant metastasis were included within the study. As part of that study, all patients in the cohort undergoing a LND underwent a lymph node dissection extending from the crus of the diaphragm inferiorly towards the bifurcation of the aorta or vena cava. In their study, the median follow-up was 12.6 years with no statistical difference noted with regards to overall survival (OS), loco-regional disease progression, or distant metastatic spread between those undergoing and not undergoing LND at time of radical nephrectomy. Only 14 (3%) of the patients undergoing a LND were found to have confirmed regional nodal metastasis.[60] By 2010, Whitson *et al.* weighed in on the subject using SEER data to retrospectively evaluate treatment patterns and outcomes among those undergoing LND in the context of RCC. Search criteria sought to identify all patients treated with radical or partial nephrectomy and concomitant LND which generated a cohort of 9,586 patients who were without evidence of distant mestastatic disease. The data clearly demonstrated a significant positive correlation between lymph node metastasis with increasing tumor size, T stage, higher nuclear grade, older age, and male gender. In this cohort, 1,265 (13.2%) of the patients exhibited node positive disease. At a median follow-up of 3.5 years, the CSS was significantly different for those with node negative disease versus node positive disease (58% and 20%, respectively). The authors also examined the effects of a more extensive LND. In those with a negative lymph node status, there was no benefit to harvesting more nodes while just the opposite was found in those with positive nodes. [61] This is suggestive but not conclusive that performing a LND in those with positive nodes is beneficial. A clinically pertinent study was published by Pantuck *et al.* who used a retrospective study in which patients were divided into 4 subgroups: 1) those without nodal or distant metastatic disease, 2) those with nodal disease in the absence of distant sites of metastasis, 3) those with both nodal and distant metastasis, and 4) those with distant metastasis without evidence of positive regional nodes. Of those deemed without clinical evidence of metastatic disease, there was only a 7.4% incidence of positive regional nodes whereas patients with M1 disease had concomitant regional nodal metastasis 26% of the time. Among the 112 patients with node positive disease who underwent LND compared with the 17 who did not undergo LND, there was a significant median OS benefit of 5 months (p = 0.0002) on univariate analysis and this OS benefit remained on multivariate analysis for those undergoing a LND who were found to be 3 times less likely to die from RCC. The multivariate analysis also demonstrated a significant OS benefit to those undergoing a LND in terms of their subsequent response to immunotherapy. [62]

Currently *in press* is a systematic review of the literature which outlines an algorithm outlining when to perform a LND based on clinical staging. Using the TNM staging system, in those with cT1-T2N0M0, evidence supports omitting a LND unless purely for staging purposes or in the presence of intraoperative suspicion of nodal involvement at which time an extended LND should be performed. In all other cases, those with T3-T4 disease, those with node positive disease, and in those exhibiting metastatic disease with intent for cytoreduction surgery, an extended LND may be warranted as well. [42,63]

Laparoscopic Radical Nephrectomy

Despite the diverse armamentarium of surgical approaches for RCC, they all remained quite invasive prior to the acceptance of laparoscopic techniques. In 1991, laparoscopic radical nephrectomy (LRN) was first described by Clayman *et al* [64] and since that time the safety [65] and efficacy with respect to cancer control[66] between ORN and LRN have been deemed equivalent. In a large meta-analysis evaluating the complications of laparoscopic renal surgery, 20 studies were identified as describing complication rates attributed to LRN. The most common complication was the need to convert to an open surgical procedure, occurring in 2.5% of the cases. Both venous (1.8%) and arterial bleeding (1.0%) were noted as common complications with a need for transfusion occurring 0.7% of the time. Colonic injury was the only other complication noted in > 1% of the procedures (1.5%) performed. [65] Lou *et al.* noted a mean CSS of 82.3 and 81.6 months for pT1 lesions managed by LRN or ORN, respectively, while the CSS related to pT2 lesions was noted to be 69.0 versus 72.1 months for the same aforementioned procedures, with no significant difference demonstrated between these two surgical approaches. [66] With the arrival of LRN, came the necessity to explore the limitations of this new technology. Just as with an open procedure, it was found that a laparoscopic nephrectomy could be performed both transperitoneally and retro-peritoneally with the same general perceived advantages and disadvantages associated with the equivalent open surgical procedure. In 2005, Desai *et al.* published a prospective randomized study comparing these two approaches in 102 patients noting that the retro-peritoneal approach allowed for significantly more expedited control of both: the renal artery and renal vein as well as a significantly shorter overall operative time. However, there was no significant difference between the 2 groups with respect to estimated blood loss (EBL), complications, hospital stay, perioperative narcotic requirement, or local cancer control. [67]

Interestingly, a recent Cochrane Review was conducted to assess the differences between the various surgical techniques currently used to manage RCC and only 3 randomized studies could be identified. [68] Thus, currently accepted standards are based, for the most part, on retrospective studies or prospective studies without randomization. However, Nabi *et al.* were able to utilize the 3 available randomized studies to conclude that there were no differences in intraoperative parameters (operative time, EBL), hospital stay, analgesia requirement, complications, or time to oral intake when comparing LRN, hand-assisted laparoscopic nephrectomy (HALN), and retroperitoneal laparoscopic nephrectomy (RLN) which is more appropriately termed reteroperineoscopic nephrectomy.

Just as in open surgery, clinical scenarios such as a significant history of prior abdominal procedures, a history of peritonitis, or the presence of an intraperitoneal device such as a peritoneal dialysis catheter or ventriculoperitoneal shunt may favor a retroperitoneal approach to the kidney which can be achieved safely laparoscopically (i.e. retroperitoneoscopically).

B. Partial Nephrectomy

The 1990s brought forth major advancements in the surgical management of RCC. Not only was the LRN gaining widespread acceptance, but the roll of open partial nephrectomy (OPN) was being actively investigated. The necessity for NSS was evident: 1) in those patients presenting with lesions involving an anatomic or functionally solitary kidney, 2) those with predisposing medical conditions associated with CKD, 3) patients with bilateral tumors, and 4) those with genetic predisposition to develop subsequent multifocal and/or bilateral renal tumors.

OPN or NSS as we know it today was described by Licht and Novick in 1993 and the first report of a laparoscopic partial nephrectomy (LPN) was reported that same year by Winfield et al.[69,70] Rapidly, studies establishing clinical safety and oncologic efficacy of partial (PN) ensued. [69,71]. By 2000, Fergany et al. reported their 10-year experience with PN for RCC. [72] The efficacy in terms of cancer control was clearly evident with a reported 10-yr CSS ranging from 67-100% among patients with pathologic T1a to T3a tumors. Only those with pT3b tumors had a significantly lower 10-yr CSS compared to the radical nephrectomy cohort.[72] In 2004, Go et al. published a study inclusive of more than 1 million patients and clearly documented an inverse relationship between glomerular filtration rate (GFR) and the incidence of hospitalizations, cardiac events, and death. [73] This was soon followed by evidence demonstrating that those undergoing PN were significantly less likely to develop CKD as defined as a GFR < 60 mL/min/1.73 m^2 as compared to those managed with RN. [20] By 2007, the publication of the European Urological Association (EUA) Guidelines on the Treatment of Cancer and the National Comprehensive Cancer 2011 Kidney Cancer Panel Treatment Guidelines established partial nephrectomy as the standard of care for SRMs as defined by a maximal cross-sectional diameter of <4cm. [42,74] OPN has also been endorsed by the American Urologic Association (AUA) as the treatment of choice for clinical stage T1a and select T1b renal tumors. [6,74]

Warm Ischemia

While small, exophytic tumors may be amenable to resection without clamping of the renal vessels, ischemia is often beneficial with more complex lesions. Ischemia affords limited intraoperative renal hemorrhage, better visualization of the tumor extent, more precise tumor specific excision, and a better opportunity to reconstruct the collecting system and perform a renorhaphy in a bloodless surgical field. However, with a goal of offering NSS, the necessity for judicious use of ischemia has been extensively examined. By identifying a cohort of 458 patients undergoing PN in the clinical context of a solitary kidney, Thompson et al. evaluated the effect of warm ischemia (WI). Ninety-six (21%) of the lesions were managed without ischemia while 362 (79%) were exposed to a median WI time of 21 minutes. The authors point out that the decision to utilize renal cooling was based on the clinical impression that a particular tumor could not be excised in less than 20 to 30 minutes. On multivariate analysis, patients exposed to WI were significantly (6 times) more apt to experience acute-onset of GFR deterioration. Despite perceived benefits allotted by better visualization; there was no significant difference between the two groups with respect to hemorrhage or urine leaks but one must remember that those lesions excised under cold ischemia (CI) were significantly larger. [75] La Rochelle *et al.* presented a prospective study of 84 anatomically solitary kidneys subjected to partial nephrectomy which demonstrated a long-term (greater than 1 month following partial nephrectomy) reduction in eGFR of 12%, 6%, and 16% in those patients undergoing no clamping, WI, and CI; respectively. [7] Of note, only 12 patients necessitated renal cooling with an average CI time of 33 minutes. Of those 22 patients exposed to WI, the average clamp time was 12 minutes. These numbers are similarly reported by Lane *et al.* in a retrospective study of 660 solitary kidneys comparing cold and warm ischemia. [76]

Renal Cooling

Traditionally, achievement of hypothermic organ preservation by means of renal cooling during OPN has been achieved by application of external ice slush. [77] The use of renal cooling allows for a slowing of the metabolic rate of renal tissue whereby limiting the hypoxic injury experienced due to renal ischemia at time of PN. In 1975, it was determined that achieving an organ temperature of 15°C is the most beneficial for renal protection during temporary renal ischemia. [78] As OPN principles have been transferred to the techniques of LPN, renal cooling has been found to be cumbersome and no optimal means of achieving organ hypothermia during LPN have been agreed upon. Continuing the time tested approach of external ice slush application, Gill *et al.* described confinement of the fully mobilized kidney within an endocatch bag along with infused ice slush before exposing the tumor for excision. Weld *et al.* reported on the simultaneous use of two standard suction-irrigators to infuse nearly frozen saline irrigation to achieve hypothermia. [79,80] Renal arterial perfusion with cold Ringer's lactate solution has also been described using both a percutaneous access via a femoral stick and by laparoscopic insertion of a 21 gauge butterfly needle directly into the renal artery. [81,82] Using the percutanous method, renal parenchymal temperatures reached 25°C. Both groups note that the use of intravascular irrigation obviates the need for venous occlusion as the perfusion pressure prevents venous back flow. Retrograde placement of an ipsilateral ureteral access sheath through which a 7.1 French pigtail catheter was inserted to perfuse the collecting system with ice-cold saline and direct laparoscopic cannulation of the renal pelvis for continuous infusion have also been described to bring parenchymal temperatures down to between 21 to 26 °C. [83,84]

While the effects of ischemia and utilization of hypothermia are well studied, [7,85,86] with the benefits of omitting ischemia and limiting warm ischemia times to <20-30 minutes described, only recently has it been noted in a multicenter study of 660 patients that the true tenant with respect to post-partial nephrectomy renal function is the simplistic reality that the more viable tissue you leave behind, the better the postoperative renal function of the remaining ipsilateral kidney. [76] To that effect, techniques such as selective segmental renal artery clamping, arterial only occlusion, and "zero ischemia" have as well been explored.

Selective Segmental Renal Artery Clamping

Shao *et al.* evaluated 75 patients managed by LPN of which 31 of the procedures were completed using selective segmental renal artery clamping. While the operative times, EBL, and WI times were all significantly longer, the reduction in eGFR attributable to the LPN was significantly less. Of note, multiple segmental arteries were occluded as needed and of the 38 renal units intended for management by selective segmental renal artery occlusion, 7 necessitated complete renal artery occlusion to safely complete the procedure.[87] A small series of OPNs were investigated in a similar fashion, however, renal cooling was applied and serum creatinine served as the surrogate for renal function as opposed to eGFR. Again, management by means of selective renal artery occlusion proved more efficacious for renal function sparing. [88] Each of the above series stipulated that arterial mapping by means of a CT angiogram or arterial angiography be performed preoperatively and neither commented on how the ipsilateral renal vein should be managed (i.e. clamped/unclamped) during the procedure.

Arterial Only Occlusion

The potential benefit of allowing for venous backflow perfusion by means of occluding only the ipsilateral artery, and not the vein, was investigated in a small prospective porcine solitary kidney model. The model examined the potential benefit of clamping only the ipsilateral renal artery as opposed to hilar clamping (inclusive of both the ipsilateral renal artery and vein) with respect to renal functional loss. The findings suggest that arterial only clamping did not offer the same protective effect on early postoperative renal function when applied laparoscopically as opposed to during an open procedure. [89] However, the same group was not as confident in this assertion when reporting on their retrospective analysis in human subjects. [90] The obvious difference being that, during laparoscopic procedures, the presence of a pneumoperitoneum may negate venous backflow perfusion.

Early Unclamping

Recently published, Nguyen and Gill described early unclamping as releasing the hilar clamp after controlling the transected intrarenal blood vessels within the pelvicaliceal system. Thus, parenchymal reconstruction is performed off-clamp. This technique was evaluated in 2 cohorts (50 patients each) of patients undergoing LPN for lesions with no significant size difference. The only difference was the time point at which the hilar clamp was released. In the cohort in which early unclamping was applied, the mean warm ischemia time (WIT) was 13.9 ± 4.8 minutes as compared to 31.1 ± 71 minutes in the comparative cohort ($p < 0.0001$). The shorter WIT was associated with a smaller change in eGFR attributable to the nephron-sparing procedure ($p < 0.03$) but the width of the median surgical margin was also significantly less in the group managed with early unclamping, potentially leaving more renal parenchyma behind. [91] Thus, one could speculate about the true benefit derived in lesions that can be managed with 20-30 minutes of WIT given that the true tenant of NSS is that the more renal parenchyma that is preserved, the better the postoperative renal function.

Zero Ischemia

Further pushing the envelope, Eisenberg *et al.* have introduced the novel concept of "zero ischemia". Using pharmacologic agents such as isoflurane, nitroglycerin, and esmolol to reduce patients' mean arterial pressure (MAP) to between 50-80mmHg at time of deep resection. The first 15 cases have been reported to be without associated cardiac or neurologic events. However, extensive invasive cardiovascular monitoring is required including use of: electrocardiogram leads, a bispectral index brain monitor, a cerebral oximeter, a central venous catheter, an arterial line, a pulmonary artery catheter, and a transesophageal echocardiogram (TEE) which are all placed at the outset of the procedure. The authors themselves foresee the potential risks of the procedure and note that the selection of patients with a low-risk for these catastrophic events is necessary. [92,93] At this point, this remains only an experimental treatment alternative and should not be applied to current standard surgical practices.

Laparoscopic Partial Nephrectomy

Familiarity with laparoscopic instrumentation and techniques has become more prevalent amongst many urologists who utilize their laparoscopic skill set to perform minimally invasive NSS. In 2007, Gill *et al.* compared the outcomes of 1,800 PNs performed using open versus laparoscopic techniques. This was not a randomized study and, hence, the patient cohorts were significantly different. The OPN subgroup was significantly older and exhibited larger, more central tumors. Further, this cohort was inclusive of patients with poorer preoperative renal function and patients with only a solitary kidney. Despite the more technically challenging aspects of the tumors in the OPN group, the WI times were 1.69 times (95% CI 1.62-1.77) longer for the laparoscopic group than in the OPN group; 30.7 versus 20.1 minutes, respectively. However, in the OPN group, a multivariate analysis found the mean operative time and intraoperative EBL to be significantly less for the LPN group. With respect to rates of complications, a multivariate analysis was not feasible due to the paucity of unforeseen events. However, evaluation of the absolute number of events suggests that LPN is more likely to be associated with positive surgical margins, intra- and postoperative complications, postoperative hemorrhage, postoperative urine leaks, as well as loss of functioning kidney within 90 days following surgery. [94]

Aware of the benefits of NSS, Hollenbeck *et al.* utilized data pertaining to 66,621 subjects who underwent either radical or partial nephrectomy between 1988 and 2002 to evaluate treatment patterns for RCC. They noted that both the utilization of PN and RN increased between 1988 and 2002; with 12.3% of those with RCC managed by PN at the end of the study. [95] However by 2001, only 42% of those patients exhibiting lesions <2 cm in size were managed with PN [96] which, again, is a current standard of care for such lesions when technically feasible. [6,13] Those institutes considered teaching hospitals, with high nephrectomy volumes, and located within an urban setting were more likely to perform PN. [95] The disparity between the incidence of SRMs and the utilization of PN seems incongruent with the standard of care despite a known consequence of chronic renal insufficiency (CRI) which is significantly more likely after enduring a RN as opposed to a PN at 3 and 5 years following surgery. In fact, of those patients undergoing PN with a normal preoperative creatinine, none developed CRI in the follow-up period. The patient characteristics predisposing for the development of renal insufficiency included: hypertension, diabetes, tobacco smoking, elevated preoperative serum creatinine, increased anesthesia risk (ASA score 3 or greater), and advanced age. [97]

C. Thermal Ablative Techniques

Originally proposed as a treatment option for SRMs among those with significant co-morbidities, advanced age, and/or personal preferences prohibitive of surgical intervention, the less invasive thermal ablative (TA) techniques such as cryoablation (Cryo) and radiofrequency ablation (RFA) have gained increasing acceptance as a front line treatment option in well selected cases. [6] In fact, in those with clinical stage T1a lesions and major co-morbitidies, thermal ablation is a recommended treatment modality that deserves consideration after relaying to such patients that PN or RN remains the gold standard from an oncological standpoint. In those without confounding health risks, ablative modalities remain only an option without conclusive evidence to either support or dismiss their use in such circumstances, particularly with its limited long-term data (>5 years) currently available. [6]

As with all evolving therapies, patient safety is at the forefront of such discussions. In a meta-analysis, the overall major complication rate of Cryo and RFA were 4.9% and 6.0%, respectively. These rates are indistinguishable from one another or to those of OPN or LRN however those electing for Cryo or RFA were substantially older. [6] In the clinical context of prior renal TA for suspected RCC, a local recurrence is defined as any persistent or recurrent disease present in the treated kidney or associated renal fossa after the initial treatment as outlined by the working group of Image-Guided Tumor Ablation. [98]

To more adequately assess the efficacy of ablative techniques, Kunkle and Uzzo conducted a meta-analysis in 2008 of 47 studies from 45 centers constituting 1375 renal lesions treated by either Cryo or RFA. Statistical analysis of patient age, tumor size, and duration of follow-up were not significantly different among those treated by Cryo and RFA. The study was restricted to SRMs with a mean tumor size of 2.6 cm. At a median follow-up of 18.7 months, 31 of 600 (5.2%) renal lesions managed with Cryo and 100 of 775 (12.9%) of those managed with RFA exhibited evidence of local progression. This represents a significant difference between the two cohorts ($p < 0.0001$).

Metastatic progression was noted in 6 of 600 (1%) patients undergoing Cryo and 19 of 775 (2.5%) treated with RFA which trends towards a statistical significant difference ($p = 0.06$) in favor of Cryo. [99] This represented an overall rate of progression to metastatic disease of 1.8% which is very similar to the 1% rate reported among those patients on active surveillance. [41,99]

When applying TA therapies, both retroperitoneal percutaneous and transperitoneal approaches can be employed. The percutaneous methods are more readily applied to posterior or laterally positioned renal lesions located within the mid to lower pole of the kidney. This allows for an unobstructed path for the insertion of ablative probes. For anterior lesions and those in the upper pole, a transperitoneal approach may be necessary to allow for safe access. Further, lesions lying in close proximity to adjacent structures that warrant retraction may also be addressed transperitoneally. However, percutaneous strategies such as hydrodistention to safely displace such structures have been described although not widely accepted among treating urologists. [100]

Radiofrequency Ablation

The use of RFA for the management of renal tumors was first reported in 1997. [101] Using percutaneously placed probes, alternating current of radiofrequency energy is delivered to the targeted lesion and the impedance offered by cells leads to the generation of hea reaching temperatures of up to 105 °C. Cell death and coagulation necrosis is demonstrated when temperatures exceed 70 °C and a necrotic lesion is formed within 24 to 48 hours, reaching a maximal size by 7 days. [102,103] The simultaneous instillation of hypertonic saline via perfusion electrodes allows for the creation of larger lesions but also leads to unpredictable patterns of ablation. [104]

Cryoablation

The surgical utility of Cryo has been long known as the modern era of Cryo techniques commenced in the 1960's with the development of automated cryosurgical equipment. However, the first description of using Cryo to manage SRMs was not until 1995. [105] The mechanisms of tissue injury are multiple and significant injury is actuallized hours after the last thaw cycle. Initially, the cooling allows for extracellular freezing, desiccation of targeted tumor cells as well as alterations of intracellular pH and protein denaturation. As temperatures near the tumoricidal -40 °C, intracellular ice crystal formation leads to mechanical destruction of the intracellular organelles as well as of the cell membrane. A slow thaw is important for the recrystallizaton process, allowing for further intracellular ice crystal expansion. Repeated cycles improve the odds of complete tumor killing/eradication. After the freeze-thaw cycles are complete, reperfusion of the damaged microcirculation leads to microthrombi formulation and microcirculatory occlusion resulting in tissue ischemia and uniform tissue destruction. [106]

D. Active Surveillance

The current trends of increasing use of abdominal cross-sectional imaging, increasing prevalence of incidentally discovered renal masses, and downward stage migration, has only intensified the active discussion regarding the most appropriate treatment of SRMs. Thus, both the AUA and EUA have recently set forth guidelines regarding such lesions; both of which advocate surgical excision as the gold standard therapy for SRMs. However, active surveillance (AS) has been explored as an appropriate course of non-action when a patient's co-morbidities, potential post-surgical need for renal replacement therapy, or personal preference obviate the role of surgical intervention. The integration of AS within our treatment armamentarium has allowed for a better understanding of the natural history of RCC.

A meta-analysis of 10 single institutional retrospective studies consisting of 286 patients without evidence of local and/or distant metastases reported a mean annual growth rate of 0.28 cm/year, with only 3 (1%) patients progressing to metastatic disease at a mean follow-up of 34 months.

Of note, the tumor size at initial diagnosis was not predictive of the growth rate of the mass. However, of those lesions that were pathologically confirmed as malignant, the growth rate was 0.4 cm/year. [41] Crispen et al. examined the tumor growth kinetics of 173 localized renal tumors and noted that 128 (74%) of the lesions demonstrated an interval growth while 45 (26%) of the lesions displayed no growth or actually diminished in size. However, the authors were unable to discern between those that would enlarge and those that would not based solely on: tumor diameter at time of diagnosis, multifocality, gender, and/or pathological characteristics. The role of percutaneous renal biopsy among patients placed on AS remains highly debated (see Section IIIC).

V. Surgical Management of Locally Advanced/Metastatic RCC

A. RCC Venous Tumor Thrombus

RCC has the unique ability to potentially propagate within the local venous system (as a tumor thrombus) within either the renal vein, inferior vena cava (IVC), and right atrium of the heart. Between 4 to 10% of patients with RCC are associated with intravenous tumor thrombus (IVTT) presenting more frequently (up to 95%) with clinical symptoms than do patients without an IVTT. [107,108] Specifically, the generally accepted signs suspicious for IVTT include: bilateral lower extremity edema, newly discovered varicoceles (especially on the right side), dilated superficial abdominal wall veins, caput medusae, and pulmonary emboli.

Using the TNM staging system previously outlined above (see Section IIIA), extension into the renal vein, the IVC below the diaphragm, and into the IVC above the level of the diaphragm correspond to the designations T3a, T3b, and T3c; respectively. All tumors exhibiting venous wall invasion are also described as clinical T3c. [109] The TNM staging system is intended to differentiate individual tumors on the basis of associated prognosis and a recent international consortium of 11 centers attempted to validate the recent staging modifications with respect to the level of venous involvement. Reviewing the data of 1048 patients with records conducive to inclusion, the 5 and 10-year CSS was 43.2% and 23%; respectively, for those with pathological T3a lesions. When the IVTT extended into the IVC below the level of the diaphragm (pathological T3b), CSS dropped to 37.3% and 21.2% at these same time points. Of those with IVTT extending above the diaphragm (pathological T3c), the 5 and 10-year CSS was to 22.2% and 13.2%, respectively. The difference in CSS between those with pathological T3b and T3c disease was noted regardless of the lymph node or metastatic tumor burden. [110]

B. Adjacent Organ Involvement (T4)

Locally advanced RCC, generally defined as tumor extending beyond Gerota's fascia, involving the ipsilateral adrenal gland, and/or involving adjacent organs or the presence of isolated regional adenopathy is rare. Historically, the reported incidence of pathological T4 RCC is 5-15%, but the majority of such encompassing lesions are associated with synchronous metastases. [111,112] Recently, a validation study of the 2010 TNM staging system (which for the first time includes ipsilateral adrenal involvement as pathological T4) reported only a 4% incidence of pathological T4 disease in a contemporary patient cohort. However, this Same patient population included a 4% and 6% incidence of regional adenopathy and metastatic disease, respectively. The potential overlap of the 3 staging categories was not addressed. Further, this study was inclusive of only patients undergoing extirpative treatment and may underestimate the true extent of locally advanced RCC. [32]

Margulis et al. recently identified 30 patients with locally advanced RCC by the 2002 TNM classification, of which 10 (33%) demonstrated regional adenopathy. All patients were managed with open radical nephrectomy, regional lymphadenectomy, en bloc resection of all involved adjacent organs, and removal of venous tumor thrombus if present. Nine (30%) of the patients were managed with prompt adjuvant therapy protocols and 17 (57%) received systemic immunotherapy and/or chemotherapy. Using multivariate Cox regression analyses, regional lymph node metastasis was a significant predictor of RFS and CSS. The 3-year RFS was 29% versus 10% in those with N0 or $\geq$N1 disease, respectively (p = 0.001) and the 3-year CSS was 66% for those with N0 disease while only 12% with $\geq$N1 status. (p <0.001). [113]

C. Cytoreductive Nephrectomy

As previously noted, there has been a downward stage migration, discovery of smaller tumors at time of diagnosis, and a rapid rise in incidentally diagnosed tumors due to the frequent use of imaging techniques, [2-5] However, 25-30% of RCCs continue to be diagnosed due to symptoms resulting from metastatic disease which is associated with a dismal prognosis (0-20% reported 5-year survival). [74,114] Thus, it is not unusual that multimodality approaches consisting of surgical resection and systemic therapies (targeted and/or immunotherapy) have been explored in this patient cohort. Specifically, the use of immunotherapy subsequent to cytoreductive nephrectomy (CN) has previously demonstrated a survival benefit in 2 prior landmark studies. [115,116] In fact, a pooled analysis of these two studies demonstrated a 6 month OS advantage in those undergoing CN followed by immunotherapy. [117] However, tyrosine kinase inhibitors (TKIs) have since proven to have a superior therapeutic effect with respect to overall response rates and PFS. [118] The utilization of targeted therapies directed at manipulation of the vascular endothelial growth factor (VEGF) pathways has rapidly expanded in recent years; shifting our current treatment paradigm. Choueiri et al. retrospectively demonstrated a continued OS benefit of CN in those falling in the good and intermediate Memorial Sloan Kettering Cancer Center (MSKCC) risk groups [118] who were subsequently placed on TKIs or VEGF monoclonal antibodies. However, an OS benefit of CN was not seen among patients within the poor MSKCC risk group. [119] Thus, risk stratification is an important parameter when considering CN and balancing the risks of surgery with the survival advantage it may entail. In addition, patient risk stratification is an important therapeutic consideration when tailoring the optimal systemic therapy. [120] Recently, multiple efforts examining the ability to stratify patients based on clinical histoy, current tumor burden, and serologic composites have identified clinical parameters prognostic of OS in metastatic RCC (mRCC). [48,119,121,122] Furthermore, potential immunosuppressive lymphocytes have been surmised to contribute to the outcomes of those with mRCC by proposed mechanisms of allowing escape of tumor cells from immunosurveillance . [123-125]

D. Metastatectomy

As previously stated, 25-30% of patients diagnosed with RCC present with metastatic disease and, in addition, up to 50% of patients will eventually develop metastatic disease following nephrectomy for localized disease. In this clinical context, the role of metastatectomy (i.e. surgical resection of an isolated local site of recurrence) is an important therapeutic consideration in such patients. [6,126] However, the wide distribution with respect to location and number of metastases present within each individual makes it difficult to create a blanket statement regarding the role of surgical management in all patients with a local/regional recurrence. What is clear is that the most common sites of distant metastasis is clearly within the lung, bone, and liver. [127] In a retrospective review of 99 consecutive patients with mRCC undergoing a standardized outpatient-cytokine protocol, 46 (46.5%) patients underwent some form of metastasectomy for pain control, management of pathological fractures, and essential clinical indications such as brain metastasis. [128] Within these 46 patients, 30% of them were treated with intent for cure and 21% were rendered free of disease. Using the Motzer criteria outlined above, [118] the majority were determined to be high-risk. On multivariate analysis of OS, metastasectomy (even incomplete) was shown to significantly improve median OS (median OS 6.6 months). [128]

VI. Postoperative Surveillance

	Months of Follow-up										
	3	6	12	18	24	30	36	48	60	84	108
Low risk:											
History + physical examination			•		•		•	•	•		
Laboratory Studies*			•		•		•	•	•		
Chest CT			•		•		•	•	•		
Abdominal CT					•			•			
Intermediate risk:											
History + physical examination		•	•	•	•	•	•	•	•	•	•
Laboratory Studies*		•	•	•	•	•	•	•	•	•	•
Chest CT†		•	•	•	•	•	•	•	•	•	•
Abdominal CT		•					•		•	•	•
High risk:											
History + physical examination		•	•	•	•	•	•	•	•	•	•
Laboratory Studies*		•	•	•	•	•	•	•	•	•	•
Chest CT†		•	•	•	•	•	•	•	•	•	•
Abdominal CT		•	•	•	•		•	•	•	•	•
Nodal disease:											
History + physical examination	•	•	•	•	•		•	•	•	•	•
Laboratory Studies*	•	•	•	•	•		•	•	•	•	•
Chest CT†	•	•	•	•	•		•	•	•	•	•
Abdominal CT	•	•	•	•	•		•	•	•	•	•

* Includes complete blood count, serum chemistries, and liver function tests.
† A chest radiograph can be alternated with a chest CT after 3 years of follow-up

Adapted with permission from Lam *et al. J Urol* 2005.[134]

Figure 1. Risk group assignment of patients with localized and locally advanced renal cell carcinoma.

Postoperatively, patients, and treating physicians alike, are very concerned about the risk of recurrence and overall disease-specific outcomes. Currently, the Fox Chase Cancer Center sponsors a website (www.cancernomograms.com) that offers multiple interactive nomograms to help accurately provide this information to patients. [129-132] As approximately 30% of those with a localized primary renal tumor managed surgically will later develop either a local or distant recurrence, patients are often concerned about the measures that will be taken to closely monitor their disease status. [130] To that effect, recent efforts have used evidenced-based medicine to define surveillance protocols. [133,134] In 2004, a multicenter Canadian study reported on 495 patients with locally confined primary renal tumors managed by either radical nephrectomy (n = 426) or partial nephrectomy (n = 69). At a median follow-up of 42 months, using protocols at each physician's discretion, the 5-year RFS was found to directly, and significantly, correlate with tumor staging. For tumors confined to the kidney, the 5-year RFS was 93% and 81% for tumors less than or greater 7cm in greatest diameter, respectively. The median time to recurrence was also stage dependent; 35 months for T1 lesions and 25 months for T2 lesions. [133] Similar findings were described by Lam *et al.* who developed the University of California-Los Angeles Integrated Staging System (UISS) which stratified patients into low, intermediate, and high risk groups based on the 1997 TNM staging, grade, and Eastern Cooperative Oncology Group (ECOG) performance status. In those deemed low-risk, no abdominal recurrence presented prior to 20 months postoperatively and the median time to recurrence was 32 months. [134] It should be noted, that while the TNM staging has been revised twice since 1997, the only major difference with respect to local disease is that ipsilateral adrenal involvement now mandates a T4 classification as opposed to T3a, leaving the UISS still quite applicable today. The surveillance protocol derived from the outcomes using the UISS system is shown in Figure 1.

Conclusions

Contemporary studies have demonstrated a downward stage migration, tumors to be of a smaller size at time of diagnosis, and a rising incidence of incidentally diagnosed tumors due to readily available imaging techniques. However, recent studies have demonstrated the significant presence of baseline CKD amongst those presenting with renal tumors and acknowledges the added morbidity and mortality experienced by individuals with underlying renal insufficiency compared to those with normal renal function. Thus, PN has become the gold standard for surgical management of amenable renal tumors and has proven equivalent with respect to patient safety and oncologic outcomes for tumors less than 7 cm. To further preserve functional renal parenchyma, multiple surgical techniques seeking to limit renal ischemia time and apply intraoperative renal cooling have been explored and published. However, methods for renal cooling remain cumbersome when performed laparoscopically. Alternatively, thermal ablative techniques such as Cryo and RFA have increasing interest in the SRM treatment algorithm for those individuals unfit for surgical extirpation. Active surveillance has also found a role in the management of SRMs in carefully selected patients and has reopened the active debate about the utility of a percutaneous renal biopsy for select SRMs. When radical nephrectomy is necessitated, laparoscopic techniques can be readily applied and have been rapidly adopted by urologists; allowing for patients to reap the benefits of minimally invasive surgery without compromising oncological outcomes. However, performing a LPN requires more advanced laparoscopic dexterity and may be a contributing factor to the fact that PN is clearly underutilized today. With respect to advanced RCC, there remains continued speculation about the benefits derived from performing a concomitant lymph node dissection as part of standard practice and about the appropriate template that should apply. However, the literature suggests that those with clinical stage T3-T4 disease, those with suspected clinical lymph node positive disease, and those exhibiting metastatic disease with intent for cytoreductive surgery, should at the very least be considered for an extended LND.

References

[1]   Jemal A, Siegel R, Xu J, Ward E. Cancer statistics, 2010. *CA Cancer J Clin.* Sep-Oct 2010;60(5):277-300.

[2]   Hollingsworth JM, Miller DC, Daignault S, Hollenbeck BK. Rising incidence of small renal masses: a need to reassess treatment effect. *J Natl Cancer Inst.* Sep 20 2006;98(18):1331-1334.

[3]   Kane CJ, Mallin K, Ritchey J, Cooperberg MR, Carroll PR. Renal cell cancer stage migration: analysis of the National Cancer Data Base. *Cancer.* Jul 1 2008;113(1):78-83.

[4]   Chow WH, Devesa SS, Warren JL, Fraumeni JF, Jr. Rising incidence of renal cell cancer in the United States. *Jama.* May 5 1999;281(17):1628-1631.

[5]   Hock LM, Lynch J, Balaji KC. Increasing incidence of all stages of kidney cancer in the last 2 decades in the United States: an analysis of surveillance, epidemiology and end results program data. *J Urol.* Jan 2002;167(1):57-60.

[6]   Campbell SC, Novick AC, Belldegrun A, et al. Guideline for management of the clinical T1 renal mass. *J Urol.* Oct 2009;182(4):1271-1279.

[7]   La Rochelle J, Shuch B, Riggs S, et al. Functional and oncological outcomes of partial nephrectomy of solitary kidneys. *J Urol.* May 2009;181(5):2037-2042; discussion 2043.

[8]   Chen DY, Uzzo RG. Evaluation and management of the renal mass. *Med Clin North Am.* Jan 2011;95(1):179-189.

[9]   Glazer A, Novick AC. Preoperative transesophageal echocardiography for assessment of vena caval tumor thrombi: a comparative study with venacavography and magnetic resonance imaging. *Urology.* Jan 1997;49(1):32-34.

[10]   Sharma V, Cusimano RJ, McNama P, Wasowicz M, Ko R, Meineri M. Intraoperative migration of an inferior vena cava tumour detected by transesophageal echocardiography. *Can J Anaesth.* May 2011;58(5):468-470.

[11]   Schallner N, Wittau N, Kehm V, Humburger F, Schmidt R, Steinmann D. Intraoperative pulmonary tumor embolism from renal cell carcinoma and a patent foramen ovale detected by transesophageal echocardiography. *J Cardiothorac Vasc Anesth.* Feb 2011;25(1):145-147.

[12]   Cywinski JB, O'Hara JF, Jr. Transesophageal echocardiography to redirect the intraoperative surgical approach for vena cava tumor resection. *Anesth Analg.* Nov 2009;109(5):1413-1415.

[13]   Ljungberg B, Cowan NC, Hanbury DC, et al. EAU guidelines on renal cell carcinoma: the 2010 update. *Eur Urol.* Sep 2010;58(3):398-406.

[14]   Bosniak MA. Problems in the radiologic diagnosis of renal parenchymal tumors. *Urol Clin North Am.* May 1993;20(2):217-230.

[15]   Curry NS. Small renal masses (lesions smaller than 3 cm): imaging evaluation and management. *AJR Am J Roentgenol.* Feb 1995;164(2):355-362.

[16]   Silverman SG, Lee BY, Seltzer SE, Bloom DA, Corless CL, Adams DF. Small (< or = 3 cm) renal masses: correlation of spiral CT features and pathologic findings. *AJR Am J Roentgenol.* Sep 1994;163(3):597-605.

[17] Davenport MS, Neville AM, Ellis JH, Cohan RH, Chaudhry HS, Leder RA. Diagnosis of renal angiomyolipoma with hounsfield unit thresholds: effect of size of region of interest and nephrographic phase imaging. *Radiology.* Jul 2011;260(1):158-165.

[18] Warren KS, McFarlane J. The Bosniak classification of renal cystic masses. *BJU Int.* May 2005;95(7):939-942.

[19] Graumann O, Osther SS, Osther PJ. Characterization of complex renal cysts: a critical evaluation of the Bosniak classification. *Scand J Urol Nephrol.* Mar 2011;45(2):84-90.

[20] Huang WC, Levey AS, Serio AM, et al. Chronic kidney disease after nephrectomy in patients with renal cortical tumours: a retrospective cohort study. *Lancet Oncol.* Sep 2006;7(9):735-740.

[21] Levey AS, Coresh J, Greene T, et al. Using standardized serum creatinine values in the modification of diet in renal disease study equation for estimating glomerular filtration rate. *Ann Intern Med.* Aug 15 2006;145(4):247-254.

[22] Levey AS, Stevens LA, Schmid CH, et al. A new equation to estimate glomerular filtration rate. *Ann Intern Med.* May 5 2009;150(9):604-612.

[23] Stacul F, van der Molen AJ, Reimer P, et al. Contrast induced nephropathy: updated ESUR Contrast Media Safety Committee guidelines. *Eur Radiol.* Aug 25 2011.

[24] Coakley FV, Panicek DM. Iodine allergy: an oyster without a pearl? *AJR Am J Roentgenol.* Oct 1997;169(4):951-952.

[25] Brockow K, Christiansen C, Kanny G, et al. Management of hypersensitivity reactions to iodinated contrast media. *Allergy.* Feb 2005;60(2):150-158.

[26] Greenberger P, Patterson R, Kelly J, Stevenson DD, Simon D, Lieberman P. Administration of radiographic contrast media in high-risk patients. *Invest Radiol.* Nov-Dec 1980;15(6 Suppl):S40-43.

[27] Lawrentschuk N, Gani J, Riordan R, Esler S, Bolton DM. Multidetector computed tomography vs magnetic resonance imaging for defining the upper limit of tumour thrombus in renal cell carcinoma: a study and review. *BJU Int.* Aug 2005;96(3):291-295.

[28] Hallscheidt PJ, Fink C, Haferkamp A, et al. Preoperative staging of renal cell carcinoma with inferior vena cava thrombus using multidetector CT and MRI: prospective study with histopathological correlation. *J Comput Assist Tomogr.* Jan-Feb 2005;29(1):64-68.

[29] Leiner T, Kucharczyk W. NSF prevention in clinical practice: summary of recommendations and guidelines in the United States, Canada, and Europe. *J Magn Reson Imaging.* Dec 2009;30(6):1357-1363.

[30] Ozulker T, Ozulker F, Ozbek E, Ozpacaci T. A prospective diagnostic accuracy study of F-18 fluorodeoxyglucose-positron emission tomography/computed tomography in the evaluation of indeterminate renal masses. *Nucl Med Commun.* Apr 2011;32(4):265-272.

[31] Edge S.B. BDR, Compton C.C., Fritz A.G., Greene F.L., Trotti A., ed *AJCC Cancer Staging Manual.* Seventh ed. New York: Springer-Verlag; 2010.

[32] Novara G, Ficarra V, Antonelli A, et al. Validation of the 2009 TNM version in a large multi-institutional cohort of patients treated for renal cell carcinoma: are further improvements needed? *Eur Urol.* Oct 2010;58(4):588-595.

[33] Kovacs G, Akhtar M, Beckwith BJ, et al. The Heidelberg classification of renal cell tumours. *J Pathol.* Oct 1997;183(2):131-133.

[34] Fuhrman SA, Lasky LC, Limas C. Prognostic significance of morphologic parameters in renal cell carcinoma. *Am J Surg Pathol.* Oct 1982;6(7):655-663.

[35] Choueiri TK, Schutz FA, Hevelone ND, et al. Thermal ablation vs surgery for localized kidney cancer: a Surveillance, Epidemiology, and End Results (SEER) database analysis. *Urology.* Jul 2011;78(1):93-98.

[36] Leveridge MJ, Finelli A, Kachura JR, et al. Outcomes of small renal mass needle core biopsy, nondiagnostic percutaneous biopsy, and the role of repeat biopsy. *Eur Urol.* Sep 2011;60(3):578-584.

[37] Volpe A, Mattar K, Finelli A, et al. Contemporary results of percutaneous biopsy of 100 small renal masses: a single center experience. *J Urol.* Dec 2008;180(6):2333-2337.

[38] Kutikov A, Fossett LK, Ramchandani P, et al. Incidence of benign pathologic findings at partial nephrectomy for solitary renal mass presumed to be renal cell carcinoma on preoperative imaging. *Urology.* Oct 2006;68(4):737-740.

[39] Schmidbauer J, Remzi M, Memarsadeghi M, et al. Diagnostic accuracy of computed tomography-guided percutaneous biopsy of renal masses. *Eur Urol.* May 2008;53(5):1003-1011.

[40] Eshed I, Elias S, Sidi AA. Diagnostic value of CT-guided biopsy of indeterminate renal masses. *Clin Radiol.* Mar 2004;59(3):262-267.

[41] Chawla SN, Crispen PL, Hanlon AL, Greenberg RE, Chen DY, Uzzo RG. The natural history of observed enhancing renal masses: meta-analysis and review of the world literature. *J Urol.* Feb 2006;175(2):425-431.

[42] NCCN. Clinical Practice Guidelines in Oncology: Kidney Cancer *Version* 22011.

[43] Gold PJ, Fefer A, Thompson JA. Paraneoplastic manifestations of renal cell carcinoma. *Semin Urol Oncol.* Nov 1996;14(4):216-222.

[44] Kim HL, Belldegrun AS, Freitas DG, et al. Paraneoplastic signs and symptoms of renal cell carcinoma: implications for prognosis. *J Urol.* Nov 2003;170(5):1742-1746.

[45] Pepper K, Jaowattana U, Starsiak MD, et al. Renal cell carcinoma presenting with paraneoplastic hypercalcemic coma: a case report and review of the literature. *J Gen Intern Med.* Jul 2007;22(7):1042-1046.

[46] Paule B. [Interleukin-6 and bone metastasis of renal cancer: molecular bases and therapeutic implications]. *Prog Urol.* Apr 2001;11(2):368-375.

[47] Weissglas MG, Schamhart DH, Lowik CW, Papapoulos SE, Theuns HM, Kurth KH. The role of interleukin-6 in the induction of hypercalcemia in renal cell carcinoma transplanted into nude mice. *Endocrinology.* May 1997;138(5):1879-1885.

[48] Motzer RJ, Bacik J, Schwartz LH, et al. Prognostic factors for survival in previously treated patients with metastatic renal cell carcinoma. *J Clin Oncol.* Feb 1 2004;22(3):454-463.

[49] Motzer RJ, Bukowski RM, Figlin RA, et al. Prognostic nomogram for sunitinib in patients with metastatic renal cell carcinoma. *Cancer.* Oct 1 2008;113(7):1552-1558.

[50] Manola J, Royston P, Elson P, et al. Prognostic Model for Survival in Patients with Metastatic Renal Cell Carcinoma: Results from the International Kidney Cancer Working Group. *Clin Cancer Res.* Aug 15 2011;17(16):5443-5450.

[51] Wilson W, Taubert KA, Gewitz M, et al. Prevention of infective endocarditis: guidelines from the American Heart Association: a guideline from the American Heart Association Rheumatic Fever, Endocarditis and Kawasaki Disease Committee, Council

on Cardiovascular Disease in the Young, and the Council on Clinical Cardiology, Council on Cardiovascular Surgery and Anesthesia, and the Quality of Care and Outcomes Research Interdisciplinary Working Group. *J Am Dent Assoc.* Jan 2008;139 Suppl:3S-24S.

[52] Antibiotic prophylaxis for urological patients with total joint replacements. *J Urol.* May 2003;169(5):1796-1797.

[53] Wolf JS, Jr., Bennett CJ, Dmochowski RR, Hollenbeck BK, Pearle MS, Schaeffer AJ. Best practice policy statement on urologic surgery antimicrobial prophylaxis. *J Urol.* Apr 2008;179(4):1379-1390.

[54] Geerts WH, Pineo GF, Heit JA, et al. Prevention of venous thromboembolism: the Seventh ACCP Conference on Antithrombotic and Thrombolytic Therapy. *Chest.* Sep 2004;126(3 Suppl):338S-400S.

[55] Forrest JB, Clemens JQ, Finamore P, et al. AUA Best Practice Statement for the prevention of deep vein thrombosis in patients undergoing urologic surgery. *J Urol.* Mar 2009;181(3):1170-1177.

[56] Robson CJ. Radical nephrectomy for renal cell carcinoma. *J Urol.* Jan 1969;89:37-42.

[57] Lane BR, Tiong HY, Campbell SC, et al. Management of the adrenal gland during partial nephrectomy. *J Urol.* Jun 2009;181(6):2430-2436; discussion 2436-2437.

[58] Kutikov A, Piotrowski ZJ, Canter DJ, et al. Routine adrenalectomy is unnecessary during surgery for large and/or upper pole renal tumors when the adrenal gland is radiographically normal. *J Urol.* Apr 2011;185(4):1198-1203.

[59] O'Malley RL, Godoy G, Kanofsky JA, Taneja SS. The necessity of adrenalectomy at the time of radical nephrectomy: a systematic review. *J Urol.* May 2009;181(5):2009-2017.

[60] Blom JH, van Poppel H, Marechal JM, et al. Radical nephrectomy with and without lymph-node dissection: final results of European Organization for Research and Treatment of Cancer (EORTC) randomized phase 3 trial 30881. *Eur Urol.* Jan 2009;55(1):28-34.

[61] Whitson JM, Harris CR, Reese AC, Meng MV. Lymphadenectomy improves survival of patients with renal cell carcinoma and nodal metastases. *J Urol.* May 2011;185(5):1615-1620.

[62] Pantuck AJ, Zisman A, Dorey F, et al. Renal cell carcinoma with retroperitoneal lymph nodes: role of lymph node dissection. *J Urol.* Jun 2003;169(6):2076-2083.

[63] Capitanio U, Becker F, Blute ML, et al. Lymph Node Dissection in Renal Cell Carcinoma. *Eur Urol.* Sep 13 2011.

[64] Clayman RV, Kavoussi LR, Soper NJ, et al. Laparoscopic nephrectomy: initial case report. *J Urol.* Aug 1991;146(2):278-282.

[65] Pareek G, Hedican SP, Gee JR, Bruskewitz RC, Nakada SY. Meta-analysis of the complications of laparoscopic renal surgery: comparison of procedures and techniques. *J Urol.* Apr 2006;175(4):1208-1213.

[66] Luo JH, Zhou FJ, Xie D, et al. Analysis of long-term survival in patients with localized renal cell carcinoma: laparoscopic versus open radical nephrectomy. *World J Urol.* Jun 2010;28(3):289-293.

[67] Desai MM, Strzempkowski B, Matin SF, et al. Prospective randomized comparison of transperitoneal versus retroperitoneal laparoscopic radical nephrectomy. *J Urol.* Jan 2005;173(1):38-41.

[68] Nabi G, Cleves A, Shelley M. Surgical management of localised renal cell carcinoma. *Cochrane Database Syst Rev.* 2010(3):CD006579.

[69] Licht MR, Novick AC. Nephron sparing surgery for renal cell carcinoma. *J Urol.* Jan 1993;149(1):1-7.

[70] Winfield HN, Donovan JF, Godet AS, Clayman RV. Laparoscopic partial nephrectomy: initial case report for benign disease. *J Endourol.* Dec 1993;7(6):521-526.

[71] Morgan WR, Zincke H. Progression and survival after renal-conserving surgery for renal cell carcinoma: experience in 104 patients and extended followup. *J Urol.* Oct 1990;144(4):852-857; discussion 857-858.

[72] Fergany AF, Hafez KS, Novick AC. Long-term results of nephron sparing surgery for localized renal cell carcinoma: 10-year followup. *J Urol.* Feb 2000;163(2):442-445.

[73] Go AS, Chertow GM, Fan D, McCulloch CE, Hsu CY. Chronic kidney disease and the risks of death, cardiovascular events, and hospitalization. *N Engl J Med.* Sep 23 2004;351(13):1296-1305.

[74] Ljungberg B, Hanbury DC, Kuczyk MA, et al. Renal cell carcinoma guideline. *Eur Urol.* Jun 2007;51(6):1502-1510.

[75] Thompson RH, Lane BR, Lohse CM, et al. Comparison of warm ischemia versus no ischemia during partial nephrectomy on a solitary kidney. *Eur Urol.* Sep 2010;58(3):331-336.

[76] Lane BR, Russo P, Uzzo RG, et al. Comparison of cold and warm ischemia during partial nephrectomy in 660 solitary kidneys reveals predominant role of nonmodifiable factors in determining ultimate renal function. *J Urol.* Feb 2011;185(2):421-427.

[77] Novick AC. Renal hypothermia: in vivo and ex vivo. *Urol Clin North Am.* Nov 1983;10(4):637-644.

[78] Ward JP. Determination of the Optimum temperature for regional renal hypothermia during temporary renal ischaemia. *Br J Urol.* Feb 1975;47(1):17-24.

[79] Gill IS, Abreu SC, Desai MM, et al. Laparoscopic ice slush renal hypothermia for partial nephrectomy: the initial experience. *J Urol.* Jul 2003;170(1):52-56.

[80] Weld KJ, Koziol S, Montiglio C, Sorenson P, Cespedes RD, Bishoff JT. Feasibility of laparoscopic renal cooling with near-freezing saline irrigation delivered with a standard irrigator aspirator. *Urology.* Mar 2007;69(3):465-468.

[81] Janetschek G, Abdelmaksoud A, Bagheri F, Al-Zahrani H, Leeb K, Gschwendtner M. Laparoscopic partial nephrectomy in cold ischemia: renal artery perfusion. *J Urol.* Jan 2004;171(1):68-71.

[82] Marley CS, Siegrist T, Kurta J, et al. Cold intravascular organ perfusion for renal hypothermia during laparoscopic partial nephrectomy. *J Urol.* Jun 2011;185(6):2191-2195.

[83] Landman J, Rehman J, Sundaram CP, et al. Renal hypothermia achieved by retrograde intracavitary saline perfusion. *J Endourol.* Sep 2002;16(7):445-449.

[84] Crain DS, Spencer CR, Favata MA, Amling CL. Transureteral saline perfusion to obtain renal hypothermia: potential application in laparoscopic partial nephrectomy. *Jsls.* Jul-Sep 2004;8(3):217-222.

[85] Becker F, Van Poppel H, Hakenberg OW, et al. Assessing the impact of ischaemia time during partial nephrectomy. *Eur Urol.* Oct 2009;56(4):625-634.

[86] Russo P. Partial nephrectomy for renal cancer: Part I. *BJU Int.* May 2010;105(9):1206-1220.

[87] Shao P, Qin C, Yin C, et al. Laparoscopic partial nephrectomy with segmental renal artery clamping: technique and clinical outcomes. *Eur Urol.* May 2011;59(5):849-855.

[88] Nohara T, Fujita H, Yamamoto K, Kitagawa Y, Gabata T, Namiki M. Modified anatrophic partial nephrectomy with selective renal segmental artery clamping to preserve renal function: a preliminary report. *Int J Urol.* Oct 2008;15(11):961-966.

[89] Orvieto MA, Zorn KC, Mendiola F, et al. Recovery of renal function after complete renal hilar versus artery alone clamping during open and laparoscopic surgery. *J Urol.* Jun 2007;177(6):2371-2374.

[90] Gong EM, Zorn KC, Orvieto MA, Lucioni A, Msezane LP, Shalhav AL. Artery-only occlusion may provide superior renal preservation during laparoscopic partial nephrectomy. *Urology.* Oct 2008;72(4):843-846.

[91] Nguyen MM, Gill IS. Halving ischemia time during laparoscopic partial nephrectomy. *J Urol.* Feb 2008;179(2):627-632; discussion 632.

[92] Eisenberg MS, Patil MB, Thangathurai D, Gill IS. Innovations in laparoscopic and robotic partial nephrectomy: a novel 'zero ischemia' technique. *Curr Opin Urol.* Mar 2011;21(2):93-98.

[93] Gill IS, Eisenberg MS, Aron M, et al. "Zero ischemia" partial nephrectomy: novel laparoscopic and robotic technique. *Eur Urol.* Jan 2011;59(1):128-134.

[94] Gill IS, Kavoussi LR, Lane BR, et al. Comparison of 1,800 laparoscopic and open partial nephrectomies for single renal tumors. *J Urol.* Jul 2007;178(1):41-46.

[95] Hollenbeck BK, Taub DA, Miller DC, Dunn RL, Wei JT. National utilization trends of partial nephrectomy for renal cell carcinoma: a case of underutilization? *Urology.* Feb 2006;67(2):254-259.

[96] Miller DC, Hollingsworth JM, Hafez KS, Daignault S, Hollenbeck BK. Partial nephrectomy for small renal masses: an emerging quality of care concern? *J Urol.* Mar 2006;175(3 Pt 1):853-857; discussion 858.

[97] McKiernan J, Simmons R, Katz J, Russo P. Natural history of chronic renal insufficiency after partial and radical nephrectomy. *Urology.* Jun 2002;59(6):816-820.

[98] Goldberg SN, Grassi CJ, Cardella JF, et al. Image-guided tumor ablation: standardization of terminology and reporting criteria. *Radiology.* Jun 2005;235(3):728-739.

[99] Kunkle DA, Uzzo RG. Cryoablation or radiofrequency ablation of the small renal mass : a meta-analysis. *Cancer.* Nov 15 2008;113(10):2671-2680.

[100] Bodily KD, Atwell TD, Mandrekar JN, et al. Hydrodisplacement in the percutaneous cryoablation of 50 renal tumors. *AJR Am J Roentgenol.* Mar 2010;194(3):779-783.

[101] Zlotta AR, Wildschutz T, Raviv G, et al. Radiofrequency interstitial tumor ablation (RITA) is a possible new modality for treatment of renal cancer: ex vivo and in vivo experience. *J Endourol.* Aug 1997;11(4):251-258.

[102] Hwang JJ, Walther MM, Pautler SE, et al. Radio frequency ablation of small renal tumors:: intermediate results. *J Urol.* May 2004;171(5):1814-1818.

[103] Schulman C, Zlotta A. Transurethral needle ablation of the prostate (TUNA): pathological, radiological and clinical study of a new office procedure for treatment of benign prostatic hyperplasia using low-level radiofrequency energy. *Arch Esp Urol.* Nov 1994;47(9):895-901.

[104] Hinshaw JL, Lee FT, Jr. Image-guided ablation of renal cell carcinoma. *Magn Reson Imaging Clin N Am.* Aug 2004;12(3):429-447, vi.

[105] Uchida M, Imaide Y, Sugimoto K, Uehara H, Watanabe H. Percutaneous cryosurgery for renal tumours. *Br J Urol.* Feb 1995;75(2):132-136; discussion 136-137.

[106] Gage AA, Baust J. Mechanisms of tissue injury in cryosurgery. *Cryobiology.* Nov 1998;37(3):171-186.

[107] Hatcher PA, Anderson EE, Paulson DF, Carson CC, Robertson JE. Surgical management and prognosis of renal cell carcinoma invading the vena cava. *J Urol.* Jan 1991;145(1):20-23; discussion 23-24.

[108] Zisman A, Pantuck AJ, Chao DH, et al. Renal cell carcinoma with tumor thrombus: is cytoreductive nephrectomy for advanced disease associated with an increased complication rate? *J Urol.* Sep 2002;168(3):962-967.

[109] Edge SB, Compton CC. The American Joint Committee on Cancer: the 7th Edition of the AJCC Cancer Staging Manual and the Future of TNM. *Ann Surg Oncol.* Jun 2010;17(6):1471-1474.

[110] Martinez-Salamanca JI, Huang WC, Millan I, et al. Prognostic impact of the 2009 UICC/AJCC TNM staging system for renal cell carcinoma with venous extension. *Eur Urol.* Jan 2011;59(1):120-127.

[111] Lam JS, Belldegrun AS, Pantuck AJ. Long-term outcomes of the surgical management of renal cell carcinoma. *World J Urol.* Aug 2006;24(3):255-266.

[112] Frank I, Blute ML, Cheville JC, Lohse CM, Weaver AL, Zincke H. An outcome prediction model for patients with clear cell renal cell carcinoma treated with radical nephrectomy based on tumor stage, size, grade and necrosis: the SSIGN score. *J Urol.* Dec 2002;168(6):2395-2400.

[113] FL Greene DP, CM Batch, ID Fleming, and M Morrow, ed *AJCC Cancer Staging Manual.* New York: Springer Verlag; 2002.

[114] Cancer Facts and Figures 2011. Atlanta: American Cancer Society; 2011.

[115] Flanigan RC, Salmon SE, Blumenstein BA, et al. Nephrectomy followed by interferon alfa-2b compared with interferon alfa-2b alone for metastatic renal-cell cancer. *N Engl J Med.* Dec 6 2001;345(23):1655-1659.

[116] Mickisch GH, Garin A, van Poppel H, de Prijck L, Sylvester R. Radical nephrectomy plus interferon-alfa-based immunotherapy compared with interferon alfa alone in metastatic renal-cell carcinoma: a randomised trial. *Lancet.* Sep 22 2001;358(9286):966-970.

[117] Flanigan RC, Mickisch G, Sylvester R, Tangen C, Van Poppel H, Crawford ED. Cytoreductive nephrectomy in patients with metastatic renal cancer: a combined analysis. *J Urol.* Mar 2004;171(3):1071-1076.

[118] Motzer RJ, Hutson TE, Tomczak P, et al. Sunitinib versus interferon alfa in metastatic renal-cell carcinoma. *N Engl J Med.* Jan 11 2007;356(2):115-124.

[119] Choueiri TK, Xie W, Kollmannsberger C, et al. The impact of cytoreductive nephrectomy on survival of patients with metastatic renal cell carcinoma receiving vascular endothelial growth factor targeted therapy. *J Urol.* Jan 2011;185(1):60-66.

[120] Schmidinger M, Zielinski CC. Defining risk status in the first-line treatment of metastatic renal cell carcinoma. *J Cancer Res Clin Oncol.* Jul 2010;136(7):961-968.

[121] Negrier S, Escudier B, Gomez F, et al. Prognostic factors of survival and rapid progression in 782 patients with metastatic renal carcinomas treated by cytokines: a report from the Groupe Francais d'Immunotherapie. *Ann Oncol.* Sep 2002;13(9):1460-1468.

[122] You D, Jeong IG, Ahn JH, et al. The value of cytoreductive nephrectomy for metastatic renal cell carcinoma in the era of targeted therapy. *J Urol.* Jan 2011;185(1):54-59.

[123] Nakano O, Sato M, Naito Y, et al. Proliferative activity of intratumoral CD8(+) T-lymphocytes as a prognostic factor in human renal cell carcinoma: clinicopathologic demonstration of antitumor immunity. *Cancer Res.* Jul 1 2001;61(13):5132-5136.

[124] Bromwich EJ, McArdle PA, Canna K, et al. The relationship between T-lymphocyte infiltration, stage, tumour grade and survival in patients undergoing curative surgery for renal cell cancer. *Br J Cancer.* Nov 17 2003;89(10):1906-1908.

[125] Siddiqui SA, Frigola X, Bonne-Annee S, et al. Tumor-infiltrating Foxp3-CD4+CD25+ T cells predict poor survival in renal cell carcinoma. *Clin Cancer Res.* Apr 1 2007;13(7):2075-2081.

[126] Bukowski RM. Natural history and therapy of metastatic renal cell carcinoma: the role of interleukin-2. *Cancer.* Oct 1 1997;80(7):1198-1220.

[127] Breau RH, Blute ML. Surgery for renal cell carcinoma metastases. *Curr Opin Urol.* Sep 2010;20(5):375-381.

[128] Vogl UM, Zehetgruber H, Dominkus M, et al. Prognostic factors in metastatic renal cell carcinoma: metastasectomy as independent prognostic variable. *Br J Cancer.* Sep 18 2006;95(6):691-698.

[129] Karakiewicz PI, Briganti A, Chun FK, et al. Multi-institutional validation of a new renal cancer-specific survival nomogram. *J Clin Oncol.* Apr 10 2007;25(11):1316-1322.

[130] Zisman A, Pantuck AJ, Wieder J, et al. Risk group assessment and clinical outcome algorithm to predict the natural history of patients with surgically resected renal cell carcinoma. *J Clin Oncol.* Dec 1 2002;20(23):4559-4566.

[131] Sorbellini M, Kattan MW, Snyder ME, et al. A postoperative prognostic nomogram predicting recurrence for patients with conventional clear cell renal cell carcinoma. *J Urol.* Jan 2005;173(1):48-51.

[132] Thompson RH, Leibovich BC, Lohse CM, et al. Dynamic outcome prediction in patients with clear cell renal cell carcinoma treated with radical nephrectomy: the D-SSIGN score. *J Urol.* Feb 2007;177(2):477-480.

[133] Stephenson AJ, Chetner MP, Rourke K, et al. Guidelines for the surveillance of localized renal cell carcinoma based on the patterns of relapse after nephrectomy. *J Urol.* Jul 2004;172(1):58-62.

[134] Lam JS, Shvarts O, Leppert JT, Pantuck AJ, Figlin RA, Belldegrun AS. Postoperative surveillance protocol for patients with localized and locally advanced renal cell carcinoma based on a validated prognostic nomogram and risk group stratification system. *J Urol.* Aug 2005;174(2):466-472; discussion 472; quiz 801.

In: Essentials and Updates in Urologic Oncology
Editor: Philippe E. Spiess

ISBN: 978-1-62081-494-9
© 2013 Nova Science Publishers, Inc.

Chapter XXIV

Systemic Therapy for Kidney Cancer

*Guru Sonpavde[1] and Toni K. Choueiri[*2]*
[1]University of Alabama at Birmingham (UAB) Comprehensive Cancer Center,
Birmingham, Alabama, US
[2]Dana Farber Cancer Institute and Harvard Medical School,
Boston, Massachusetts, US

Abstract

Better knowledge of the critical role of angiogenesis has yielded significant advances in the therapy of advanced renal cell carcinoma (RCC). Sunitinib, pazopanib, and the combination of bevacizumab plus interferon (IFN)-α improved outcomes as first-line therapy in trials mostly enrolling good and intermediate risk RCC. Temsirolimus improved outcomes in patients with poor risk RCC and high dose (HD) interleukin (IL)-2 plays a role in good-risk clear cell-RCC based on durable complete responses in a small fraction of patients. Following VEGF inhibitors, second-line axitinib or everolimus have both demonstrated similar long-term outcomes. Optimal patient selection for specific agents is undergoing investigation. A commitment to clinical trials and comprehensive understanding of mechanisms of resistance to current therapies will generate further advances.

Introduction

An understanding of the role of angiogenesis has led to the addition of multiple agents to the therapeutic armamentarium for clear-cell renal cell carcinoma (RCC). The loss of VHL (Von Hippel Lindau) at the germline or somatic level upregulates the transcription factor, hypoxia inducible factor (HIF), which leads to the production of multiple proangiogenic

* Correspondence: Toni K. Choueiri, MD, Dana Farber Cancer Institute and Harvard Medical School, 450 Brookline Ave, Boston, Massachusetts 02215

molecules including vascular endothelial growth factor (VEGF).[1, 2] Both VEGF inhibitors and inhibitors of mTOR, a component of the survival pathway, have conferred extensions in progression-free survival (PFS). The median overall survival (OS) has also been extended to ~ 2 years from the historical benchmark of ~1 year in the era of cytokines.[3-6]

Tumor Biology

An important study demonstrated 3 groups of tumors with distinct molecular characteristics [7]. Tumors with intact VHL or pVHL-deficient and HIF-1α/HIF-2α-expression demonstrated upregulated Akt/mTOR and ERK/MAPK signaling. Tumors with pVHL-deficiency and only HIF-2α expression displayed elevated c-Myc activity, leading to enhanced proliferation and resistance to replication stress. Several lines of evidence suggest that deregulation of HIF-α, and especially HIF-2α rather than HIF-1α, contributes to pVHL-defective renal carcinogenesis with the former playing the role of an oncogene, while the latter exerting the function of a tumor-suppressor gene[8]. Two subtypes of RCC, clear cell type A (ccA) and type B (ccB), were identified in another study based on gene expression profiling[9]. The genes associated with ccA were involved in angiogenesis, β-oxidation, organic acid metabolism, fatty acid metabolism and pyruvate metabolism. Conversely, ccB tumors overexpressed genes associated with cell differentiation, epithelial to mesenchymal transition (EMT), the mitotic cell cycle, transforming growth factor-beta, response to wounding and Wnt.

While tumors may exhibit denovo/intrinsic resistance, exposure to VEGF inhibition may trigger multiple acquired mechanisms of resistance, although VEGF receptor mutations appear unlikely to mediate resistance[10]. Activation of alternative pro-angiogenic pathways (e.g. interleukin-8, FGF, ephrin and angiopoietin-Tie pathways), recruitment of bone marrow-derived pro-angiogenic cells, increased pericyte coverage of tumor vasculature and enhancement of invasion and metastasis (e.g. by hepatocyte growth factor-MET and insulin-like growth factor pathways) may continue to drive angiogenesis[1, 2]. Immune mechanisms may be mediated by intratumoral myeloid derived suppressor cells[11]. mTORC1 inhibition upregulates the PI3K/AKT pathway, which may activate compensatory mTORC2 signaling. Additionally, differences in drug metabolism due to host factors may engender poor activity or toxicities.

Prognostic Factors

A retrospective study analyzed prognostic factors in patients receiving VEGF inhibitors (sunitinib, sorafenib or bevacizumab), of whom approximately a third had received prior cytokines [[12]. Adverse prognostic factors were anemia, hypercalcemia, Karnofsky Performance Status (KPS) < 80%, time from diagnosis to treatment < 1 year, neutrophilia and thrombocytosis. The favorable (no factors), intermediate (1-2 factors) and poor-risk groups (≥3 factors) exhibited a 2-year OS of 75%, 53% and 7%, respectively. These prognostic factors and longer time on first-line therapy were also prognostic following prior VEGF inhibitors in a population receiving subsequent VEGF or mTOR inhibitors[13]. These prognostic factors in the setting of VEGF inhibitors are similar to those identified in the setting of IFN except that elevated LDH is replaced by neutrophilia and thrombocytosis[14, 15]. Prognostic models incorporating molecular markers may refine the prediction of outcomes.

First-Line Therapy

Sunitinib

Sunitinib 50 mg orally daily for 4 of every 6 weeks, a multitargeted oral tyrosine kinase inhibitor (TKI) targeting the VEGF, platelet derived growth factor (PDGF) and Kit receptors among other molecular targets, yielded a median progression-free survival (PFS) of 11 months compared with 5 months for IFN-α (P < .001). The median OS also demonstrated extension (26.4 vs. 21.8 months, P = .051), which attained statistical significance after censoring patients' crossing over from IFN to sunitinib. Objective response rate (RR) was 47% for sunitinib compared with 12% for IFN-α (P < .001). The most common grade 3 adverse events included hypertension, fatigue, diarrhea, hand-foot syndrome and hypothyroidism[16]. All clinical risk-groups appeared to benefit, although ~93% of patients exhibited good or intermediate risk disease. In a recent presentation of the renal EFFECT randomized phase II trial, the conventional 50 mg daily for 4 of every 6 weeks regimen was superior to the alternative schedule of 37.5 mg daily continuously when employing a composite endpoint including death, progression and patient-reported outcomes[17].

Pazopanib

A Phase III placebo-controlled study of pazopanib, a VEGF receptor TKI, enrolled patients with generally good and intermediate risk patients with RCC that were either treatment naïve or exposed to prior cytokines [[18]. The overall median PFS improved with pzopanib to 9.2 months (versus 4.2 months, p<0.0001) and for treatment naïve patients was 11.1 months (vs. 2.8 months for placebo, p<0.0001). The RR for pazopanib was 30% and extensive crossover confounded survival assessment. The common severe adverse events were diarrhea, hypertension, hair depigmentation, nausea, anorexia and vomiting. Liver enzymes (ALT or AST) elevations were occasionally severe. Myelosuppression and hand-foot syndrome appeared less common when comparing with sunitinib or sorafenib across trials, which has been attributed potentially to a smaller number of receptor tyrosine kinase targets, especially less potent Flt3 inhibition. Interestingly, a randomized phase II trial (N=168), PISCES, demonstrated that patients preferred pazopanib over sunitinib [19]. In this blinded trial, patients were randomized to receive first line pazopanib for 10 weeks followed by a 2-week washout and then sunitinib for 10 weeks or vice versa. Pazopanib was preferred by 70%, sunitinib by 22% and 8% of patients had no preference. Patients on pazopanib had fewer dose reductions (13% vs 20%) and interruptions (6% vs 12%) compared to sunitinib. The results of a completed open-label phase III trial (COMPARZ, N=1110) comparing pazopanib and sunitinib in untreated patients were recently reported[20]. This important trial demonstrated the non-inferiority of pazopanib for PFS (primary endpoint) by independent review (median 8.4 vs.9.5 monthsThe safety profile of pazopanib was differentiated from sunitinib and exhibited a lower incidence of hand-foot syndrome, fatigue and mucositis. Conversely, the incidence of liver enzyme abnormalities was higher with pazopanib. Overall, quality of life scores favored pazopanib.

Bevacizumab Plus Interferon

The AVOREN (Avastin for renal cell cancer) trial randomized 649 patients with RCC to frontline IFN-α 2a plus placebo or IFN-α 2a plus bevacizumab (monoclonal antibody against VEGF), which was administered intravenously every 2 weeks[21]. The addition of bevacizumab to IFN-α 2a significantly extended median PFS (10.2 v 5.4 months, p<0.0001) and RR (30.6% vs. 12.4%; p<0.0001). A trend toward improved OS was also observed (p=0.0670), although survival analysis was confounded by subsequent exposure to other active agents. The contribution of IFN-α 2a to the efficacy of the combination is unclear, and the small subset of poor-risk patients did not appear to benefit from this combination. The similar (but not placebo-controlled) Cancer and Leukemia Group-B trial also demonstrated a similar extension of median PFS with the combination of bevacizumab and IFN (8.5 vs. 5.2 months, p<0.0001)[22]. The most common adverse events attributable to bevacizumab were fatigue, proteinuria and hypertension. The value of IFN in this combination is unclear. Notably, a randomized phase II trial evaluated first-line bevacizumab alone or with erlotinib and demonstrated a similar median PFS of 8.5-9.9 months in both arms containing bevacizumab[23].

Temsirolimus

Temsirolimus, a relatively specific mTOR inhibitor and a sirilomus analogue, administered as a weekly intravenous infusion, prolonged median OS (10.9 vs. 7.3 months, p=0.008) compared to IFN-α in patients with poor risk RCC, i.e. ≥3 poor risk factors[24]. A third arm receiving combination temsirolimus and IFN did not demonstrate superiority over IFN alone probably partly due to lower administered doses. Notably, this trial allowed the accrual of patients without a clear cell component (~ a third of patients) and a larger fraction (~ a third) had not undergone prior nephrectomy compared to the aforementioned trials evaluating VEGF inhibitors (where ~90% had undergone prior nephrectomy). Rash, peripheral edema, hyperglycemia, and hyperlipidemia were more common with temsirolimus.

High Dose Interleukin-2

High dose (HD) Interleukin (IL)-2 may retain a role in selected patients (good risk CC-RCC, alveolar features and the absence of papillary or granular features, high CAIX expression, genomic signatures) with good performance status due to an ~7% durable complete remissions and apparent cures[3, 5, 6]. The severe cardiovascular, pulmonary and renal toxicities of HD-IL-2 also render it an option only for relatively young patients without significant comorbidities. Unfortunately, the recent prospective SELECT trial could not validate tumor CAIX expression as a predictive factor for response[25].

Second-Line Therapy

Therapy Following Prior Cytokines

The use of sorafenib, pazopanib and axitinib following cytokines is supported by level-1 evidence. The phase III Treatment Approaches in Renal cancer Global Evaluation Trial (TARGET) randomized patients with good or intermediate risk RCC who had progressed within 8 months after one first-line regimen to sorafenib or placebo (81-83% had received cytokine-based therapy) . The overall median PFS improved with sorafenib (5.5 vs. 2.8 months) independent of age, risk score, previous cytokine, lung or liver metastases and time since diagnosis (<1.5 or ≥1.5 years). An extension of OS was observed when patients who crossed-over from placebo to sorafenib were censored (17.8 vs. 14.3 months, HR = 0.78; P = .029)[26].

In the aforementioned randomized, double-blind phase III trial, pazopanib extended median PFS (7.4 vs. 4.2 months) following prior cytokines [[27]. Axitinib, a novel investigational TKI that inhibits all VEGF receptors, has demonstrated activity following cytokines in a phase II trial (median TTP 15.7 months and median survival 29.9 months), which was confirmed by the recently reported AXIS phase III trial[28, 29]. This randomized, open-label, phase III trial enrolled 723 patients and compared axitinib versus sorafenib as second-line therapy after 1 prior systemic therapy. Patients were stratified for performance status and type of prior therapy, and randomized 1:1 to axitinib 5 mg orally twice daily (titrated to 7 mg and then 10 mg twice daily as tolerated) or sorafenib 400 mg twice daily. Prior therapy included most of the approved agents at the time the trial was designed: sunitinib (54%), cytokine (35%), bevacizumab (8%) or temsirolimus (3%). The overall median PFS was 6.7 months for axitinib vs. 4.7 months for sorafenib (HR 0.665, p<0.0001) and the RR was 19.4% vs. 9.4% (P=0.0001). PFS also favored axitinib in the prior cytokine group (12.1 vs. 6.5 months; P<0.0001). The benefit for axitinib was preserved across prognostic factors and quality of life was similar in both groups. AEs of all grades more frequent with axitinib were hypertension, fatigue, dysphonia and hypothyroidism. AEs more frequent with sorafenib were hand-foot syndrome, rash, alopecia and anemia. The regulatory approval of axitinib is anticipated.

In phase II trials, sunitinib exhibited activity after cytokine therapy, yielding a median PFS of ~8 months and partial responses (PR) in 20-34%[30, 31]. Another investigational TKI with potent VEGF receptor targeting activity, tivozanib, has demonstrated similar activity in a large phase II trial that enrolled untreated or post-cytokine patients[32]. Similarly, both bevacizumab and temsirolimus have demonstrated modest activity following prior cytokines in phase II trials[33, 34]. It is likely that the number of patients in the post-cytokine setting will decline, given that cytokines will be confined to a small group qualifying for HD IL-2.

Therapy Following Prior VEGF Inhibitors

Everolimus

Everolimus was evaluated in the phase III randomized, double-blind, placebo-controlled RECORD-1 trial in patients with PD within 6 months following sunitinib, sorafenib, or both[35]. Previous therapy with bevacizumab, interleukin 2, or IFN was also permitted. Patients were randomly assigned in a 2:1 ratio to receive everolimus 10 mg once daily (n=272) or placebo (n=138) and stratification was by risk group and 1 vs. 2 prior TKIs. Of all patients, 21% had received 1 prior TKI, 53% had received 1 TKI and at least 1 other agent (commonly a cytokine), and 26% had received both TKIs with or without additional therapy. The median PFS was 4.9 months with everolimus vs. 1.9 months with placebo (HR 0.33, P < 0.001). The benefit was observed across different prognostic risk groups and regardless of the prior TKI administered. Declines in tumor size were observed in 47% of patients receiving everolimus versus 10.0% with placebo, although RECIST defined response rates were low (1% vs.0%). The median OS was 14.8 versus 14.4 months (HR, 0.87; P = 0.162), which was confounded by 80% of patients in the placebo arm crossing over to everolimus. The survival corrected for crossover was 1.9-fold longer with everolimus. Stomatitis, rash, fatigue and pneumonitis were the notable toxicities. Metabolic toxicities (hyperlipidemia, hyperglycemia) were manageable. A retrospective review examined 87 patients treated previously with at least one TKI and subsequent temsirolimus[36]. The majority of patients had either intermediate or poor-prognosis disease. The RR was 5% and was accompanied by a stable disease rate of 65%. The median TTP and OS were 3.9 and 11.2 months, respectively. Patients in the poor-prognosis group had a shorter TTP (2.6 months), while the degree of prior treatment did not appear to have an impact.

Axitinib

A phase II trial evaluated axitinib in 62 patients following sorafenib, of whom 74.2% had received ≥2 prior treatments[37]. The RR was 22.6%, and the median PFS and OS were 7.4 months and 13.6 months, respectively, which led to the phase III AXIS trial[29]. In the AXIS trial, in addition to the improvement in overall and post-cytokine outcomes, PFS favored axitinib in the prior sunitinib subgroup (4.8 vs. 3.4 months; P=0.0107).

Sequencing of VEGF Inhibitors

While all of the approved TKIs inhibit VEGF and platelet derived growth factor (PDGF) receptors and Kit, there are differences in potencies and the spectrum of molecular targets. The differences in toxicity profiles may also be partly explained by these differences. Data corroborate the lack of complete cross-resistance between the different TKIs and between initial bevacizumab and subsequent TKIs. The median PFS for the second agent in the sequence varies between ~4-7 months. Sorafenib and sunitinib in sequence has been examined in retrospective and phase II trials, and both sequences demonstrating modest activity for the second agent in the sequence[38-40]. Prospective evaluation of the sequencing of sorafenib and sunitinib is ongoing (Table 2). Similarly, pazopanib has demonstrated activity following sunitinib or bevacizumab in a phase II trial[41]. Moreover, sunitinib has demonstrated activity in patients with bevacizumab-refractory RCC[42]. An unplanned exploratory analysis from the AVOREN trial demonstrated that median OS was numerically longer (38.6 *vs.* 33.6 months, HR = 0.80, p=0.20) in patients receiving TKI after bevacizumab-IFN compared with those receiving TKIs after IFN[43, 44].

Rechallenge

In a retrospective study, 23 patients who were rechallenged with sunitinib after PD on prior sunitinib were retrospectively identified[45]. Upon rechallenge, 5 patients (22%) attained a PR. The median PFS with initial sunitinib was 13.7 months and 7.2 months with rechallenge. Patients with >6-month interval between sunitinib treatments had a longer PFS with rechallenge (median PFS, 16.5 vs. 6.0 months, p=.03). There was no significant difference in outcomes based on number or mechanisms of activity of intervening treatments. These data, although retrospective and subject to selection bias, suggest a resetting of sensitivity to sunitinib in a proportion with longer duration of time off sunitinib. Data for the strategy of rechallenging when employing other TKIs are necessary.

VEGF or mTOR Inhibitors Following VEGF Inhibitors?

A retrospective study of 645 patients with metastatic RCC analyzed outcomes with VEGF or mTOR inhibitors following VEGF inhibitors. Patients who received first-line VEGF-targeted therapy of whom, 216 received second-line VEGF-targeted therapy (majority were receiving sunitinib or sorafenib) or mTOR-inhibitors (temsirolimus or everolimus) were analyzed[46]. On multivariate analysis, a higher baseline KPS before first-line therapy predicted the likelihood of receiving second-line therapy. The median time to failure (TTF) of second-line therapy was 4.9 months for anti-VEGF therapy and 2.5 months for mTOR inhibitors (P = .014) after adjusting for prognostic factors. The difference remained after adjusting for an imbalance in sarcomatoid histology. However, OS from start of second-line therapy was not significantly different (14.2 vs. 10.6 months, p = 0.38).

Another retrospective study examined patients treated with first-line anti-VEGF therapy that had primary resistance, i.e. PD as the best response[47]. Of 1056 patients, 272 (26%) patients had PD as the best response to sunitinib (n=203), sorafenib (n=51) or bevacizumab (n=18). The predictors of PD were KPS < 80%, diagnosis to treatment < 1 year, neutrophilia, thrombocytosis and anemia[12]. The median PFS and OS in patients with primary refractory disease vs. other patients was 2.4 vs. 11 months (p<0.0001) and 6.8 vs. 29 months (p<0.0001), respectively. Only 108 (40%) patients proceeded to receive second-line therapy. The overall RR, PFS and OS of second-line therapy were 9%, 2.5 months and 7.4 months, respectively. Second-line mTOR inhibitors did not appear better than alternative anti-VEGF agents with similar RR, PFS and OS for VEGF inhibitors vs. mTOR inhibitors of 10% vs. 6% (p=NS), 2.8 vs. 2.0 months (p=0.069) and 7.9 vs. 4.7 months (p=0.40), respectively. Another retrospective study examined whether second-line therapy could be potentially selected based on the type of response to first-line VEGF therapy[48]. The counterintuitive finding was that no correlation was observed between first-line and second-line PFS (p=0.59) or response (p=0.17). Recently, the INTORSECT multicenter, randomized, open-label phase 3 trial (N=512) compared temsirolimus versus sorafenib in patients who progressed following prior sunitinib therapy [49]. The vast majority of patients had clear-cell histology and favorable or intermediate risk disease. This trial did not demonstrate an extension in the primary endpoint, PFS, with temsirolimus (median ~4 months for both). Intriguingly, the sorafenib arm had a longer survival (median 16.6 vs. 12.3 months, P=0.014). Safety data were as expected with both agents.

Immunotherapy Following VEGF Inhibitors

There is a lack of evidence for this strategy and no clinical trials available. One retrospective study examined HD IL-2 after prior TKIs (sorafenib or sunitinib) and/or bevacizumab[50]. The efficacy of HD IL-2 was dismal in this population, with no patients experiencing a response, and only 13% achieving stable disease (SD). Moreover, 6 of the 23 patients (26%) experienced severe cardiac toxicities (including 1 sudden cardiac death), all of whom had received a prior TKI.

Therapy Following Prior mTOR Inhibitors

Comprehensive data are unavailable to guide therapy following mTOR inhibitors. The AXIS trial included few patients (n=24) who received second-line axitinib following temsirolimus[29]. In a retrospective cohort study, third-line sorafenib appeared modestly active and safe after first-line sunitinib and second-line everolimus or temsirolimus[51]. The RR was 23.5% coupled with a median PFS of 4 months and a median OS of 7 months. Cross-resistance in sequential employment of the mTOR inhibitors, everolimus and temsirolimus, has not been assessed.

Therapy of Non-Clear Cell And Sarcomatoid RCC

A standard of therapy has not been established for non-clear cell RCC and clinical trials should be preferred. Among the phase III trials, only the trial comparing temsirolimus with IFN allowed patients bearing tumors without a clear cell component[24]. Indeed, the subset of non-clear cell patients exhibited better hazard ratios for extension of survival from temsirolimus. Retrospective studies have demonstrated activity for VEGF targeting TKIs in papillary and chromophobe RCC, although the activity appears less robust than in clear cell RCC[52]. Randomized phase II trials are comparing everolimus with sunitinib for non-clear cell RCC. Additionally, the RECORD-III trial (Table 2) allowed such patients and may yield complementary information. Similarly, less robust activity for VEGF inhibitors has been observed in sarcomatoid RCC, with better activity in those with a smaller sarcomatoid component (<20%)[53]. Chemotherapeutic regimens in patients with a sarcomatoid component demonstrate modest activity and combination with VEGF inhibitors are undergoing early phase II evaluation (e.g. capecitabine, gemcitabine plus bevacizumab, sunitinib plus gemcitabine).

Role of Cytoreductive Nephrectomy and Perioperative Therapy

In the era of cytokines, cytoreductive nephrectomy (CN) before the institution of cytokines was demonstrated to improve outcomes significantly in patients with metastatic clear cell RCC[54-56]-[57] Notably, there are no data to definitively support the role of CN in patients with non-clear cell-RCC[58, 59]. The vast majority of patients on phase III trials that led to the approval of novel agents over the last 5 years had undergone prior nephrectomy. A recent retrospective report of 314 patients suggests that CN may continue to play a role in the setting of anti-angiogenic agents although the limitations of a retrospective study do not allow firm conclusions[60]. The value of performing a CN is being evaluated in prospective trials. The CARMENA trial is designed as a non-inferiority trial comparing sunitinib therapy alone versus CN followed by sunitinib.

Data have demonstrated the feasibility and activity of VEGF inhibitors as neoadjuvant therapy before CN, and may render resectable a proportion of tumors initially considered unresectable[61, 62]. Trials have performed CN after 12 or 16 weeks of sunitinib and within 1 day to 14 days after stopping sunitinib, followed by resumption of sunitinib at least 2 weeks after CN[63, 64]. A slight increase in perioperative complications following neoadjuvant sunitinib (hemorrhage, delayed wound healing and altered surgical field), and progression of disease during the treatment break entailed by surgery have been observed, most of whom responded or stabilized on continued post-operative sunitinib[65, 66]. No difference was noted in a small dataset for stopping sunitinib within 1 day or 14 days before CN[64]. Data reassuringly indicate no compromise of long-term outcomes in patients receiving either neoadjuvant sunitinib (2 or 3 cycles) or bevacizumab-based therapy preceding CN.[63, 67] In the trial evaluating neoadjuvant bevacizumab, high nephrectomy tumor AMPK (which regulates the PI3K pathway) and low PI3K pathway expression (low pAkt, low pS6K, high PTEN) correlated with longer survival, which may be a candidate pathway that interacts with the VEGF pathway and a potential resistance mechanism. The investigators hypothesized that agents targeting the PI3K pathway may provide clinical benefits in bevacizumab treated patients.[68, 69]. Thus, neoadjuvant therapy may facilitate the analysis of tumor tissue following therapy and the discovery of mechanisms of resistance, which may expedite rational drug development. The SURTIME phase III trial is evaluating the timing of therapy and CN and will compare either post-CN sunitinib with or without 2-3 cycles of pre-CN sunitinib. The role of adjuvant therapy is undergoing vigorous evaluation. Both TKIs (sunitinib, sorafenib, pazopanib) and mTOR inhibitors (everolimus) are being studied in placebo-controlled trials. Most of these trials evaluate a duration of 1 year of therapy, except the placebo-controlled SORCE trial, which compares 1 versus 3 years of sorafenib.

Individualized Therapy: Consideration of Clinical and Molecular Factors and Toxicity Profiles

It is unclear if second-line therapy could be tailored based on prognostic risk-grouping similar to first-line therapy (Table 1). For example, given the demonstrated extension of survival with temsirolimus for poor-risk RCC, patients with poor-risk disease who receive a first-line VEGF targeting agent may preferentially warrant a second-line mTOR inhibitor rather than another VEGF targeting agent. Second line change of class may provide relief from a panel of toxicities, which is particularly relevant for patients discontinuing for toxicities. All of the VEGF targeting agents have been associated to some extent with hypertension, cardiac toxicities, hand-foot syndrome, hypothyroidism and arterial thrombotic events, which are not commonly seen with mTOR inhibitors[70]. Hence, switching to an mTOR inhibitor may confer toxicity benefits in such patients. However, TKIs have incompletely overlapping toxicity profiles and those experiencing prohibitive toxicities with a TKI may tolerate a different TKI. Conversely, hypertension appears to be a pharmacodynamic marker correlating with outcomes in the setting of VEGF inhibitors and dose modifications probably should be pursued before discontinuation in such patients[71]. The primarily hepatic metabolism and excretion of mTOR inhibitors suggests feasibility in those with renal dysfunction.

Additionally, mTOR inhibitors have unique adverse effects, such as hyperglycemia, hyperlipidemia and interstitial pneumonitis, which may limit tolerance in select populations. Furthermore, given the cost of these agents, patients may make choices driven by financial considerations[72]. In this retrospective study, patients receiving bevacizumab incurred higher costs compared to sunitinib or sorafenib patients due to higher drug and intravenous administration costs, while those who received sunitinib incurred the highest cost for adverse event management.

Optimal selection of patients based on molecular factors is still in its infancy. Prognostic molecular panels have been discovered, but have not been demonstrated to facilitate selection of therapy[73, 74]. Lower baseline levels of sVEGFR-3 and VEGF-C were associated with better RR and PFS in a phase II trial that evaluated sunitinib following bevacizumab[42]. Germline variants in angiogenesis (IL-8, HIF1α, VEGF-A) and exposure-related genes (NR1I2) may predict treatment response to pazopanib[75].

One study did not find a significant increase in response to VEGF targeting agents in patients with tumor VHL inactivation, although loss of function mutations appeared to identify more sensitive tumors[76]. Similarly, tumor pS6 and pAkt expression may be promising predictive biomarkers for response to temsirolimus based at least on one small retrospective study[77].

Table 1. Algorithm for Management of Advanced RCC.

Setting	Patients	Primary Therapy (level 1 evidence)	Other Options (≥ level 2 evidence)
First-line	Good or Intermediate risk	Sunitinib Bevacizumab + IFN Pazopanib	HD IL-2 Sorafenib Observation
	Poor risk	Temsirolimus	Sunitinib Pazopanib
Second-line	Post-Cytokine	Sorafenib Pazopanib Axitinib	Sunitinib, Bevacizumab Temsirolimus
	Post-VEGF inhibitor	Everolimus Axitinib	Other VEGF inhibitors Temsirolimus
	Post-mTOR inhibitor	Trial	VEGF inhibitors
Third-line	Post TKI→TKI	Everolimus	Temsirolimus
	Post mTOR→TKI or Post TKI→mTOR	Trial	Different TKI Rechallenge TKI

Index: HD IL-2- high dose interleukin-2, IFN- interferon, VEGF- vascular endothelial growth factor, mTOR- mammalian target of rapamycin, TKI- tyrosine kinase inhibitor

Intermediate Surrogates for Outcomes

Early radiographic changes may predict long-term outcomes but require validation. In a retrospective study that compared 4 radiographic alterations with first-line VEGF inhibitors, a 10% reduction in the sum of longest unidimensional diameters was an optimal early predictor of survival[78]. In another study, changes in morphology, attenuation, size and structure (accounting for central necrosis) by MASS Criteria correlated better with outcomes than conventional criteria[79]. The development of functional imaging as a prognostic or predictive parameter is of paramount importance although still in its infancy. mTOR inhibitors decrease glucose uptake and may be expected to down-regulate FDG-PET uptake. An ongoing phase II trial is evaluating early FDG-PET changes to predict clinical benefit from second-line everolimus. Baseline high FDG PET uptake and increased number of positive lesions appeared to yield prognostic information and PET-CT progression at 16 weeks was associated with poor survival in patients receiving sunitinib[80]. DCE-US changes may facilitate the prediction of efficacy of sunitinib[81].

Ongoing Trials Evaluating Novel Approaches and Novel Agents

Another VEGF receptor TKI, tivozanib, is anticipated to be approved based on the results of a recently presented phase III trial [82]. Tivozanib demonstrated significant improvement in PFS (median 11.9 vs. 9.1 months) as well as secondary endpoints when compared with sorafenib as first-line therapy. The results of a phase III trial comparing axitinib and sorafenib as first-line therapy are awaited. Combinations of angiogenesis inhibitors and/or mTOR inhibitors have been plagued by toxicities, e.g. bevacizumab plus sunitinib, temsirolimus plus bevacizumab, sunitinib plus temsirolimus[83-86]. However, optimal first-line combinations may, in principle, delay the emergence of resistance. Preliminary data indicate that the combination of bevcizumab with either temsirolimus or everolimus does not improve outcomes. The INTORACT phase III trial compared first-line bevacizumab combined with either interferon or temsirolimus [87]. The primary endpoint, PFS appeared similar (9.1 months vs. 9.3 months) and secondary endpoints also appreared similar (RR 27-28%, median OS 25-26 months). Moreover, the randomized phase II RECORD-2 trial also did not demonstrate an improvement in PFS (median ~9-10 months for both arms) with bevacizumab plus everolimus when compared to bevacizumab plus interferon as first-line therapy [88]. Ongoing trials are evaluating new agents as salvage therapy. A key phase III trial is comparing sorafenib versus dovitinib (TKI targeting VEGF and FGF receptors) following 1 prior VEGF and 1 prior mTOR inhibitor.Other randomized trials are comparing the first→second-line sequence of sorafenib→sunitinib versus sunitinib→sorafenib and sunitinib→everolimus versus everolimus→sunitinib (Table 2). Multiple phase II trials are also underway to evaluate other novel agents and synergistic non-toxic rational combinations (Table 2). Immunotherapy is resurging as a viable class of agents, with the recent demonstration of activity of both the CTLA-4 inhibiting monoclonal antibody, ipilimumab, and the PD-1 monoclonal antibody, BMS-936558. Indeed, a phase III trial will compare everolimus with BMS-936558 in those with advanced clear-cell RCC that have received prior anti-angiogenic therapy.

**Table 2. Ongoing Randomized Trials of Systemic Therapy
for Advanced Clear Cell RCC**

Phase	Design	Standard arm	Experimental arm	Primary endpoint
III	First-line	Sorafenib	Axitinib	PFS
III	First-line	Sunitinib	Sunitinib-AGS003 (dendritic cells electroporated with CD40L and tumor mRNA)	PFS
III	First-line	Bevacizumab-IFN	Bevacizumab-everolimus	PFS
III	Sequencing first→second	Sunitinib → Sorafenib	Sorafenib → Sunitinib	PFS
III	Second-line following VEGF TKI	Everolimus + Placebo	Everolimus + Bevacizumab	PFS
III	Third line VEGF and mTOR inhibitor	Sorafenib	Dovitinib (FGF and VEGF receptor TKI)	PFS
II	Sequencing first→second	Sunitinib → Everolimus	Everolimus → Sunitinib	PFS
II	Second-line following VEGF inhibitor	Everolimus	MK-2206 (PI3K inhibitor)	PFS
II	Second-line following VEGF inhibitor	Everolimus	Everolimus + BNC-105P (vascular disrupting agent)	PFS
II	Second-line following VEGF inhibitor	Axitinib	Axitinib + CVX-060 (Angiopoietin inhibitor)	PFS
III	Following VEGF inhibitors	Everolimus	BMS-936558 (PD1 inhibitor)	OS

Index: IFN- interferon, PFS- progression-free survival, IMA901- autologous tumor-associated peptides, TKI- tyrosine kinase inhibitor, VEGF- vascular endothelial growth factor

Conclusion

Current therapy for metastatic clear cell RCC may be tailored based on risk grouping (Table 1). Current clinical decision making is also governed by comorbidities, patient preferences and toxicity profiles. Robust data to support an optimal sequence of therapy are unavailable at this time. Given the similar activity of mTOR inhibitors and VEGF inhibitors following first-line VEGF inhibitors, both VEGF inhibiting TKIs and mTOR inhibitors are viable strategies as second-line therapy, i.e. a sequence of TKI→TKI→mTOR inhibitor or TKI→mTOR inhibitor→TKI may both be reasonable. The spectrum of VEGF targeting TKIs appears poised to expand with the probable addition of tivozanib in the near future. Additionally, novel immunotherapeutic agents appear highly promising and enrollment on trials evaluating such agents should be a priority. Data gathered from ongoing research and the development of predictive factors will hopefully facilitate better patient selection for optimal sequences and combinations. Given that novel antiangiogenic agents are not generally curative and require chronic suppressive therapy associated with toxicities, clinical trials should continue to be vigorously supported.

References

[1]   Paez-Ribes M, Allen E, Hudock J et al. Antiangiogenic therapy elicits malignant progression of tumors to increased local invasion and distant metastasis. Cancer cell 2009; 15: 220-231.

[2]   Huang D, Ding Y, Zhou M et al. Interleukin-8 mediates resistance to antiangiogenic agent sunitinib in renal cell carcinoma. Cancer research 2010; 70: 1063-1071.

[3]   McDermott DF, Regan MM, Clark JI et al. Randomized phase III trial of high-dose interleukin-2 versus subcutaneous interleukin-2 and interferon in patients with metastatic renal cell carcinoma. Journal of clinical oncology : official journal of the American Society of Clinical Oncology 2005; 23: 133-141.

[4]   Negrier S, Escudier B, Lasset C et al. Recombinant human interleukin-2, recombinant human interferon alfa-2a, or both in metastatic renal-cell carcinoma. Groupe Francais d'Immunotherapie. The New England journal of medicine 1998; 338: 1272-1278.

[5]   Fyfe G, Fisher RI, Rosenberg SA et al. Results of treatment of 255 patients with metastatic renal cell carcinoma who received high-dose recombinant interleukin-2 therapy. Journal of clinical oncology : official journal of the American Society of Clinical Oncology 1995; 13: 688-696.

[6]   Fisher RI, Rosenberg SA, Fyfe G. Long-term survival update for high-dose recombinant interleukin-2 in patients with renal cell carcinoma. The cancer journal from Scientific American 2000; 6 Suppl 1: S55-57.

[7]   Gordan JD, Lal P, Dondeti VR et al. HIF-alpha effects on c-Myc distinguish two subtypes of sporadic VHL-deficient clear cell renal carcinoma. Cancer cell 2008; 14: 435-446.

[8]   Li L, Kaelin WG, Jr. New insights into the biology of renal cell carcinoma. Hematology/oncology clinics of North America 2011; 25: 667-686.

[9]   Brannon AR, Reddy A, Seiler M et al. Molecular Stratification of Clear Cell Renal Cell Carcinoma by Consensus Clustering Reveals Distinct Subtypes and Survival Patterns. Genes and cancer 2010; 1: 152-163.

[10] Bergers G, Hanahan D. Modes of resistance to anti-angiogenic therapy. Nature reviews. Cancer 2008; 8: 592-603.

[11] Finke J, Ko J, Rini B et al. MDSC as a mechanism of tumor escape from sunitinib mediated anti-angiogenic therapy. Int Immunopharmacol 11: 856-861.

[12] Heng DY, Xie W, Regan MM et al. Prognostic factors for overall survival in patients with metastatic renal cell carcinoma treated with vascular endothelial growth factor-targeted agents: results from a large, multicenter study. Journal of clinical oncology : official journal of the American Society of Clinical Oncology 2009; 27: 5794-5799.

[13] Heng DY, Xie W, Bjarnason GA, et al. A unified prognostic model for first- and second-line targeted therapy in metastatic renal cell carcinoma (mRCC): Results from a large international study. J Clin Oncol 28:15s, 2010 (suppl; abstr 4523).

[14] Motzer RJ, Bacik J, Murphy BA et al. Interferon-alfa as a comparative treatment for clinical trials of new therapies against advanced renal cell carcinoma. Journal of clinical oncology : official journal of the American Society of Clinical Oncology 2002; 20: 289-296.

[15] Motzer RJ, Bacik J, Schwartz LH et al. Prognostic factors for survival in previously treated patients with metastatic renal cell carcinoma. Journal of clinical oncology : official journal of the American Society of Clinical Oncology 2004; 22: 454-463.

[16] Motzer RJ, Hutson TE, Tomczak P et al. Overall Survival and Updated Results for Sunitinib Compared With Interferon Alfa in Patients With Metastatic Renal Cell Carcinoma. J Clin Oncol 2009.

[17] Motzer RJ, Hutson T, Olsen MR, et al. Randomized phase II multicenter study of the efficacy and safety of sunitinib on the 4/2 versus continuous dosing schedule as first-line therapy of metastatic renal cell carcinoma: Renal EFFECT Trial. J Clin Oncol 29: 2011 (suppl 7; abstr LBA308).

[18] Sternberg CN, Davis ID, Mardiak J et al. Pazopanib in Locally Advanced or Metastatic Renal Cell Carcinoma: Results of a Randomized Phase III Trial. J Clin Oncol 2010; 28: 1061-1068.

[19] Escudier BJ, Porta C, Bono P, et al Patient preference between pazopanib and sunitinib: Results of a randomized double-blind, placebo-controlled, cross-over study in patients with metastatic renal cell carcinoma—PISCES study. J Clin Oncol 30, 2012 (suppl; abstr CRA4502).

[20] Motzer RJ, Hutson T, Reeves J, et al. Randomized, open label, phase III trial of pazopanib versus sunitinib in first-line treatment of patients with metastatic renal cell carcinoma (mRCC); Results of the COMPARZ trial. Proc European Society of Medical Oncology Congress LBA8, Vienna, Austria September 28-October 2, 2012.

[21] Escudier B, Pluzanska A, Koralewski P et al. Bevacizumab plus interferon alfa-2a for treatment of metastatic renal cell carcinoma: a randomised, double-blind phase III trial. Lancet 2007; 370: 2103-2111.

[22] Rini BI, Halabi S, Rosenberg JE et al. Bevacizumab plus interferon alfa compared with interferon alfa monotherapy in patients with metastatic renal cell carcinoma: CALGB 90206. J Clin Oncol 2008; 26: 5422-5428.

[23] Bukowski RM, Kabbinavar FF, Figlin RA et al. Randomized phase II study of erlotinib combined with bevacizumab compared with bevacizumab alone in metastatic renal cell cancer. J Clin Oncol 2007; 25: 4536-4541.

[24] Hudes G, Carducci M, Tomczak P et al. Temsirolimus, interferon alfa, or both for advanced renal-cell carcinoma. N Engl J Med 2007; 356: 2271-2281.

[25] McDermott DF, Ghebremichael MS, Signoretti S, et al The high-dose aldesleukin (HD IL-2) "SELECT" trial in patients with metastatic renal cell carcinoma (mRCC). J Clin Oncol 28:15s, 2010 (suppl; abstr 4514)

[26] Escudier B, Eisen T, Stadler WM et al. Sorafenib for treatment of renal cell carcinoma: Final efficacy and safety results of the phase III treatment approaches in renal cancer global evaluation trial. J Clin Oncol 2009; 27: 3312-3318.

[27] Sternberg CN, Davis ID, Mardiak J et al. Pazopanib in locally advanced or metastatic renal cell carcinoma: results of a randomized phase III trial. Journal of clinical oncology : official journal of the American Society of Clinical Oncology 2010; 28: 1061-1068.

[28] Rixe O, Bukowski RM, Michaelson MD et al. Axitinib treatment in patients with cytokine-refractory metastatic renal-cell cancer: a phase II study. Lancet Oncol 2007; 8: 975-984.

[29] Rini BI, Escudier B, Tomczak P, Kaprin A, Hutson TE, Szczylik C, et al. Axitinib versus sorafenib as second-line therapy for metastatic renal cell carcinoma: Results of phase III AXIS trial. Lancet;378(9807):1931-9.

[30] Motzer RJ, Rini BI, Bukowski RM et al. Sunitinib in patients with metastatic renal cell carcinoma. JAMA : the journal of the American Medical Association 2006; 295: 2516-2524.

[31] Escudier B, Roigas J, Gillessen S et al. Phase II study of sunitinib administered in a continuous once-daily dosing regimen in patients with cytokine-refractory metastatic renal cell carcinoma. Journal of clinical oncology : official journal of the American Society of Clinical Oncology 2009; 27: 4068-4075.

[32] Bhargava P, Esteves B, Lipatov ON, et al. Activity and safety of AV-951, a potent and selective VEGFR1, 2 and 3 kinase inhibitor, in patients with renal cell carcinoma (RCC): Interim results of a phase II randomized discontinuation trial. . In Genitourinary Cancer Symposium, Edition Orlando, Florida: 2009; Abstract 283.

[33] Yang JC, Haworth L, Sherry RM et al. A randomized trial of bevacizumab, an anti-vascular endothelial growth factor antibody, for metastatic renal cancer. N Engl J Med 2003; 349: 427-434.

[34] Atkins MB, Hidalgo M, Stadler WM et al. Randomized phase II study of multiple dose levels of CCI-779, a novel mammalian target of rapamycin kinase inhibitor, in patients with advanced refractory renal cell carcinoma. Journal of clinical oncology : official journal of the American Society of Clinical Oncology 2004; 22: 909-918.

[35] Motzer RJ, Escudier B, Oudard S et al. Phase 3 trial of everolimus for metastatic renal cell carcinoma : final results and analysis of prognostic factors. Cancer 2010; 116: 4256-4265.

[36] Mackenzie MJ, Rini BI, Elson P et al. Temsirolimus in VEGF-refractory metastatic renal cell carcinoma. Ann Oncol 2010, 22: 145-148.

[37] Rini BI, Wilding G, Hudes G et al. Phase II study of axitinib in sorafenib-refractory metastatic renal cell carcinoma. Journal of clinical oncology : official journal of the American Society of Clinical Oncology 2009; 27: 4462-4468.

[38] Sablin MP, Negrier S, Ravaud A et al. Sequential sorafenib and sunitinib for renal cell carcinoma. J Urol 2009; 182: 29-34; discussion 34.

[39] Dudek AZ, Zolnierek J, Dham A et al. Sequential therapy with sorafenib and sunitinib in renal cell carcinoma. Cancer 2009; 115: 61-67.

[40] Garcia JA, Hutson TE, Elson P et al. Sorafenib in patients with metastatic renal cell carcinoma refractory to either sunitinib or bevacizumab. Cancer 2010; 116: 5383-5390.

[41] Reeves JA, Spigel DR, Daniel DB, Friedman EK, Burris HA, Hainsworth JD. Pazopanib in patients with metastatic renal cell carcinoma previously treated with sunitinib or bevacizumab: A Sarah Cannon Research Institute phase II trial. J Clin Oncol 29: 2011 (suppl; abstr 4659)

[42] Rini BI, Michaelson MD, Rosenberg JE et al. Antitumor activity and biomarker analysis of sunitinib in patients with bevacizumab-refractory metastatic renal cell carcinoma. J Clin Oncol 2008; 26: 3743-3748.

[43] Escudier B, Bellmunt J, Negrier S et al. Phase III trial of bevacizumab plus interferon alfa-2a in patients with metastatic renal cell carcinoma (AVOREN): final analysis of overall survival. J Clin Oncol 28: 2144-2150.

[44] Bracarda S, Bellmunt J, Melichar B et al. Overall survival in patients with metastatic renal cell carcinoma initially treated with bevacizumab plus interferon-alpha2a and subsequent therapy with tyrosine kinase inhibitors: a retrospective analysis of the phase III AVOREN trial. BJU international 2011; 107: 214-219.

[45] Zama IN, Hutson TE, Elson P et al. Sunitinib rechallenge in metastatic renal cell carcinoma patients. Cancer 2010; 116: 5400-5406.

[46] Vickers MM, Choueiri TK, Rogers M et al. Clinical outcome in metastatic renal cell carcinoma patients after failure of initial vascular endothelial growth factor-targeted therapy. Urology 2010; 76: 430-434.

[47] Heng DY, MacKenzie M, Vaishampayan UN, Knox JJ, Bjarnason GA, TanM, et al Primary anti-VEGF-refractory metastatic renal cell carcinoma (mRCC): Clinical characteristics, risk factors, and subsequent therapy. J Clin Oncol 29: 2011 (suppl 7; abstr 305)

[48] Al-Marrawi MY, Rini B, Harshman LC, et al. The association of clinical outcome to front-line VEGF-targeted therapy with clinical outcome to second-line VEGF-targeted therapy in metastatic renal cell carcinoma (mRCC) patients. J Clin Oncol 29: 2011 (suppl; abstr 4555).

[49] Escudier B, Hutson T, Esteban E, et al Temsirolimus vs Sorafenib as Second Line Therapy in Metastatic Renal Cell Carcinoma: Results From the INTORSECT Trial. Proc European Society of Medical Oncology Congress Abstract LBA22, Vienna, Austria September 28-October 2, 2012.

[50] Cho DC, Puzanov I, Regan MM et al. Retrospective analysis of the safety and efficacy of interleukin-2 after prior VEGF-targeted therapy in patients with advanced renal cell carcinoma. Journal of immunotherapy 2009; 32: 181-185.

[51] Di Lorenzo G, Buonerba C, Federico P et al. Third-line sorafenib after sequential therapy with sunitinib and mTOR inhibitors in metastatic renal cell carcinoma. European urology 2010; 58: 906-911.

[52] Choueiri TK, Plantade A, Elson P et al. Efficacy of sunitinib and sorafenib in metastatic papillary and chromophobe renal cell carcinoma. Journal of clinical oncology : official journal of the American Society of Clinical Oncology 2008; 26: 127-131.

[53] Golshayan AR, George S, Heng DY et al. Metastatic sarcomatoid renal cell carcinoma treated with vascular endothelial growth factor-targeted therapy. Journal of clinical oncology : official journal of the American Society of Clinical Oncology 2009; 27: 235-241.

[54] Flanigan RC, Salmon SE, Blumenstein BA et al. Nephrectomy followed by interferon alfa-2b compared with interferon alfa-2b alone for metastatic renal-cell cancer. N Engl J Med 2001; 345: 1655-1659.

[55] Mickisch GH, Garin A, van Poppel H et al. Radical nephrectomy plus interferon-alfa-based immunotherapy compared with interferon alfa alone in metastatic renal-cell carcinoma: a randomised trial. Lancet 2001; 358: 966-970.

[56] Lara PN, Jr., Tangen CM, Conlon SJ et al. Predictors of survival of advanced renal cell carcinoma: long-term results from Southwest Oncology Group Trial S8949. J Urol 2009; 181: 512-516; discussion 516-517.

[57] Pantuck AJ, Belldegrun AS, Figlin RA. Nephrectomy and interleukin-2 for metastatic renal-cell carcinoma. N Engl J Med 2001; 345: 1711-1712.

[58] Kassouf W, Sanchez-Ortiz R, Tamboli P et al. Cytoreductive nephrectomy for metastatic renal cell carcinoma with nonclear cell histology. J Urol 2007; 178: 1896-1900.

[59] Shuch B, Said J, La Rochelle JC et al. Cytoreductive nephrectomy for kidney cancer with sarcomatoid histology--is up-front resection indicated and, if not, is it avoidable? J Urol 2009; 182: 2164-2171.

[60] Choueiri TK, Xie W, Kollmannsberger CK, et al. The impact of cytoreductive nephrectomy in patients with metastatic renal cell carcinoma (mRCC) treated with

vascular endothelial growth factor (VEGF)-targeted therapy. Genitourinary Cancer Symposium 2010, San Francisco, CA: abstract 311.

[61] van der Veldt AA, Meijerink MR, van den Eertwegh AJ et al. Sunitinib for treatment of advanced renal cell cancer: primary tumor response. Clin Cancer Res 2008; 14: 2431-2436.

[62] Thomas AA, Rini BI, Lane BR et al. Response of the primary tumor to neoadjuvant sunitinib in patients with advanced renal cell carcinoma. J Urol 2009; 181: 518-523; discussion 523.

[63] Powles T, Blank C, Chowdhury S et al. The outcome of patients treated with sunitinib prior to planned nephrectomy in metastatic clear cell renal cancer. European urology 2011; 60: 448-454.

[64] Powles T, Kayani I, Blank C et al. The safety and efficacy of sunitinib before planned nephrectomy in metastatic clear cell renal cancer. Annals of oncology : official journal of the European Society for Medical Oncology / ESMO 2011; 22: 1041-1047.

[65] Powles T, Kayani I, Blank C, et al The safety and efficacy of sunitinib prior to planned nephrectomy in metastatic clear cell renal cancer. Genitourinary Cancer Symposium 2010, San Francisco, CA, abstract 369.

[66] Harshman LC, Yu R, Gill HS, et al. Surgical complications associated with presurgical tyrosine kinase inhibition for advanced renal cell carcinoma (RCC). Genitourinary Cancer Symposium 2010, San Francisco, CA, abstract 404.

[67] Jonasch E, Wood CG, Matin SF et al. Phase II presurgical feasibility study of bevacizumab in untreated patients with metastatic renal cell carcinoma. J Clin Oncol 2009; 27: 4076-4081.

[68] Jonasch E, Tsavachdidou D, Wood CG, et al. Phase II presurgical study of bevacizumab plus erlotinib in untreated patients with metastatic renal cell carcinoma. J Clin Oncol 27:15s, 2009 (suppl; abstr 5004)

[69] Cowey CL, Amin C, Pruthi RS et al. Neoadjuvant Clinical Trial With Sorafenib for Patients With Stage II or Higher Renal Cell Carcinoma. J Clin Oncol 28: 1502-1507.

[70] Choueiri TK, Schutz FA, Je Y et al. Risk of arterial thromboembolic events with sunitinib and sorafenib: a systematic review and meta-analysis of clinical trials. Journal of clinical oncology : official journal of the American Society of Clinical Oncology 2010; 28: 2280-2285.

[71] Rini BI, Cohen DP, Lu DR et al. Hypertension as a biomarker of efficacy in patients with metastatic renal cell carcinoma treated with sunitinib. Journal of the National Cancer Institute 2011; 103: 763-773.

[72] Choueiri TK, McDermott D, Sheng Duh M et al. Costs associated with angiogenesis inhibitor therapies for metastatic renal cell carcinoma in clinical practice: Results from a medical chart review study. Urologic oncology 2010.

[73] Pena C, Lathia C, Shan M et al. Biomarkers predicting outcome in patients with advanced renal cell carcinoma: Results from sorafenib phase III Treatment Approaches in Renal Cancer Global Evaluation Trial. Clinical cancer research : an official journal of the American Association for Cancer Research 2010; 16: 4853-4863.

[74] Jiang Z, Chu PG, Woda BA et al. Analysis of RNA-binding protein IMP3 to predict metastasis and prognosis of renal-cell carcinoma: a retrospective study. The lancet oncology 2006; 7: 556-564.

[75] Xu CF, Bing NX, Ball HA et al. Pazopanib efficacy in renal cell carcinoma: evidence for predictive genetic markers in angiogenesis-related and exposure-related genes. J Clin Oncol 29: 2557-2564.

[76] Choueiri TK, Vaziri SA, Jaeger E et al. von Hippel-Lindau gene status and response to vascular endothelial growth factor targeted therapy for metastatic clear cell renal cell carcinoma. The Journal of urology 2008; 180: 860-865; discussion 865-866.

[77] Cho D, Signoretti S, Dabora S et al. Potential histologic and molecular predictors of response to temsirolimus in patients with advanced renal cell carcinoma. Clinical genitourinary cancer 2007; 5: 379-385.

[78] Krajewski KM, Guo M, Van den Abbeele AD et al. Comparison of four early posttherapy imaging changes (EPTIC; RECIST 1.0, tumor shrinkage, computed tomography tumor density, Choi criteria) in assessing outcome to vascular endothelial growth factor-targeted therapy in patients with advanced renal cell carcinoma. European urology 2011; 59: 856-862.

[79] Smith AD, Shah SN, Rini BI et al. Morphology, Attenuation, Size, and Structure (MASS) criteria: assessing response and predicting clinical outcome in metastatic renal cell carcinoma on antiangiogenic targeted therapy. AJR. American journal of roentgenology 2010; 194: 1470-1478.

[80] Katani I, Avril NE, Bomanji J et al. Sequential FDG-PET/CT as a biomarker of response to sunitinib in metastatic clear cell renal cancer. Clinical cancer research : an official journal of the American Association for Cancer Research 2011.

[81] Lassau N, Koscielny S, Albiges L et al. Metastatic renal cell carcinoma treated with sunitinib: early evaluation of treatment response using dynamic contrast-enhanced ultrasonography. Clinical cancer research : an official journal of the American Association for Cancer Research 2010; 16: 1216-1225.

[82] Motzer RJ, Nosov D, Eisen T, Bondarenko IN, Lesovoy V, Lipatov ON, et al. Tivozanib versus sorafenib as initial targeted therapy for patients with advanced renal cell carcinoma: Results from a phase III randomized, open-label, multicenter trial. J Clin Oncol 30, 2012 (suppl; abstr 4501)

[83] Negrier S, Gravis G, Perol D et al. Temsirolimus and bevacizumab, or sunitinib, or interferon alfa and bevacizumab for patients with advanced renal cell carcinoma (TORAVA): a randomised phase 2 trial. The lancet oncology 2011.

[84] Patel PH, Senico PL, Curiel RE, Motzer RJ. Phase I study combining treatment with temsirolimus and sunitinib malate in patients with advanced renal cell carcinoma. Clinical genitourinary cancer 2009; 7: 24-27.

[85] Feldman DR, Baum MS, Ginsberg MS et al. Phase I trial of bevacizumab plus escalated doses of sunitinib in patients with metastatic renal cell carcinoma. Journal of clinical oncology : official journal of the American Society of Clinical Oncology 2009; 27: 1432-1439.

[86] Rini BI, Garcia JA, Cooney MM et al. Toxicity of sunitinib plus bevacizumab in renal cell carcinoma. Journal of clinical oncology : official journal of the American Society of Clinical Oncology 2010; 28: e284-285; author reply e286-287.

[87] Rini BI, Bellmunt J, Clancy J, et al. Randomized Phase IIIb Trial of Temsirolimus and Bevacizumab versus Interferon and Bevacizumab in Metastatic Renal Cell Carcinoma: Results from INTORACT. Proc European Society of Medical Oncology Congress LBA21, Vienna, Austria September 28-October 2, 2012.

[88] Ravaud A, Barrios C, Anak O, et al. Randomized phase II study of first-line everolimus plus bevacizumab versus interferon alfa-2A plus bevacizumab in patients with metastatic renal cell carcinoma: RECORD-2. Proc European Society of Medical Oncology Congress Abstract 7830, Vienna, Austria September 28-October 2, 2012.

Section 6. Testis Cancer

Stephen D.W. Beck and Richard S. Foster
Section Editors

In: Essentials and Updates in Urologic Oncology
Editor: Philippe E. Spiess

ISBN: 978-1-62081-494-9
© 2013 Nova Science Publishers, Inc.

Chapter XXV

Epidemiology, Clinical Manifestations, and Staging of Germ Cell Tumours

Yaron Ehrlich[1], Ofer Yossepowitch[2] and Jack Baniel[2]
[1]Department of Urology Auckland City Hospital, Auckland, New Zealand.
[2]Department of Urology, Rabin Medical Centre Beilinson Campus, Petah Tiqwa, Israel

Germ cell tumors (GCTs) are relatively uncommon, accounting for only 1% of male malignancies in the United States. It has become an important oncological disease for several reasons. Firstly, it is the most common malignancy in young men 15–35 years old, and thus has the potential to greatly shorten productive years of life. Secondly, GCTs are among a unique numbers of neoplasms where biochemical markers play a critical role. Serum tumour markers are an integral part of patient management. They play a role in diagnosis, staging, risk assessment, evaluation of response to therapy and detection of relapse. It is also a model of curable cancer, and a triumph of modern oncology. Current chemotherapy protocols and surgery yield cure rates exceeding 95% [1].

There are three major subsets of male GCTs: 1) Teratomas and yolk-sac tumors that occur primarily in neonates and infants, usually have a benign nature; 2) spermatocytic seminoma, which is typically diagnosed in older men; and 3) pure seminoma, and nonseminomatous germ cell tumours (NSGCT) – affecting predominantly young men. This chapter will focus on the latter group.

Epidemiology

GCTs affect young adults with median age at diagnosis of 34. The age-adjusted incidence rate in the United States is 5.4 per 100,000 men per year. These rates are based on cases diagnosed in 2003-2007 by the Surveillance, Epidemiology and End Results (SEER) Program. The SEER database includes information on incidence and survival from specific geographic areas representing 26 percent of the US population.

It is estimated that 7920 new cases of testis cancer were diagnosed in the United States in 2007 while only 380 (5%) patients died of their disease. Improved survival in the last 30 years is attributed to the development of cisplatin combination chemotherapy. High cure rate coupled with the young age at diagnosis, result in a growing population of testicular cancer survivors. In 2007 there were approximately 200,000 men alive in the US with a history of testicular cancer.

For unknown reasons, the incidence of GCT, particularly in Caucasian populations, is increasing throughout the world. The lifetime risk of GCTs in US Caucasian men is estimated to be 1 in 230. In countries with the highest rate of GCTs, such as Demark, lifetime risk exceeds 1%. The SEER data indicates that between 1975 and 2004, the age-adjusted incidence rate of testicular cancer for males aged 15-49 years increased from 2.9 to 5.1 per 100,000 [2]. This increase was more pronounced in seminoma compared to NSGCT. The trend appears to be influenced by a birth cohort effect, where people born in a specific time interval show different risk compared to people born immediately earlier or later. For example, men born in Denmark and Norway during World War II have a lower risk of testicular cancer than either previous or subsequent birth cohorts [3].

Overall, rates of testicular cancer in the industrialized countries are five times higher than those in the less developed regions of the world. Yet there are considerable differences between neighbouring countries and within regions of the same country. For example, Denmark, Germany and Austria report age-standardised rates of around 10 per 100,000, while in Lithuania, Estonia, Spain and Latvia cancer incidence is around 2 per 100,000. Immigrant populations tend to carry the risk of their country of birth in the first generation.

However, the risk of the second generation immigrants shifts toward the adopting population incidence. These observations coupled with the young age at presentation suggest an environmental risk factor acting in-utero or early in life. No specific etiological factors have yet been identified.

The incidence of testicular cancer varies, with respect to race. The highest rates are seen in Caucasian populations. The US incidence among white men has been, on average, five times higher than the incidence among African Americans. Recently rates of testicular cancer for African Americans appear to be increasing [4]. Pacific Islanders, Asian, American Indian and Alaskan Natives have an intermediate risk. New Zealand native Maori are an exception. Their testicular cancer incidence is one of the highest in the world exceeding the local white European population [5].

Although most patients will be cured, there are potential dangers that loom over the future of these young patients. The contralateral testis may produce a second primary GCT in 2-5%. Late relapse of GCT affects approximately 3% of patients with NSGCT [6]. Non-germ cell cancers are becoming an increasing problem following treatment of GCT. The 40-year cumulative incidence of second malignant neoplasm may reach approximately one in three [7].

In addition, survivors are at increased risk of developing delayed cardiovascular disease [8]. Other treatment-related complications include nephrotoxicity, neuropathy, ototoxicity, and pulmonary toxicity. Additionally, sexual dysfunction and sub-fertility post treatment represent significant long-term morbidity in this young patient population [9]

Risk Factors

Testicular Intratubular Germ Cell Neoplasia Unclassified (ITGCNU)

TIGCNU is the precursor lesion of adult GCTs. It is frequently identified in the testicular parenchyma adjacent to an invasive cancer. Autopsy studies of young men who died of other causes show a prevalence of ITGCNU that is consistent with the life time risk of GCT [10]. TIGCNU carries a 50% risk of progression to an invasive cancer in 5 years [11]. This rate of progression is likely to increase with longer follow-up.

Men with testicular GCT are at an increased risk of developing a second primary GCT in the remaining testis. When a contralateral biopsy is obtained in men with testicular cancer, ITGCNU is diagnosed in 5%. Detection rates may be higher with associated testicular atropy [12]. Open testicular biopsies of the unaffected testis can accurately detect ITGCNU and therefore identify patients at risk of interval invasive cancer development. However the need for a routine biopsy is debatable.

ITGCNU responds well to low dose radiation (20 Gy). Post-radiation biopsies consistently show eradication of ITGCNU, thus greatly reducing but not eliminating the chance of progression to an invasive cancer [13] There is evidence that systemic chemotherapy may also reduce the risk of ITGCNU progression however to a lesser extent than radiation. Despite this there is no evidence of an overall survival benefit with early treatment of ITGCNU compared with deferred treatment in the subgroup of patients who develop GCT. Furthermore, infertility is almost a certain consequence of testicular irradiation, and endocrine function may also be compromised.

A European consensus has recently recommended testicular biopsy in selected cases [14]. Patients with testicular atrophy who presents with stage I testicular GCT, not likely to receive systemic chemotherapy, may be the best candidates of testicular biopsy for reasons stated above. In the US the estimated 15-year cumulative rate of metachronous testicular cancer is 2% [15]. Because of the low risk of a second primary testicular cancer, and the uncertain survival benefit with early testicular radiation, routine biopsy of the unaffected testicle is not generally recommended in North America.

Cryptorchidism

Undescended testis occurs in two to five percent of boys born at term. It is associated with impaired fertility and is an established risk factor for testicular cancer. Patients with cryptorchidism have two to eight fold increase risk for developing GCT. Five to ten percent of all men with testicular cancer have a history of cryptorchidism. Both testes are at risk, about 20% of testicular tumours in men with unilateral cryptorchidism occur in the normally descended testicle.

Bringing the undescended testis to the scrotum facilitates physical examination and early detection of cancer. This may also lower the risk of GCT. In a cohort of Swedish patients who underwent orchiopexy for treatment of undescended testis before age 13 the relative risk of subsequent testicular cancer was reduced from 5.4 to 2.2 compared to boys who were treated at 13 years or older [16].

Family History

The most consistent chromosomal anomaly in GCT is gain in the short arm of chromosome 12. Genetic syndromes linked to GCTs include Klinefelter syndrome which is associated with primary mediastinal GCT, and in Down's syndrome in which an increased rate of testicular seminoma has been observed.

It is estimated 1.4% of men with newly diagnosed GCT have a positive family history. This rate exceeds the degree expected by chance alone. Sons of men with TGCT have a four- to sixfold increase in GCT risk, while siblings of men with GCT have an increased risk of eight- to tenfold [17].

The International Testicular Cancer Linkage Consortium is collaboration of multiple sites around the globe that holds the largest database of familial GCT published to date. 985 patients from 461 families have been studied thus far. Clinical and pathologic characteristics were similar to those generally described for non-familial cases. However, an increased prevalence of testicular microlithiasis on ultrasound was found in men with familial testicular cancer and their relatives [18].

Unlike other hereditary cancers most GCT families consist of only two affected cases making genetic studies more difficult. Efforts are underway to find susceptibility genes for GCT within this unique group of familial cancers. Whether familial clusters of GCT are due to inherited mutations or simply reflect a shared environmental risk factor remains to be proven.

Acquired Immune Deficiency Syndrome (AIDS)

In addition to three AIDS-defining tumours; Kaposi's sarcoma, non-Hodgkin's lymphoma, and invasive cervical cancer, HIV-infected patients are at increased risk of certain other tumours collectively known as non-AIDS-defining cancers. Among the non-AIDS-defining cancers testicular cancer incidence is modestly increased compared to the general population [19]. The natural history of GCTs is comparable to patients not infected with HIV and as such, cancer management follows the same principles.

Infertility

Approximately half of testicular cancer patients have a poor semen quality at the time of GCT diagnosis [20]. This may be related to a pre-existing condition or to the local and systemic effects of the cancer. Testicular atrophy has been associated with the development of GCT.

A large US retrospective study demonstrated that men evaluated for infertility were at an increased risk for a subsequent diagnosis of testicular cancer [21]. Men with known male factor infertility were 2.8 times more likely to develop testicular cancer relative to the general population. Similar results were reported in a cohort of men from Denmark [22].

Testicular Microlithiasis

Testicular microlithiasis refers to a sonographic pattern of hyperechoic multiple, 1-mm to 3-mm foci distributed randomly throughout the testicular parenchyma. In a cohort of 1504 healthy young volunteers age 18-35 from the US army, 84 (5.6%) harbored testicular microlithiasis. None of these 84 patients had a testicular tumour. The prevalence of microlithiasis in this cohort far exceeded the lifetime risk of GCTs. Findings were typically bilateral and were more frequent in African Americans than Caucasian volunteers. These results suggest that in a healthy population microlithiasis is not associated with GCTs [23]. In a followup study [24] 63 men (of the original 84 volunteers with microlithiasis) were identified after 5 years, and one developed testicular tumour 5 years after initial screening. The low rate of cancer detected argued against long term followup of healthy men with microlithiasis however self-awareness is advised.

Unlike asymptomatic screened volunteers, the finding of microlithiasis in patients who undergo testicular ultrasound for a cause may be associated with testicular cancer. Testes involved with intratubular germ cell neoplasia frequently contain intratubular microcalcifiations that can be detected by ultrasound. Individuals with microlithiasis and associated risk factors for testicular cancer, may have an increased risk of concurrent diagnosis of testicular cancer or ITGCNU of approximately eight-fold. [25].

Histologic Classification

GCTs are diagnosed in 99% of adult testicular cancer. The remaining 1% are non-germ cell tumours including most commonly sex cord tumours and lymphomas. GCTs are classified based on pathologic and clinical features into two broad histologic groups: seminomas and non-seminomatous germ cell tumours (NSGCT). Approximately 60% of testicular GCT are pure seminomas with the remainder comprised of NSGCT. Four major cell types are seen in NSGCT: embryonal carcinomas, yolk sac tumours, choriocarcinomas, and teratomas. Most NSGCT are composed of two or more cell types. Mixed tumour containing seminoma and non-seminoma element is classified as NSGCT.

The peak frequency for NSGCT occurs in the 20-29 year age group whereas seminoma incidence peeks at a decade later. Three-quarters of all men with testicular GCT are diagnosed with localized disease (Stage I), however the frequency of metastatic disease at presentation changes according to histologic type. According to the SEER database, 86% of all seminomas and 62% of NSGCT are stage one at initial diagnosis.

Classic seminoma is composed of sheet-like arrangement of clear cells with well-defined cytoplasmic borders. The tumour is subdivided into nests or clusters by lymphocyte-bearing, fibrovascular septa. Syncytiotrophoblast cells are occasionally seen. Spermatocytic seminomas may occasionally be confused with classic seminoma. The distinction between the two is important as spermatocitic seminomas are generally benign. Therefore, orchidectomy alone is mostly curative. Spermatocytic seminoma is composed of three cell types, small, intermediate and large cells that are evenly distributed. Spermatocitic seminoma occurs in older men (mean age 55) and is not associated with intratubular germ cell neoplasia.

Embryonal carcinoma is relatively common among NSGCT. It is usually seen in a mixed GCT alongside other histologies, while10% of are pure embryonal carcinomas. Its distinctive features include sheets, glands, and papillary structures composed of primitive epithelial cells with crowded, pleomorphic nuclei.

Yolk sac tumour, also known as endodermal sinus tumour, is a common component of mixed germ cell tumors. Pure yolk sac tumors are rare in adults but are the most common testicular germ cell tumor in children. There are numerous patterns of yolk sac tumor. The more common subtypes are microcystic, myxomatous, hepatoid, and solid patterns.

Choriocarcinoma may be seen as part of a mixed NSGCT. Pure choriocarcinoma is rare tumour with unique biology. It usually present with hematogenous metastasis and is rarely diagnosed in an early stage. Patients may present with disseminated disease, very high serum levels of hCG, and a small (at times non-palpable) testicular tumour. The typical histologic pattern is a plexiform arrangement of syncytiotrophoblast and cytotrophoblast cells around foci of hemorrhage.

Teratoma is seen as component of mixed GCT. It contains tissue resembling normal derivatives of two or three of the germ layers: ectoderm, endorem and mesoderm. Mature teratoma resembles benign structures, whereas immature teratoma usually manifest as immature neuroepithelium. Pure testicular teratoma is a rare tumour. Unlike mature ovarian teratoma and prepubertal testicular teratoma which are uniformly benign, postpubertal teratoma of the testis is considered malignant. Metastases, often as non-teratomatous GCT, occur in 20% to 40% of the patients.

Extragonadal GCT

Most GCTs originate for the testis but five percent arise in extragonadal sites such as the mediastinum, retroperitoneum, pineal gland and suprasellar regions. Prognosis and treatment algorithms are similar for primary retroperitoneal and testicular GCTs. Indeed, some patients contain microscopic GCT or evidence of a burned-out tumour in the testis when orchiectomy is performed following chemotherapy for an assumed primary retroperitoneal disease [26].

Unlike primary retroperitoneal GCT, primary mediastinal GCTs represent a distinct clinical entity, with a clinical behaviour that suggests it is biologically different from testicular GCTs. Primary mediastinal germ-cell tumours are associated with several unique syndromes, including Klinefelter's syndrome and acute megakaryocytic leukemia. Although histologically identical to testicular GCT, primary mediastinal tumours have inferior survival. In addition, mediastinal tumours have a propensity to develop into non–germ-cell malignant histology such as sarcomas and carcinomas that are highly resistant to chemotherapy.

Clinical Manifestation

Local Signs and Symptoms

Painless scrotal swelling is the typical finding leading to a diagnosis of testicular cancer, although non-tender testicular mass (rather than painless) better describes the standard presenting symptom. We reviewed 145 consecutive patients treated for GCT between 1995 and 2006 [27]. 67 patients (46%) had associated scrotal pain and 78 (54%) had a truly painless mass. Patients usually complain of dull pain but on examination the affected testis is not tender. Acute pain at presentation mimicking testicular torsion is rare.

The tumour can be felt as a firm area within the testis, harder in consistency compared to the unaffected testis. It may involve part of or replace the entire testis. At times it can reach the size of a grapefruit with little or no associated symptoms. The mass arises from the testicle and may involve the epididymis and cord, but should be differentiated from paratesticular masses. Most intratesticular solid lesions are malignant, whereas extratesticular lesions are usually benign.

The differential diagnosis for scrotal masses includes testicular cancer, epididymo-orchitis, para-testicular tumours, torsion, hydrocele, hernia and varicocele. Genitourinary TB with involvement of the epididymis may present as testicular tumour. Bilateral testicular masses in men with congenital adrenal hyperplasia are most likely to be adrenal rest. This should be kept in mind before proceeding to radical treatment. These lessons may regress during glucocorticoid therapy [28]

The distinction between testicular cancer and other causes of scrotal mass usually becomes apparent after thorough history taking and careful physical examination. In the presence of a definite testicular mass especially when serum tumour markers are elevated there is no need for testicular imaging to establish the diagnosis. When available, scrotal ultrasound is frequently performed. It is indicated if the testicle cannot be adequately examined as in the case of surrounding hydrocele, or when a testicular tumour is suspected but no definite mass is noted on examination.

High-resolution sonography, with colour or power Doppler can distinguish testicular from extra-testicular lesions and solid versus cystic lesions. Testicular solid lesion should be considered malignant until proven otherwise. Nonetheless, in one series 10% of all testicular lesions surgically removed for testicular tumour were found to be benign [29]. Ultrasound cannot accurately predict cancer histology, although pure seminomas are often described as homogeneous hypoechoic lesion. NSGCT may show mixed signals including hyperechoic and isoechoic areas. Cystic components in an otherwise solid tumour are commonly seen with teratoma. Simple testicular cysts without solid component are usually benign. With high frequency transducers testicular lesions as small as one to two millimetre can be detected. The frequency of benign lesions in incidental non-palpable testicular lesions diagnosed by ultrasound is high [30].

Systemic Signs and Symptoms

The primary metastatic site of testicular GCT is the retroperitoneum by way of the lymphatics. The majority of retroperitoneal lymphadenopathy goes unnoticed by the patient; however large retroperitoneal masses can become symptomatic. Masses can cause back pain due to nerve involvement or renal obstruction. Rarely, compression and occasional penetration of the upper gastrointestinal tract by retroperitoneal mass may cause related symptoms of intestinal obstruction and gastrointestinal bleeding. An eroding gastric or duodenal GCT may be misdiagnosed as gastric carcinoma leading to unnecessary laparotomy and delay in appropriate treatment [31].

With advanced disease dissemination to more distant sites via lymphatics or blood stream is not uncommon. Mediastinal and supraclavicular adenopathy represents direct lymphatic spread from the retroperitoneum. This is typically asymptomatic and most commonly identified and the time of systemic staging. Hematogenous spread is most frequent to the lungs and may cause shortness of breath, hemoptysis and cough. Other manifestations include bone pain, neurological changes depending on the site of metastasis.

On examination, a large retroperitoneal mass can be felt in a thin patient. The neck, especially the left supraclavicular area where the thoracic duct joins the left subclavian vein should be inspected for masses. Swelling of the lower extremities may be caused by iliac vein or inferior vena caval compression or may be a sign of deep vein thrombosis. In the absence of scrotal violation, inguinal adenopathy is rare.

Gynecomastia, usually bilateral, occurs in 5% to 7% of patients with GCT and is more frequent in patients with testicular leyding cell tumour (up to 20%). It results from an imbalance between oestrogen or its precursors and androgens. Gynecomastia is frequently associated with elevated hCG [32]. In patients evaluated for gynecomastia testicular cancer is recognized in 2% to 4%. There have been reports of patients in whom gynecomastia preceded the identification of palpable testicular mass [33]. As such, testicular examination should be performed in all patients evaluated for gynecomastia and repeated in 3-6 months if no other cause is found.

Paraneoplastic Syndromes

Compared to other urological cancers such as renal cell carcinoma, testicular cancer is not commonly associated with paraneoplastic syndromes. The most common paraneoplastic syndrome in patients with metastatic NSGCT is hyperthyroidism. It is probably related to the ability of hCG to activate the TSH receptor. Patients usually present with very high hCG (>50000 mIU/ml) and thyroid function tests consistent with hyperthyroidism. Some patients will clearly manifest signs of thyrotoxicosis but most symptoms like fatigue and weight loss overlap with those of metastatic disease. Free thyroxin levels normalize with successful chemotherapy. In one study as many as 50% of patients presenting with metastatic NSGCT and HCG >50000 mIU/ml had biochemical evidence hyperthyroidism [34]. With this in mind, thyroid function should be assessed in patients with high HCG levels and symptomatic hyperthyroidism may temporarily require treatment with beta-blockade or antithyroid medication.

A less common syndrome linked to testicular cancer is paraneoplastic limbic encephalitis. It is characterized by rapid development of irritability, depression, sleep disturbances, seizures, hallucinations and short term memory loss. Clinically, Ma-2 antibodies have been correlated with symptoms associated with limbic, diencephalic, or brainstem encephalopathy. The detection of Ma-2 antibodies is important as it represents a paraneoplastic syndrome with the most common malignancy being testicular cancer. Furthermore, the neurologic complications respond to eradication of the tumour in over one third of the patients. The diagnosis of testicular cancer may be difficult as this paraneoplastic syndrome can predate the occurrence of palpable testicular mass [35].

Delay in Diagnosis

Diagnosis delay may be due to patient denial, embarrassment, and lack of self-awareness. Another cause of delay is misdiagnosis. As discussed earlier, GCT is frequently associated with scrotal pain leading to a wrong initial diagnosis of epididymo-orchitis, trauma or hydrocele. Failure to examine the genitalia in patients presenting with back pain, gynecomastia or neck mass is another concerning cause of delay.

GCTs are heterogeneous cancers. Some grow at a rapid rate and present with advanced disease albeit a small primary tumour. Others grow slowly and remain confined to the testis despite long diagnostic delay. As such a prolonged time to diagnosis may not necessarily correlate with a more advance disease. On an individual patient basis however, the longer the delay the higher the tumour burden is likely to be. With modern chemotherapy cure is possible for the majority of patients making the prognostic disadvantage associated with long diagnostic delay even more difficult to prove. Nonetheless, some centres were able to show that a delay in diagnosis was associated with a more advanced disease [36, 37]. Researchers from Toulouse France recently presented data from 542 patients diagnosed with GCT [38]. Diagnostic delay was associated with more advanced disease and decreased survival for patients with NSGCT but not for patients with seminoma. The study had shown that some testicular tumors especially seminomas grow slowly over several months without causing much discomfort. Diagnostic delay was longer for seminoma than for NSGCT (Mean delay of 4.9 ± 6.1 mo vs. 2.8 ± 4.0 mo) and local symptoms (e.g. scrotal pain) where more often observed with NSGCT.

Serum Tumour Markers

A-Fetoprotein (AFP)

AFP is single-chain glycoprotein with a molecular weight of 70,000 Da. In the fetus, AFP is a major serum binding protein produced by the fetal yolk sac, hepatic cells, and the gastrointestinal tract. The highest concentrations approach 3 mg/ml during the 12th to 14th weeks of gestation and decline to < 40 ng/ml 1 year after birth. In the adult patient the upper limit is 10-15 ng/ml. The metabolic half-life of AFP is between 5 - 7 days.

AFP is secreted by embryonal cell carcinoma and yolk sac tumour but not by pure choriocarcinoma or pure seminoma. Yolk sac tumours appear to be the primary source of AFP with more than 90% of tumours reacting positively to anti-AFP antibody.

Excluding GCT, the most impressive serum AFP levels are seen in patients with hepatocellular carcinoma. AFP has been found to be elevated in other neoplasms including pancreatic cancer (23%), gastric cancer (20%), colorectal cancer (5%), and bronchial cancer (7%) [39]. Non-neoplastic liver diseases are also associated with an elevated serum AFP including viral hepatitis, cirrhosis, and liver trauma. AFP levels secondary to benign liver disease rarely exceed 500 ng/ml. The AFP gene is located on chromosome 4 and a hereditary persistence of an elevated AFP through an autosomal dominant trait has been reported [40].

The carbohydrate moiety of AFP exhibits heterogeneity due to post-translational modifications in which different carbohydrates are added to the polypeptide backbone [41].

Based on the difference in their binding affinity to various lectins and particularly concanvalin-A it is possible to distinguish with very high sensitivity and specificity AFP of GCT and liver origin [42]. Despite initial promising results [43, 44] wide acceptance awaits the results of further clinical trials, as the technique has not been standardized, and false negative results have been published [45].

Human Chorionic Gonadotropin (hCG)

Primary production of hCG occurs during pregnancy by the syncytiotrophoblastic cells of the placenta which maintains the corpus luteum. In GCT, synctytiotrophoblastic cells are responsible for the production of hCG. All patients with choriocarcinoma and 40% to 60% of patients with embryonal cell carcinoma have raised serum hCG. Approximately 10-20% of patients with pure seminoma have elevated serum hCG though the level is typically below 500 mIU/ml. The serum half-life of hCG is between 24 - 36 hours. For most assays the upper limit of normal is between 5-10 mIU/ml.

hCG is a glycoprotein with a molecular weight of 38,000 Da composed of α and β subunits. The α subunit closely resembles that of other pituitary hormones including luteinizing hormone (LH), follicular stimulating hormone, and thyroid stimulating hormone. The β subunit contains a 24 amino acid C-terminal extension making it antigenic distinct from the other pituitary hormones allowing production of antibodies used in radio-immunoassay.

Some cross reactivity with the β subunit of LH may occur resulting in a false positive test in conditions where LH is elevated. LH commonly elevated due to hypogonadism associated with testicular cancer. With the development of more sensitive and specific assays it became evident that the pituitary gland is capable of producing hCG [46]. Furthermore, hypogonadism can induce LH as well as hCG production by the pituitary gland [47]. Short course of testosterone replacement suppresses pituitary LH and hCG secretion allowing for a "true" measure of serum hCG of potential germ cell origin.

Marijuana use has been attributed to a falsely elevated serum hCG, although conflicting data has been reported [48, 49] Various tumours can produce hCG elevation including: liver, pancreas, stomach, breast, kidney, and bladder cancer. False-positive hCG measurements resulting from heterophile antibodies interference with commercial immunoassays have been described [50].

Lactate Dehydrogenase (LDH)

LDH is a cytoplasmatic enzyme with a molecular weight of 134,000 Da found in all living cells. LDH catalyzes the reduction of pyruvate to lactate and is measured in the serum by enzymatic activity assays. The normal levels are highly variable and depends on assay conditions. It is considered elevated if > 1.5 times the lab-specific upper limit of the normal. LDH measured in the serum is a mixture of five isoenzymes each as a tetramer formed by a combination of two different subunits encoded by structurally distinct genes, LDHA and LDHB [51]. GCT patients typically express high levels of LDH isoenzyme 1 [52].

Dying and dead cells leak LDH which can be measured in the serum. As such the test has low specificity. There is a direct relationship between GCTs burden and LDH levels thus its levels after orchiectomy correlate with prognosis. Different factors may cause may cause LDH elevation during or following GCT treatment. Therefore, serum LDH levels must be incorporated with other clinical findings when making management decisions [53].

Placental Alkaline Phosphatase

Placental alkaline phosphatase is fetal isoenzyme that is frequently elevated in patients with seminoma (60%–70%). Its serum concentrations are increased up to 10-fold in smokers [54]. With this, as well as the limited commercial assays, it is not routinely utilized in the management of GCT.

Markers and Prognosis in Metastatic GCT

Serum tumour markers levels should be determined prior to radical orchiectomy for several reasons. Firstly, when the nature of a testicular mass is questioned, raised serum tumour markers will establish the diagnosis of a GCT and confirm the need for orchiectomy. Secondly, the classification of GCT into seminoma and NSGCT is based on histologic examination. However, if pre-orchiectomy AFP is elevated in a tumour diagnosed as seminoma based on histology, nonseminomatous component can be presumed to be present in a metastatic lesion or occult in the testis primary. This is because seminoma does not produce AFP. With this in mind the tumour should be reclassified as NSGCT and treated accordingly. Thirdly, if all cancer cells are removed by orchiectomy, as is expected in a true stage I disease, serum tumour markers should decline according to their half life. For patients with clinical stage I disease in whom markers fail to normalize following removal of the primary tumour recategorization as clinical stage Is should be made. These patients are considered to have metastatic disease.

In metastatic NSGCT, the degree of marker elevation before chemotherapy (following orchiectomy) correlates with prognosis. The International Germ Cell Cancer Collaborative Group (IGCCCG) has incorporated serum concentrations of hCG, AFP and LDH into a prognostic classification system with high, intermediate, and low risk disease (Table 1,2) [55]. The fifth edition of the TNM classification by the American Joint Committee on Cancer and the International Union against Cancer [56] was based on the validated IGCCCG model. Primary tumour, lymph node and distant metastasis were supplemented by a new category of serum tumour marker. Accordingly three categories were defined:

- S1: AFP<1000 ng/mL, and hCG<5000 mIU/mL, and LDH<1.5 upper limit of normal
- S2: AFP=1000-10,000 ng/mL, or hCG=5000-50,000 mIU/mL, or LDH=1.5-10 upper limit of normal
- S3: AFP>10,000 ng/mL, or hCG>50,000 mIU/mL, or LDH>10 upper limit of normal

Table 1. TNM Staging

Primary Tumour (T)	
TX	Primary tumor cannot be assessed
T0	No evidence of primary tumour
Tis	Intratubular germ cell neoplasia
T1	Tumor limited to the testis and epididymis without lymphatic/vascular invasion; tumor may invade into the tunica albuginea but not the tunica vaginalis
T2	Tumor limited to the testis and epididymis with vascular/lymphatic invasion, or tumor extending through the tunica albuginea with involvement of the tunica vaginalis
T3	Tumor invades the spermatic cord with or without vascular/lymphatic invasion
T4	Tumor invades the scrotum with or without vascular/lymphatic invasion
Regional lymph nodes (N) clinical staging	
Nx	Regional lymph nodes cannot be assessed
N0	No regional lymph node metastasis
N1	Metastasis with a single or multiple lymph node masses ≤ 2 cm in greatest dimension
N2	Metastasis with a single or multiple lymph node masses 2 to 5 cm in greatest dimension
N3	Metastasis with a single or multiple lymph node masses ≥ 5 cm in greatest dimension
Regional lymph nodes (N) pathological staging	
pNx	Regional lymph nodes cannot be assessed
pN0	No regional lymph node metastasis
pN1	Metastasis in 1 to 5 lymph nodes and mass ≤ 2 cm in greatest dimension
pN2	Metastasis in more than 5 nodes all less than 5 cm in greatest dimension; or metastasis in 1 to 5 nodes 2 to 5 cm in greatest dimension, or extranodal extension of tumour
pN3	Metastasis with a single or multiple lymph node mass ≥ 5 cm in greatest dimension
Distant metastasis (M)	
M0	No distant metastasis
M1a	Nonregional nodal or pulmonary metastasis
M1b	Distant metastasis other than to nonregional lymph nodes and lungs
Serum tumor markers (S) measured post-orchiectomy	
S1	AFP<1000 ng/mL, and hCG<5000 mIU/mL, and LDH<1.5 of the upper limit of normal.
S2	AFP=1000-10,000 ng/mL, or hCG=5000-50,000 mIU/mL, or LDH=1.5-10 of the upper limit of normal.
S3	AFP>10,000 ng/mL, or hCG>50,000 mIU/mL, or LDH>10 of the upper limit of normal.

Metastatic NSGCT to non-pulmonary visceral sites and primary mediastatinal NSGCT are classified as poor risk regardless of the degree of serum tumour marker elevation. All other patients with metastatic NSGCT, i.e. patients with lymph node metastasis (retroperitoneal or non regional lymph nodes) and pulmonary metastasis, are categorized based on post-orchiectomy tumour marker levels. Patients with markers category S1, S2, S3 are thus assigned a good, intermediate and poor prognosis respectively. In a recent meta-analysis the 5-year survival rates for low, intermediate, and high risk NSGCT are 94%, 83%, and 71% respectively [57].

Patients with pure seminoma metastatic to non-pulmonary visceral sites are classified as intermediate risk, all others are classified as low risk. For the purpose of model simplification, marker levels were not incorporated in the seminoma IGCCCG risk model. However, other studies have emphasized the importance of LDH level in patients with metastatic seminoma. In a multi-institutional study an elevated LDH level (≥ 2 upper limit) and the presence of non-pulmonary visceral metastases were independent adverse prognostic factors in patients with advanced seminoma [58]. Another prospective multicenter trial evaluated the significance of hCG elevation in 726 patients with metastatic pure seminoma [59]. While hCG elevation was associated with a larger tumour mass (primary tumour and/or metastases), predictors of recurrence included stage of disease and elevation of LDH but not hCG elevation.

Table 2. International Germ Cell Consensus Classification Prognostic Groups in Patients with Metastatic Disease Treated with First Line Chemotherapy

	NSGCT	Seminoma	5-year survival*
Good Prognosis	Primary site: Testis or RP *and* Metastases: Nodal or pulmonary *and* Marker level: S1	Primary site: All *and* Metastases: Nodal or pulmonary *and* Marker level: any LDH, any hCG	Seminoma 86% NSGCT 94%
Intermediate Prognosis	Primary site: Testis or RP *and* Metastases: Nodal or pulmonary *and* Marker level: S2	Primary site: All *and* Metastases: Non-pulmonary visceral *and* Marker level: any LDH, any hCG	Seminoma 72% NSGCT 83%
Poor Prognosis	Primary site: Mediastinal *or* Metastases: Non-pulmonary visceral *or* Marker level: S3	No patients classified as poor prognosis	NSGCT 71%

Abbreviation: **NSGCT**: Nonseminomatous germ cell tumor; **S1**: a-fetoprotein (AFP)<1000 ng/ml, and human chorionic gonadotrophin (hCG)<5000 mIU/ml, and lactic dehydrogenase (LDH)<1.5 upper limit of normal; **S2**: AFP=1000-10,000 ng/ml, or hCG=5000-50,000 mIU/ml, or LDH=1.5-10 upper limit of normal; **S3**: AFP>10,000 ng/ml, or hCG>50,000 mIU/ml, or LDH>10 upper limit of normal; **RP**: Retroperitoneum
*Survival data for Seminoma patients based on IGCCCG study [55]. Survival for NSGCT patients is based on a more recent meta-analysis [57].

References

[1]   Einhorn LH. Curing metastatic testicular cancer. *Proc Natl Acad Sci U S A.* 2002;99(7):4592-5.

[2]   Holmes L Jr, Escalante C, Garrison O, Foldi BX, Ogungbade GO, Essien EJ, et al. Testicular cancer incidence trends in the USA (1975-2004): plateau or shifting racial paradigm? *Public Health.* 2008 ;122:862-72.

[3]   Bergström R, Adami HO, Möhner M, Zatonski W, Storm H, Ekbom A et al. Increase in testicular cancer incidence in six European countries: a birth cohort phenomenon. *J Natl Cancer Inst.* 1996;88:727-33.

[4]   McGlynn KA, Devesa SS, Graubard BI, Castle PE. Increasing incidence of testicular germ cell tumors among black men in the United States. *J Clin Oncol.* 2005 ;23:5757-61

[5]   Sarfati D, Shaw C, Blakely T, Atkinson J, Stanley J. Ethnic and socioeconomic trends in testicular cancer incidence in New Zealand. *Int J Cancer*. 2010 Jun 1. [Epub ahead of print]

[6]   Baniel J, Foster RS, Gonin R, Messemer JE, Donohue JP, Einhorn LH. Late relapse of testicular cancer. *J Clin Oncol*. 1995;13:1170-6.

[7]   Travis LB, Fosså SD, Schonfeld SJ, McMaster ML, Lynch CF, Storm H, et al. Second cancers among 40,576 testicular cancer patients: focus on long-term survivors. *J Natl Cancer Inst*. 2005 ;97:1354-65.

[8]   Haugnes HS, Wethal T, Aass N, Dahl O, Klepp O, Langberg CW, et al.Cardiovascular Risk Factors and Morbidity in Long-Term Survivors of Testicular Cancer: A 20-Year Follow-Up Study. *J Clin Oncol*. 2010 Sep 20. [Epub ahead of print]

[9]   Travis LB, Beard C, Allan JM, Dahl AA, Feldman DR, Oldenburg J, et al. Testicular cancer survivorship: research strategies and recommendations. *J Natl Cancer Inst*. 2010;102:1114-30

[10]   Linke J, Loy V, Dieckmann KP. Prevalence of testicular intraepithelial neoplasia in healthy males. *J Urol*. 2005;173:1577-9.

[11]   von der Maase H, Rørth M, Walbom-Jørgensen S, Sørensen BL, Christophersen IS, Hald T, Jacobsen GK et al. Carcinoma in situ of contralateral testis in patients with testicular germ cell cancer: study of 27 cases in 500 patients. *Br Med J* (Clin Res Ed). 1986;293:1398-401.

[12]   Dieckmann KP, Loy V. Prevalence of contralateral testicular intraepithelial neoplasia in patients with testicular germ cell neoplasms. *J Clin Oncol*. 1996;14:3126-32.

[13]   Dieckmann KP, Lauke H, Michl U, Winter E, Loy V. Testicular germ cell cancer despite previous local radiotherapy to the testis. *Eur Urol*. 2002;41:643-9

[14]   Krege S, Beyer J, Souchon R, Albers P, Albrecht W, Algaba F et al. European consensus conference on diagnosis and treatment of germ cell cancer: a report of the second meeting of the European Germ Cell Cancer Consensus group (EGCCCG): part I. *Eur Urol*. 2008;53:478-96.

[15]   Fosså SD, Chen J, Schonfeld SJ, McGlynn KA, McMaster ML, Gail MH, et al. Risk of contralateral testicular cancer: a population-based study of 29,515 U.S. men. *J Natl Cancer Inst*. 2005;97:1056-66.

[16]   Pettersson A, Richiardi L, Nordenskjold A, Kaijser M, Akre O. Age at surgery for undescended testis and risk of testicular cancer. *N Engl J Med*. 2007;356:1835-41.

[17]   Greene MH, Kratz CP, Mai PL, Mueller C, Peters JA, Bratslavsky G, et al. Familial testicular germ cell tumors in adults: 2010 summary of genetic risk factors and clinical phenotype. *Endocr Relat Cancer*. 2010;17:R109-21

[18]   Korde LA, Premkumar A, Mueller C, Rosenberg P, Soho C, Bratslavsky G, et al. Increased prevalence of testicular microlithiasis in men with familial testicular cancer and their relatives. *Br J Cancer*. 2008;99:1748-53.

[19]   Grulich AE, van Leeuwen MT, Falster MO, Vajdic CM. Incidence of cancers in people with HIV/AIDS compared with immunosuppressed transplant recipients: a meta-analysis. *Lancet*. 2007;370:59-67.

[20]   Williams DH 4th, Karpman E, Sander JC, Spiess PE, Pisters LL, Lipshultz LI. Pretreatment semen parameters in men with cancer. *J Urol*. 2009;181:736-40.

[21]   Walsh TJ, Croughan MS, Schembri M, Chan JM, Turek PJ. Increased risk of testicular germ cell cancer among infertile men. *Arch Intern Med*. 2009;169:351-6.

[22] Jacobsen R, Bostofte E, Engholm G, Hansen J, Olsen JH, Skakkebaek NE, et al. Risk of testicular cancer in men with abnormal semen characteristics: cohort study. *BMJ*. 2000;321:789-92.

[23] Peterson AC, Bauman JM, Light DE, McMann LP, Costabile RA. The prevalence of testicular microlithiasis in an asymptomatic population of men 18 to 35 years old. *J Urol*. 2001;166:2061-4.

[24] DeCastro BJ, Peterson AC, Costabile RA. A 5-year followup study of asymptomatic men with testicular microlithiasis. *J Urol*. 2008;179:1420-3.

[25] Tan IB, Ang KK, Ching BC, Mohan C, Toh CK, Tan MH. Testicular microlithiasis predicts concurrent testicular germ cell tumors and intratubular germ cell neoplasia of unclassified type in adults: a meta-analysis and systematic review. *Cancer*. 2010 Jun 24. [Epub ahead of print]

[26] Brown JA, Bihrle R, Foster RS. Delayed orchiectomy at postchemotherapy retroperitoneal lymph node dissection due to laterality of retroperitoneal metastatic pattern consistent with testicular primary: assessment of pathologic findings. *Urology*. 2008;71:911-4.

[27] Ehrlich Y, Konichezky M, Yossepowitch O, Baniel J. Multifocality in testicular germ cell tumors. *Urol*. 2009;181:1114-9

[28] Stikkelbroeck NM, Otten BJ, Pasic A, Jager GJ, Sweep CG, Noordam K, et al. High prevalence of testicular adrenal rest tumors, impaired spermatogenesis, and Leydig cell failure in adolescent and adult males with congenital adrenal hyperplasia. *J Clin Endocrinol Metab* 2001;86:5721-8.

[29] Elert A, Olbert P, Hegele A, Barth P, Hofmann R, Heidenreich A. Accuracy of frozen section examination of testicular tumors of uncertain origin. *Eur Urol*. 2002;41:290-3.

[30] Carmignani L, Gadda F, Gazzano G, Nerva F, Mancini M, Ferruti M, et al. High incidence of benign testicular neoplasms diagnosed by ultrasound. *J Urol*. 2003;170:1783-6.

[31] Mesa H, Rawal A, Rezcallah A, Iwamoto C, Niehans GA, Druck P, et al. "Burned out" testicular seminoma presenting as a primary gastric malignancy. *Int J Clin Oncol*. 2009;14:74-7.

[32] Hassan HC, Cullen IM, Casey RG, Rogers E. Gynaecomastia: an endocrine manifestation of testicular cancer. *Andrologia*. 2008;40:152-7.

[33] Harris M, Rizvi S, Hindmarsh J, Bryan R. Testicular tumour presenting as gynaecomastia. *BMJ*. 2006;332:837

[34] Oosting SF, de Haas EC, Links TP, de Bruin D, Sluiter WJ, de Jong IJ, et al. Prevalence of paraneoplastic hyperthyroidism in patients with metastatic non-seminomatous germ-cell tumors. *Ann Oncol*. 2010 Jan;21(1):104-8.

[35] Tenner L, Einhorn L. Ma-2 paraneoplastic encephalitis in the presence of bilateral testicular cancer: diagnostic and therapeutic approach. *J Clin Oncol*. 2009;27:e57-8.

[36] Moul JW, Paulson DF, Dodge RK, Walther PJ. Delay in diagnosis and survival in testicular cancer: impact of effective therapy and changes during 18 years. *J Urol*. 1990;143:520-3.

[37] Bosl GJ, Vogelzang NJ, Goldman A, Fraley EE, Lange PH, Levitt SH, et al. Impact of delay in diagnosis on clinical stage of testicular cancer. *Lancet*. 1981;2:970-3.

[38] Huyghe E, Muller A, Mieusset R, Bujan L, Bachaud JM, Chevreau C, et al. Impact of diagnostic delay in testis cancer: results of a large population-based study. *Eur Urol.* 2007;52:1710-6.

[39] Waldmann TA, McIntire KR. The use of a radioimmunoassay for alpha-fetoprotein in the diagnosis of malignancy. *Cancer* 1974;34:suppl:1510-15.

[40] Schefer H, Mattmann S, Joss RA. Hereditary persistence of alpha-fetoprotein. Case report and review of the literature. *Ann Oncol* 1998;9:667-72.

[41] Johnson PJ, Poon TC, Hjelm NM, et al. Glycan composition of serum alpha-fetoprotein in patients with hepatocellular carcinoma and non-seminomatous germ cell tumour. *Br J Cancer* 1999;81:1188-95.

[42] Mora J, Gascon N, Tabernero JM, Germa JR, Gonzalez F. Alpha-fetoprotein-concanavalin A binding as a marker to discriminate between germ cell tumours and liver diseases. *Eur J Cancer* 1995;3:2239-42.

[43] Kawai K, Kojima T, Miyanaga N, et al. Lectin-reactive alpha-fetoprotein as a marker for testicular tumor activity. *Int J Urol* 2005;12:284-9.

[44] Mora J, Garrido A, Antonijuan A, Martinez S, Gonzalez-Sastre F. Applicability of alpha-fetoprotein-concanavalin A (AFP-ConA) binding to discriminate between germinal or hepatic origin of AFP in germ cell tumour patients during chemotherapy or follow-up. *Clin Chem Lab Med* 2007;45:932-3.

[45] de Takats PG, Jones SR, Penn R, Cullen MH. Alpha-foetoprotein heterogeneity: what is its value in managing patients with germ cell tumours? *Clin Oncol* (R Coll Radiol) 1996;8:323-6.

[46] Odell WD, Griffin J. Pulsatile secretion of human chorionic gonadotropin in normal adults *N Engl J Med.* 1987;317:1688-91.

[47] Stenman UH, Alfthan H, Ranta T, Vartiainen E, Jalkanen J, Seppala M. Serum levels of human chorionic gonadotropin in nonpregnant women and men are modulated by gonadotropin-releasing hormone and sex steroids. *J Clin Endocrinol Metab* 1987;64:730-6.

[48] Garnick MB. Spurious rise in human chorionic gonadotropin induced by marihuana in patients with testicular cancer. *N Engl J Med* 1980;303:1177.

[49] Braunstein GD, Thompson R, Gross S, Soares JR. Marijuana use does not spuriously elevate serum human chorionic gonadotropin levels.*Urology* 1985;25:605-6.

[50] Gallagher DJ, Riches J, Bajorin DF. False elevation of human chorionic gonadotropin in a patient with testicular cancer. *Nat Rev Urol.* 2010;7:230-3

[51] Markert CL. Lactate dehydrogenase isozymes: dissociation and recombination of subunits. *Science* 1963;140:1329-30.

[52] von Eyben FE. Laboratory markers and germ cell tumors. *Crit Rev Clin Lab Sci* 2003;40:377-427.

[53] Gilligan TD, Seidenfeld J, Basch EM, Einhorn LH, Fancher T, Smith DC et al. American Society of Clinical Oncology Clinical Practice Guideline on Uses of Serum Tumor Markers in Adult Males With Germ Cell Tumors. *J Clin Oncol.* 2010;28:3388-404.

[54] Weissbach L, Bussar-Maatz R, Mann K. The value of tumor markers in testicular seminomas. Results of a prospective multicenter study. *Eur Urol.* 1997;32:16-22.

[55] International Germ Cell Cancer Collaborative Group. International germ cell consensus classification. A prognostic factor-based staging system for metastatic germ cell cancers. *J Clin Oncol* 1997;15:594–603.

[56] *AJCC (American Joint Committee on Cancer) Cancer Staging Manual*, 5th ed, Fleming, ID, Cooper, JS, Henson, DE, et al (Eds), Lippincott-Raven, Philadelphia, 1997, p225.

[57] van Dijk MR, Steyerberg EW, Habbema JD. Survival of non-seminomatous germ cell cancer patients according to the IGCC classification: An update based on meta-analysis. *Eur J Cancer*. 2006;42:820-826.

[58] Fossa SD, Oliver RT, Stenning SP, Horwich A, Wilkinson P, Read G, et al. Prognostic factors for patients with advanced seminoma treated with platinum-based chemotherapy. *Eur J Cancer*. 1997;33:1380-1387.

[59] Weissbach L, Bussar-Maatz R, Lohrs U, Schubert GE, Mann K, Hartmann M, et al. Prognostic factors in seminomas with special respect to HCG: results of a prospective multicenter study. Seminoma Study Group. *Eur Urol*. 1999;36:601-608.

In: Essentials and Updates in Urologic Oncology   ISBN: 978-1-62081-494-9
Editor: Philippe E. Spiess   © 2013 Nova Science Publishers, Inc.

Chapter XXVI

Seminomatous Germ Cell Testis Tumors

Gary Mok, Michael Jewett
and Padraig Warde[*]

Princess Margaret Hospital and University of Toronto, Toronto, Ontario, Canada

Abstract

Although testicular is an uncommon cancer, it remains the most common solid malignancy in young men between the ages of 20 and 35. Primary germ cell tumors are the most common histology in the vast majority of testicular tumors, although other histologies such as lymphomas or sarcomas are possible. Seminomas comprise 60% of germ cell tumors, 30% are non-seminomas and 10% are mixed seminomas, which contain both seminomatous and non-seminomatous elements.

With cure rates approaching 100%, testicular seminoma is a model for curable malignancies. Over the past twenty to thirty years, remarkable progress has been made in the treatment of testicular seminoma. For stage I seminoma, adjuvant radiation was the standard treatment with excellent disease free and overall survival. Single-agent carboplatin had also been demonstrated to be an effective alternative. However, concerns in regards to the potential late toxicities of these adjuvant treatments have led to active surveillance as the management option of choice in stage I testicular seminoma.

Treatment options for Stage II disease are largely dependent on size of the metastatic lymph nodes. Large bulky tumors are typically treated with chemotherapy as the risk of occult systemic disease is higher, while smaller tumors are treated with radiation targeted to the retroperitoneal lymph nodes. Stage III disease is best treated with chemotherapy.

_____

[*] Correspondence:Dr. P. Warde, Princess Margaret Hospital, Department of Radiation Oncology, 610 University Avenue, Toronto, Ontario, Canada, M5G 2M9, Tel: 416-946-2122, Fax: 416-946-4586, email address: padraig.warde@rmp.uhn.on.ca

Introduction

The American Caucasian male has a 0.2% estimated cumulative lifetime risk of developing testicular cancer and consequently comprises only 1 – 2% of all male cancers [1]. Despite the rarity of this tumor, it is the most common solid tumor in young men aged 20 to 35 and the incidence has increased by 61% from 1973 to 2003 with the majority of the rise due to seminomas compared to non-seminomas [2]. An estimated 8,480 new diagnoses and 350 deaths from testicular cancer occurred in the United States in 2010 [3]. Approximately 60% of these new diagnoses will be seminomatous germ cell tumors [4].

After histological confirmation of a testicular seminoma, management decisions are made based on disease extent. Although seminoma is a highly radiosensitive tumor and highly curable in the early stages, advances in chemotherapy, imaging and multidisciplinary care have led to improvements in outcome over the past three decades. In this chapter, we will discuss the management principles for all stages of seminomatous testicular germ cell tumors.

Initial Evaluation

The initial management of a testicular mass or suspected testicular seminoma includes a full history and physical examination. A testicular ultrasound is helpful in differentiating a solid mass from a hydroceole. After confirmation of a solid testicular mass, an inguinal orchidectomy is the recommended management approach over testicular biopsy. Histological and pathological confirmation of a testicular seminoma should prompt staging studies including an abdominal-pelvic CT scan and a chest x-ray. In the context of metastatic retroperitoneal lymph nodes, a CT scan of the thorax should be included to better evaluate for mediastinal and lung metastases.

Tumor markers including β-human chorionic gonadotropin (β-HCG), α-fetoprotein (AFP) and lactase dehydrogenase (LDH) should be taken pre-operatively in order to monitor decline after treatment. β-HCG is produced in 15% of seminomas and has a half-life of 22 hours. It may be falsely elevated by the use of marijuana or its derivatives. AFP is not elevated in pure seminomatous tumors and an elevated AFP should raise suspicion of non-seminomatous elements. LDH is a general tumor marker, but can be elevated in advanced seminomas.

In patients with bulky stage II or stage III disease, a bone scan should be performed. Evaluation of the brain by CT or MRI is indicated in patients with extensive metastatic disease, non-pulmonary visceral metastasis, or very elevated tumor markers who are at high risk for brain metastasis [5]. Renal and pulmonary function tests should be performed for patients who will undergo chemotherapy.

Stage I Seminoma

Approximately 80% of all seminomatous germ cell tumors have normal staging investigations after surgery and are classified as stage I seminoma. Treatment options include surveillance, adjuvant radiotherapy, adjuvant chemotherapy and rarely, retroperitoneal lymph node dissection. Survival approaches 100% regardless of the post-orchidectomy management option selected. Consequently, there has been a shift away from adjuvant treatments to placing these patients on surveillance protocols to minimize potential long-term toxicities.

Surveillance

There is now mature data demonstrating relapse rates of approximately 15 to 20% in stage I seminoma patients enrolled into surveillance protocols (table 1) [6-14]. The Princess Margaret Hospital (PMH) demonstrated a 5 year relapse-free rate of 85.5% for 421 patients with a median follow-up of 8.2 years [7].

**Table 1. Outcomes of Stage I Patients Managed with Surveillance,
Radiotherapy and Chemotherapy**

Author		Median FU (months)	Patients (n)	Relapse (%)	Cause specific Survival (%)
Surveillance					
Horwich (1992)		62	103	16.5	100%
Ramakrishnan (1992)		44	72	18	100%
Von der Maase (1993)		48	261	18.8	98.9%
Oliver (2001)		98	110	19	100%
Germa-Lluch (2002)		33	233	16	100%
Daugaard (2003)		60	394	17.5	100%
Warde (2005)		98	421	15.2	99.7%
Yoshida (2009)		124	64	11	98.4%
Kamba (2010)		45	186	10	100%
Retroperitoneal radiotherapy					
Bayens (1992)		88	132	4.5	99%
Hültenschmidt (1996)		N/A	188	1.0	100%
Coleman (1998)		> 120	144	4.2	100%
Fossa (1999)		54	242	3.7	100%
Santoni (2003)		105	487	4.3	99.4%
Warde (2005)		122	283	5.0	100%
Kamba (2010)		61	182	4.9	99.5%
Adjuvant Carboplatin					
Oliver (1994)	1 cycle	29	25	0.0	100%
	2 cycles	51	53	1.9	100%
Krege (1997)	2 cycles	28	43	0.0	100%
Dieckmann (2000)	1 cycle	48	93	8.6	91.1%
	2 cycles	45	32	0.0	100%
Oliver (2001)	1 cycle	52	146	0.7	100%
	2 cycles	128	57	1.8	96.5%
Aparicio (2003)	2 cycles	52	60	3.3	96.6%
Oliver (2005)	1 cycle	48	560	5.2	94.8%
Aparicio (2005)	2 cycles	34	214	3.3	100%
Argirovic (2005)	2 cycles	48	163	1.8	100%

Similarly, the Danish Testicular Cancer Study Group (DATECA) reported a relapse rate of 17% in 394 patients over a median follow-up of 60 months [8]. Two independent Japanese studies have reported slightly lower relapse rates of 10 – 11%, although these studies had fewer patients than the Canadian and Danish studies [13-14].

The para-aortic lymph nodes represent the most common site of relapse in 82 – 85% of the relapsed patients in the Danish and Canadian studies [7-8]. Relapse typically occurs at 12 to 18 months following orchidectomy, although late relapses more than 4 years after diagnosis have been reported [14-15]. Radiotherapy or chemotherapy is very effective for salvage of relapsed disease and excellent survival rates approaching 100% are expected for patients managed with surveillance.

Risk Adapted Models

The Spanish Germ Cell Cancer Cooperative Study Group has adopted a risk-adapted management approach for stage I seminoma [16]. This is based upon a prognostic model using tumor size > 4 cm and rete testis invasion as risk factors to estimate the risk of relapse. Patients with no risk factors were considered low-risk and were placed on a surveillance protocol. Patients with a single-risk factor had an intermediate-risk of relapse, while patients with both risk factors were considered to be at high-risk for relapse. Both intermediate and high-risk groups were treated with 2 cycles of adjuvant carboplatin. This study confirmed findings of the multi-institutional pooled analysis that low-risk patients managed with surveillance had a low risk of relapse [17].

Unfortunately this risk-adapted approach is problematic because it is not sufficiently powerful to identify stage I seminoma patients at very high risk of relapse to justify adjuvant treatment. The current prognostic model predicts relapse in 30% for high-risk patients, resulting in unnecessary adjuvant treatments in 70% of patients. A recent multi-institutional pooled analysis was unable to validate the prognostic model used for this approach and rete testis invasion was no longer found to be a predictor of relapse [18]. At PMH where all patients are placed on a surveillance protocol, treatment is avoided in the majority of patients. A recent review demonstrated a 6-fold decrease in treatment-episodes-per-patient in patients managed with surveillance (0.16 vs. 1.05) compared to patients managed with adjuvant RT [19].

Surveillance Schedule

There is no universal consensus in regards to an optimal surveillance schedule following orchidectomy. However, evidence-based recommendations have been published in an attempt to design an appropriate follow-up schedule based on the risk of relapse per year. In the first year of surveillance, CT scan frequency may be appropriate at every four months, as the PMH has estimated that the median time to radiological relapse is 4.4 months after orchidectomy and the estimated lymph node growth rate is 1.35 mm/month [20]. A Canadian publication has recommended abdominal/pelvic CT imaging at a frequency of every 4 months during the first 2 years of surveillance for stage I seminoma, when the annual risk of relapse is greater than 5%. The frequency of CT imaging decreases as the risk of relapse decreases to twice a year for years 3 and 4 when the risk is 1 – 5%. CT imaging becomes annual until 10 years of follow-up and can be discontinued thereafter when the risk of relapse is less than 0.3% per year [21]. The European Germ Cell Cancer Consensus Group (EGCCCG) has adopted these recommendations [22-23]. The NCCN guidelines are quite similar with 3 – 4 abdominopelvic

CT scans annually for the first 3 years, then every 6 months for years 4 – 7 and then annually until 10 years of follow-up have been completed [24].

CT Screening Radiation Exposure

Over the course of 10 years of follow-up with the EGCCCG program, a patient would receive 15 CT scans, while a patient on the NCCN guidelines would receive up to 21 CT scans. An average abdominopelvic CT scan exposes a patient to approximately 10 – 20 mSV [25-26]. Over the course of follow-up, a patient may receive up to 420 mSV of radiation on a surveillance protocol. There are valid concerns in regards to the potential effects of low-dose radiation exposure in a young patient population.

The stochastic effect of radiation is defined as the induction of cancer or a germ line mutation. The probability of stochastic effects increase with increasing dose of radiation, but no threshold dose exists below which the risk is zero. Thus, a risk of carcinogenesis is thought to exist even in individuals exposed to low doses of radiation. Data from Japanese atomic bomb survivors have been used to approximate organ dose from radiation exposure and have estimated that 0.6 – 2.0% of all cancers in the United States are attributable to CT studies [27-28]. Although this data has been criticized as an over-estimation, it represents the best available estimate for CT scan radiation exposure and the risk of carcinogenesis and mortality.

Ongoing research efforts to reduce radiation exposure in seminoma survivors are underway in both Europe and North America. The Medical Research Council is conducting the TE24 clinical study to evaluate MRI screening as an alternative to conventional CT scans for detection of relapse. The PMH has established an investigational low-dose CT scan protocol, which decreases radiation exposure for each CT scan by approximately 50% [29]. The reduction of radiation exposure comes at the expense of degraded image quality, but in the large majority of cases the image quality is sufficient to detect relapse. In the future, low-dose CT scans or MRI scans may be employed in future surveillance protocols. "Targeted imaging" with imaging of the para-aortic lymph nodes and elimination of routine imaging of low-risk regions such as the pelvic lymph nodes may further reduce radiation exposure. There may also be a role for MR lymphography for surveillance in the future as this modality becomes increasingly accessible. Early studies indicate that MR lymphography demonstrates increased sensitivity and specificity in the detection of lymph node metastasis for a variety of cancer sites, but it remains to be validated for testicular seminoma [30-32].

Adjuvant Radiotherapy

Adjuvant retroperitoneal radiotherapy was the standard adjuvant treatment for Stage I seminoma. Most institutional series report 10-year overall survival rates of approximately 92 – 99%, although cause-specific survival approaches 100%. Relapse rates are low and consistently range from 3.5 – 5% in large single institutional or multi-institutional experiences (table 1) [7, 13, 33-37] . Relapses are typically outside of the para-aortic radiation field in the mediastinum, lungs and the left supraclavicular fossa. A minority of patients may relapse in the inguinal lymph nodes and typically have predisposing risk factors, such as prior inguinal or scrotal surgery. In-field relapses are rare and a biopsy should be performed to rule-out a second malignancy.

Treatment Volume

Traditional adjuvant radiation volumes for Stage I testicular seminoma include the para-aortic and pelvic lymph nodes. The low incidence of pelvic lymph node involvement resulted in a randomized controlled trial by the Medical Research Council Testicular Study Group comparing para-aortic and pelvic irradiation (extended field) to para-aortic irradiation in 478 patients with stage I seminoma [35]. There was a 4% relapse rate in patients treated with para-aortic radiation compared to 3.4% in patients treated with para-aortic and pelvic lymph node irradiation. All relapses in the extended field arm were in supra-diaphragmatic sites, while 1.6% of patients in the para-aortic radiation arm relapsed in the pelvis.

The MRC trial demonstrated that, although para-aortic radiation provides excellent results, a small risk of pelvic failure remains. Data from the Christie Hospital in Manchester, where there is no routine evaluation of the pelvic lymph nodes after para-aortic radiation, demonstrates that that the median size of the pelvic lymph nodes at time of detection of relapse is 5 cm (range 2.5 – 9 cm) [38]. In order to ensure a pelvic relapse is detected at an early stage for effective salvage treatments, interval CT imaging of the pelvis is required if only the para-aortic lymph nodes are irradiated.

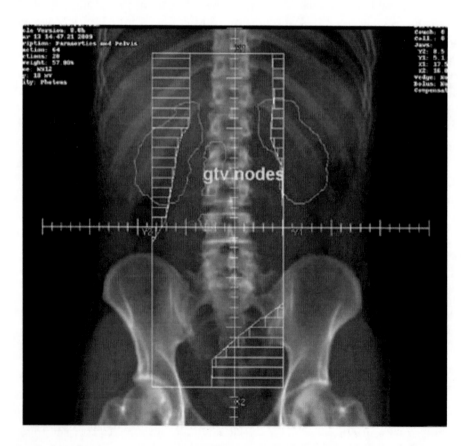

Figure 1. Radiotherapy field covering the para-aortic and ipsilateral common iliac lymph nodes.

If a patient is to be treated with adjuvant radiotherapy to the para-aortic lymph nodes, the superior field limit is to superior aspect of the T11 vertebral body and extends inferiorly to the L5/S1 intervertebral space. A compromise between traditional RT fields which placed the inferior border at the obturator foramen and para-aortic RT alone is to treat the para-aortic and ipsilateral common iliac lymph nodes by positioning the inferior border of the radiation fields at mid-pelvis (figure 1). This encompasses the lymph nodes that are typically removed at lymphadenectomy in patients with non-seminomatous tumors and also covers the vast majority of pelvic nodal recurrences in patients treated with para-aortic radiotherapy alone [39]. Left-sided testicular tumors have a propensity for relapse in the left renal hilum and this region should be included in the fields. This field will cover the para-aortic and the ipsilateral common iliac lymph node chains. Cardiac tissue should be avoided in the field of treatment. Appropriate shielding can be use to shape radiation beams to avoid critical structures, such as the kidneys and liver.

Dose of Radiation

Adjuvant radiation doses for stage I testicular seminoma have ranged from 25 to 35 Gy. The Medical Research Council conducted a randomized clinical trial (TE18) comparing 30 Gy in 15 fractions to 20 Gy in 10 fractions in 625 patients. The majority of patients received para-aortic irradiation only (88.1% in the 30Gy group and 88.7% in the 20Gy group). Relapse rates at 5 years were essentially identical with a relapse rate of 3% for the 30 Gy arm and 3.6% in the 20 Gy arm [40].

An additional 469 patients were added from a second trial comparing adjuvant chemotherapy to adjuvant radiotherapy (TE19/30982) for a total of 1,094 patients. In this trial, patients randomized to adjuvant radiotherapy arm, underwent a second randomization to either 30 Gy or 20 Gy. The 5-year relapse rates of 4.9% and 3%, for the 30Gy and 20Gy groups respectively [41]. Mature results after 7 years of median follow-up demonstrated that 20 Gy was non-inferior to 30 Gy of radiation (HR of relapse = 0.63; 90% CI .38 – 1.04) [42]

If adjuvant radiotherapy is to be used for stage I seminoma, 20 Gy in 10 fractions or an equivalent fractionation schedule, is adequate and provides excellent results. Alternative equivalent fractionation schedules may be used, which may provide higher biologically effective doses and minimize acute nausea due to less dose per fraction (table 2).

Table 2. Commonly Prescribed Retroperitoneal Radiation Doses in Testicular Seminoma

Fractionation Regimen	BED Tumor Control	BED Late Normal Tissue effects
20Gy in 10 fractions (2Gy / fraction)	24	40
25Gy in 20 fractions (1.25Gy / fraction)	28.1	40.6
25Gy in 15 fractions (1.67Gy / fraction)	29.2	45.8
20Gy in 8 fractions (2.5Gy / fraction)	25	45

BED = biologically equivalent dose

Radiation Toxicity

There is mounting evidence, in spite of the excellent results achieved with adjuvant radiation, that the risks associated with adjuvant radiation outweigh the potential benefits. Data from the M.D. Anderson, the Royal Marsden Hospital and the collective Norwegian experience have demonstrated increased risks in cardiac disease or cardiac associated mortality in seminoma survivors treated with adjuvant radiation [43-45]. The M.D. Anderson experience reported mortality rates for 453 men treated with infra-diaphragmatic radiotherapy with at least 15 years of follow-up. The cardiac specific standardized mortality risk ratio 15 years after treatment was 1.80 (95% C.I. 1.01 – 2.98) [43]. The cardiovascular mortality risk ratio was 2.4 (95% C.I. 1.04 – 5.45) in 992 men treated with infra-diaphragmatic radiotherapy compared to men monitored with surveillance at the Royal Marsden Hospital [44]. The Norwegian data, after 18 years of follow-up in 386 irradiated seminoma patients demonstrated hazard ratios of 2.1 and 2.3 for coronary artery disease and atherosclerotic disease, respectively [45]. Although the pathogenesis of cardiac disease in irradiated seminoma survivors is largely unknown, early evidence suggests that low grade inflammation and elevated levels of C-reactive protein detected in irradiated patients may play a role in the atherosclerotic process [46].

The testicular germinal epithelium is highly sensitive to ionizing radiation and scatter radiation from adjuvant treatments may impair spermatogenesis and impact fertility in the future. Testicular shielding has been shown to decrease radiation dose to the contra-lateral testis regardless if para-aortic and pelvic radiation or para-aortic radiation alone is used for treatment [47]. A Norwegian study found that reducing the radiation treatment volume from an extended field to a para-aortic field reduces the mean radiation dose to the remaining testicle from 0.32 Gy to 0.09 Gy. In this study, sperm counts remained depressed one year following extended field radiation, but not in those treated with para-aortic radiation [48]. Similarly, in the MRC randomized trial comparing radiation field size, sperm count recovery was longer in patients treated with extended field compared to para-aortic radiation (20 months vs. 13 months). However, this difference declined over time and after 3 years of follow-up sperm counts were not significantly different between the two groups [35]. Ultimately, total protection of the contra-lateral testis can not be guaranteed and sperm-banking should be offered to all men undergoing radiotherapy who wish to preserve fertility.

An increased risk in second malignancies in seminoma survivors treated with adjuvant radiation has been documented by a number of studies. The National Cancer Institute compiled 10,534 seminoma patients (all stages) treated with radiotherapy from 14 population-based registries [49]. The overall relative risk of a second non-testicular malignancy was estimated at 2.0 (95% C.I. 1.8-2.2) compared to matched cohorts from the general population. These results were confirmed by a Dutch study involving 1,354 patients treated with infra-diaphragmatic radiotherapy. The risk of a second cancer was 2.6 fold higher than the average population with a median survival after diagnosis of 1.4 years [50]. A dose-modeling study has suggested that the risk of second malignancy may be reduced by treating the para-aortic lymph nodes alone and excluding the pelvis [51]. However, a risk of second malignancy still exists and represents an unnecessary risk in the light of excellent outcomes with surveillance programs.

Adjuvant Chemotherapy

One or two cycles of carboplatin has been studied as a potentially viable alternative to adjuvant treatment to radiotherapy for stage I seminoma. Historically, dosing of carboplatin was by body surface area (400 mg/m^2), but contemporary studies have used the dosing regimen of Area under the Curve (AUC) of 7. This is largely because the AUC formula more reliably delivers the intended dose of carboplatin compared to dosing calculations using body surface area [52].

Adjuvant carboplatin was first used in stage I seminoma in a phase I trial treating 78 patients. In this study, 53 patients received 2 cycles of carboplatin and 25 received 1 cycle. During a median 44 month follow-up time, there was 1 relapse for the entire group [53]. Later studies have confirmed the effectiveness of adjuvant carboplatin with reported relapse rates ranging from 1.8% to 8.6% (table 1) [6, 16, 53-58]

A randomized controlled trial by the Medical Research Council compared single-cycle carboplatin to adjuvant radiotherapy in 1,477 men with stage I seminoma. This trial had a 5:3 randomization ratio with 904 patients treated with radiotherapy and 573 treated with carboplatin. Patients randomized to radiotherapy were further randomized to either 30 Gy or 20 Gy. Radiation fields were not randomized and 85% of patients received para-aortic radiation, while 15% received extended field irradiation. The chemotherapy consisted of a single-cycle of carboplatin using an AUC of 7 [54].

The updated results of this data demonstrate 5-year relapse rates of 4% for radiotherapy and 5.3% for single-cycle carboplatin. The 5-year rate of contralateral germ cell tumors was lower in the carboplatin arm at 0.2% compared to 1.2% in the radiotherapy arm [59]. The retroperitoneal nodes were the most common sites of relapse in 67% of the carboplatin patients [60]. Although the risk of relapse is small in patients treated with carboplatin, abdominal/pelvic CT imaging is still required to detect early relapse.

Chemotherapy Toxicity

The primary acute side-effects of carboplatin are typically myelodysplasia, nausea and vomiting. The long-term toxicities of carboplatin are less well understood, since the emergence of carboplatin as a viable adjuvant treatment option has been relatively recent. One prospective study with a median follow-up of 9 years for 199 seminoma patients treated with adjuvant carboplatin reported no increased risk of cardiovascular disease or second malignancy compared to the general UK population [61]. In comparison, 564 seminoma survivors treated with cisplatin-based chemotherapy, a median follow-up of 19 years was required to demonstrate an increased risk of cardiovascular disease (hazard ratio = 5.7) [45]. Similarly, there are multiple reports from radiotherapy data that have demonstrated large numbers and patient follow-up of up to 20 years will be required to adequately assess cardiovascular and second malignancy risk [43-44, 49-50].

Almost two decades earlier, adjuvant radiotherapy was thought not to be associated with an excess risk of second malignancy [62]. However, adequate follow-up and analysis of large databases have now demonstrated otherwise. Clinical oncologists should take care to not misinterpret early carboplatin toxicity data as clear evidence that carboplatin is not associated with long-term toxicity. Longer follow-up will be required to better understand the long-term consequences of carboplatin adjuvant therapy.

Management of Relapse

Following surveillance, the majority of patients will present with relapsed disease in the para-aortic lymph nodes within the first 2 years of treatment. Radiotherapy is typically sufficient to cure relapsed patients. In the Danish and PMH experiences, approximately 10%

of patients treated with salvage radiotherapy had a second relapse [7, 12]. Smaller relapses less than 5 cm are most suitable for salvage radiotherapy, which depends on frequent CT scans during the surveillance protocol. Large, bulky tumors are best treated with chemotherapy and are typically treated with 3 cycles of bleomycin, etoposide and cisplatin (BEP). Certain scenarios, such as horseshoe kidneys, recurrent disease situated close to a kidney or a large portion of the liver may be best treated with chemotherapy in order to avoid complications associated with irradiation of large volumes of normal tissue.

Recurrent stage I seminoma that is limited in size can be successfully treated with extended radiation fields encompassing the para-aortic and pelvic lymph nodes as described in the "Adjuvant Radiotherapy" section (figure 1). The dose of radiation at the PMH is 25 Gy in 20 fractions to para-aortic and pelvic lymph nodes, while gross recurrent disease is concomitantly boosted to an additional 10 Gy for a total of 35 Gy. However, there are a wide variety of different dose prescriptions used in practice and table 2 provides a few common dose prescriptions.

Following adjuvant radiotherapy, relapsed disease is typically found in the mediastinum, lungs and left supraclavicular fossa. In the scenario of a supradiaphragmatic relapse, patients are best treated with cisplatin-based chemotherapy and can expect close to a 100% cure rate. Isolated inguinal lymph node relapses can be successfully treated with radiotherapy [63]. It is exceedingly rare that relapses are found within the field of treatment. In this scenario biopsy should be performed to rule-out a non-seminomatous histology or a potential second malignancy.

Following adjuvant chemotherapy, the majority of relapses are found in the retroperitoneum. In these patients salvage radiotherapy as previous described or salvage cisplatin-based chemotherapy can be considered.

Summary

Stage I seminoma represents a model of curable malignancy with survival rates approaching 100% regardless of the post-orchidectomy management strategy selected. Surveillance is now the management option of choice for stage I testicular seminoma. This approach has been adopted by the Canadian Germ Cell Cancer Consensus Group, Société International d'Urologie (SIU), European Germ Cell Cancer Consensus Group (EGCCCG) and the European Society of Medical Oncology (ESMO) [22, 64-66]. An effective surveillance program allows for the early detection of relapse, which maximizes the chance of cure; however, this requires long-term participation and co-operation from both the patient and the health care team.

Stage II Seminoma

At the time of diagnosis, approximately 15-20% of patients will have metastatic para-aortic lymph nodes and are classified as having stage II disease. Stage II patients are sub-divided into three groups based on the diameter in the largest dimension of the largest retroperitoneal lymph node mass: ≤ 2 cm (stage IIA), 2.1 to 5 cm (stage IIB), and >5 cm (stage IIC). Approximately 70% of stage II patients have retroperitoneal lymph nodes ≤ 5 cm. Due to the rarity of the presentation stage II seminomas, management options are largely based on retrospective reports and institutional experiences.

The size of retroperitoneal disease, measured in the largest diameter, has been identified as the most important prognostic factor in stage II seminoma. From 1981 to 1999, ninety-five stage II seminoma patients were treated with radiotherapy at the PMH. The 5-year relapse-free rate in 79 stage IIA/B patients was 91% compared to 44% in 16 patients with stage IIC disease. The cause-specific survival was 97.5% indicating that the majority of patients are still curable [67]. The most common sites of relapse are the mediastinal or supraclavicular lymph nodes, lung or bone. These results are similar to other series in the literature and support the continued use of primary radiotherapy in stage IIA/B patients (table 3) [67-71]. Stage IIC testicular seminomas are generally best treated with chemotherapy, since radiotherapy is associated with a high failure rate and not all patients with relapsed disease are successfully salvaged.

Table 3. Results of Retroperitoneal RT in Stage II A/B Seminoma

	Patients (n)	Years of Study	# Relapse (%)	Cause-Specific Survival
Bayens (1992)	29	1975-1985	7 (24%)	93%
Vallis (1995)	48	1974-1989	3 (6%)	98%
Zagars (2001)	37	1984-1999	5 (13.5%)	100%
Classen (2003)	87	1991-1994	4 (4.6%)	100%
Chung (2004)	79	1981-1999	7 (8.8%)	97.5%

The Royal Marsden Hospital has reported a series of 62 Stage IIA/B patients treated with one to two cycles of carboplatin preceding para-aortic radiotherapy by four to six weeks. Since 1997, 29 patients have been treated with a single cycle of carboplatin and radiotherapy and no relapses have been observed with a median follow-up of 3 years. In comparison, the institution's relapse free survival is 80.7% for patients treated in the 1980's with radiation alone [72]. This approach is promising as it appears to improve the results of radiotherapy alone and decreases the amount of normal tissue irradiation by excluding pelvic lymph nodes from the radiation field. However, it is difficult to accept this approach as standard practice without further study.

Aside from the stage of disease, other factors may influence treatment decisions for stage II seminoma, such as location of disease in relation to critical organs or anatomical variations. In patients with lateralized disease or a horseshoe kidney may be best treated with chemotherapy in order to avoid toxicities from irradiation to large volumes of functional kidney. In the rare patient, in whom both radiotherapy and chemotherapy are contraindicated or if the diagnosis is uncertain, a retroperitoneal lymph node dissection should be considered.

The standard technique of radiation in stage II seminoma is similar to that used in the extended field irradiation including the para-aortic and ipsilateral pelvic lymph nodes as described in the stage I "Adjuvant Radiotherapy" section (figure 1). If chemotherapy is selected as primary treatment or used as salvage after radiotherapy relapse, 3 cycles of bleomycin, etoposide and cisplatin (BEP) or 4 cycles of etoposide and cisplatin (EP) should be considered as standard options. In older patients or those with poor pulmonary function, omission of bleomycin may be considered, particularly since the role of bleomycin has not been defined clearly.

After treatment for stage II disease, regular follow-up with clinical exam and chest x-ray are important to maximize the success of salvage therapy for patients that may relapse. CT imaging of the abdomen and pelvis is not necessary for routine evaluation once the resolution of retroperitoneal disease has been confirmed.

Residual Retroperitoneal Mass

In the majority of cases a stable, persistent mass on follow-up CT scans following treatment represents fibrosis or necrotic tumor. However, the presence of active tumor is a possibility and the existence of a non-seminomatous component should also be entertained. The current role of PET imaging for the detection of residual tumor is unclear. Management options should not be based solely on the presence of a positive PET scan, since false-positives have been reported [73-74]. Management approaches for patients with residual masses following treatment include: observation; surgical resection; and occasionally radiotherapy in the post-chemotherapy setting.

The Memorial Sloan Kettering published their experience in 55 seminoma patients with residual masses post-chemotherapy. Thirty-two patients underwent a RPLND, while the remaining 23 patients underwent intra-operative biopsies due to unresectability [75]. No viable tumor was found in residual masses less than 3 cm. In 27 patients with masses greater than 3 cm, 8 (30%) were found to have viable residual tumor. Seminoma was present in 6 of the patients, but teratoma was found in 2 patients. Given these findings, the authors have recommended biopsy or resection of masses 3 cm or larger. An alternative approach has been suggested by Culine and Droz where observation may be reasonable in residual retroperitoneal masses that continue to decrease in size following initial treatment [76].

There does not appear to be a role for routine radiotherapy for residual masses following radiotherapy. Horwich and colleagues published the experience at the Royal Marsden Hospital and found no difference in recurrences if residual masses were observed or treated with salvage radiotherapy [77]. The MRC Testicular Tumor Working Party published the findings from a retrospective pooled analysis of post-chemotherapy residual masses in 123 seminoma patients. Similar to Horwich's findings, there was no significant difference in outcome among patients who received or did not receive radiotherapy. Given these findings, it was concluded that routine radiotherapy is not indicated for a post-chemotherapy residual mass.

It is now widely accepted that patients with a residual mass of 3 cm or less can safely be observed. For patients with larger masses, surgery or observation should be considered depending on the stability of tumor size. If the mass is biopsied and confirmed to be viable residual seminoma, surgical resection should be considered as standard management.

Summary

Smaller lymph nodes can be treated successfully with radiotherapy to the retroperitoneal and ipsilateral pelvic lymph nodes, while large and bulky lymph nodes are generally best treated with multi-agent chemotherapy. Certain clinical scenarios may favor one treatment modality over another, regardless of the size of the tumor. Following initial therapy, residual disease greater than 3 cm can be either be surgically resected or observed.

Stage III Seminoma

It is unusual for patients to present with distant metastases and stage III patients comprise less than 5% of all seminoma patients. Testicular seminoma is exquisitely chemosensitive and the use of cisplatin-based regimens results in high cure rates. According to the International Germ Cell Cancer Collaborative Group Classification, patients with stage III seminoma are classified into good or intermediate prognostic groups [78]. Good prognosis disease comprises 90% of metastatic seminomas, while intermediate prognosis disease makes up the remaining 10%. Good prognosis patients are identified as patients with a seminoma from any primary site, no non-pulmonary visceral metastases and normal AFP (HCG and LDH can be any value). Intermediate prognosis patients only differed from good prognosis patients by the presence of non-pulmonary visceral metastases. A poor prognosis classification does not exist for seminoma and is reserved for the non-seminomatous histology.

Patients in the good prognosis group should be treated with 3 courses of 5-day BEP, which is considered the standard of care by the European Germ Cell Cancer Consensus group [23]. Patients who are unsuitable candidates for bleomycin can be alternatively treated with 4 courses of EP [23, 79]. Overall survival in good prognosis patients range from 85 – 90%, while intermediate prognosis patients have an overall survival rate of approximately 75% warranting more aggressive treatment [78]. Consequently, intermediate prognosis disease is generally treated with 4 courses of 5-day BEP [23].

Summary

Metastatic stage III seminoma is classified into good and intermediate prognosis disease depending on the presence of non-pulmonary visceral metastases. The prognostic group dictates the number of cycles of chemotherapy and all patients are ideally treated with BEP chemotherapy. However, omission of bleomycin can be considered in unsuitable patients.

Conclusion

The majority of seminomatous germ cell tumors present with stage I disease and the overall outcomes for these men are excellent. The primary area of controversy involves the management of stage I disease. Mature data from surveillance, radiotherapy and chemotherapy series indicate that survival rates for stage I disease approaches 100% regardless of the selected management approach. Surveillance should be the management option of choice, to avoid the potential long-term toxicities of adjuvant radiotherapy or chemotherapy. However, change within the medical community has been slow and there is still a considerable proportion of genitourinary oncologists that do not routinely discuss the option of surveillance with their patients [80].

Patients with stage II may be treated with either radiotherapy or chemotherapy depending on the clinical scenario. Generally, smaller tumors are best treated with radiotherapy, while bulkier tumors are treated with chemotherapy; however, exceptions may arise requiring the clinician to make decisions on a case-by-case basis. Residual masses greater than 3 cm following initial treatment are managed either by resection or observation. Metastatic stage III seminoma is generally treated with 3 to 4 cycles of multi-agent chemotherapy.

Current research efforts are primarily focused in stage I seminoma. The identification of suitable biomarkers to more accurately identify patients at risk for relapse would be useful for the design of a risk-adapted protocol to individually tailor adjuvant management strategies for patients. Efforts are underway to develop surveillance protocols incorporating MRI or low-dose CT screening to minimize radiation exposure from routine radiological screening.

In more advanced disease, the significance of residual masses remains unclear and better methods of identifying residual disease from fibrotic or necrotic tissue is required. Refinements in chemotherapeutic strategies are needed to better identify sub-groups of patients who may be treated with fewer cycles of chemotherapy or where bleomycin may be safely omitted. Finally, new drugs with less toxicity, but with similar clinical efficacy would be a welcome addition to the current treatments available n the treatment of testicular seminoma.

References

[1]   Sokoloff, M., G. Joyce, and M. Wise, Testis cancer. *J Urol,* 2007. 177(6): p. 2030-41.
[2]   Shah, M., et al., Trends in testicular germ cell tumours by ethnic group in the United States. *Int J Androl,* 2007. 30(4): p. 206-13.
[3]   Jemal, A., et al., Cancer statistics, 2010. *CA Cancer J Clin,* 2010. 60(5): p. 277-300.
[4]   Warde, P., J. Sturgeon, and M. Gospodarowicz, Testicular Cancer, in *Clinical Radiation Oncology*, L. Gunderson and J. Tepper, Editors. 2000, Churchill Livingstone: Philadelphia. p. 844-62.
[5]   Sohaib, A., D. Koh, and J. Husband, The role of imaging in the diagnosis, staging, and management of testicular cancer. *AJR,* 2008. 191: p. 387-95.
[6]   Oliver, R., L. Boubilkova, and J. Ong, Fifteen-year follow-up of Anglian Germ Cell Cancer group adjuvant studies of carboplatin as an alternative to radiation or surveillance for stage I seminoma. *J Clin Oncol,* 2001. 19(Abstract 780).
[7]   Warde, P., et al., Should surveillance be considered the standard of care in stage I seminoma? *J Clin Oncol* (Meeting abstracts), 2005. 23(16): p. 4520.
[8]   Daugaard, G., P. Petersen, and M. Rorth, Surveillance in stage I testicular cancer. *Apmis,* 2003. 111(1): p. 76-85.
[9]   Germa-Lluch, J., et al., Clinical pattern and therapeutic results achieved in 1490 patients with germ-cell tumors of the testis: The experience of the Spanish Germ-Cell Cancer Group (GG). *European Urology,* 2002. 42(6): p. 553-62.
[10] Horwich, A., et al., Surveillance following orchidectomy for stage I testicular seminoma. *Br J Cancer,* 1992. 65(5): p. 775-8.

[11] Ramakrishnan, S., et al., Stage I seminoma of the testis: Is post-orchiectomy surveillance a safe alternative to routine postoperative radiotherapy? *Clin Oncol* (R Coll Radiol), 1992. 4(5): p. 284-6.

[12] von der Maase, H., et al., Surveillance following orchidectomy for stage I seminoma of the testis. *Eur J Cancer*, 1993. 29A(14): p. 1931-4.

[13] Kamba, T., et al., Outcome of different post-orchiectomy management for stage I seminoma: Japanese multi-institutional study including 425 patients. *Int J Urol*, 2010. 17: p. 980-88.

[14] Yoshida, T., et al., Surveillance following orchiectomy for stage I testicular seminoma: long-term outcome. *Int J Urol*, 2009. 16: p. 756-9.

[15] Chung, P., et al., Surveillance in stage I testicular seminoma - risk of late relapse. *Can J Urol*, 2002. 9(5): p. 1637-40.

[16] Aparicio, J., et al., Risk-adapted management for patients with clinical stage I seminoma: the second Spanish Germ Cell Cancer Cooperative Group study. *J Clin Oncol*, 2005. 23(34): p. 8717-23.

[17] Warde, P., et al., Prognostic factors for relapse in stage I seminoma managed by surveillance: A pooled analysis. *J Clin Oncol*, 2002. 20(22): p. 4448-52.

[18] Chung, P., et al., Prognostic factors for relapse in stage I seminoma managed with surveillance: A validation study. *J Clin Oncol*, 2010. 28(15s): p. A4535.

[19] Leung, E., et al., Total treatment burden in stage 1 seminoma patients. *J Clin Oncol*, 2010. 28(15s): p. A4534.

[20] Marzani, W., et al., Lymph node growth rate in testicular germ cell tumors: Implications for computed tomography surveillance frequency. *Clin Oncol*, 2010.

[21] Martin, J., et al., Evidence-based guidelines for following stage I seminoma. *Cancer Res,* 2007. 109(11): p. 2248-56.

[22] Krege, S., et al., European consensus conference on diagnosis and treatment of germ cell cancer: A report of the second meeting of the European Germ Cell Cancer Consensus Group (EGCCCG) part I. *Eur Urol*, 2008. 53(3): p. 478-96.

[23] Krege, S., et al., European consensus conference on diagnosis and treatment of germ cell cancer: a report of the second meeting of the European Germ Cell Cancer Consensus Group (EGCCCG): Part II. *Eur Urol*, 2008. 53(3): p. 496-513.

[24] Motzer, R., NCCN Clinical Practice Guidelines in Oncology: Testicular Cancer v.1. *National Comprehensive Cancer Network,* 2010.

[25] Schrimpton, P., et al., National survey of doses from CT in the UK: 2003. *Br J Radiol*, 2006. 79: p. 968-80.

[26] Mettler, F., et al., Effective doses in radiology and diagnostic nuclear medicine: a catalog. *Radiology*, 2008. 248: p. 254-63.

[27] Brenner, D. and H. EJ, Computed tomography - an increasing sourve of radiation exposure. *N Engl J Med*, 2007. 357(22): p. 2277-84.

[28] Berrington de Gonzalez, A. and S. Darby, Risk of cancer from diagnostic X-rays: estimates for the UK and 14 other countries. *Lancet*, 2004. 363: p. 345-51.

[29] O'Malley, M., et al., Comparison of low dose with standard dose abdominal/pelvic multidetector CT in patients with stage I testicular cancer under surveillance. *Eur Radiol*, 2010. 20: p. 1624-30.

[30] Narayanan, P., et al., Pearls and pitfalls of MR lymphography in gynecologic malignancy. *Radiographics*, 2009. 29(4): p. 1057-69.

[31] Desemo, W., et al., Comparison of nodal risk formula and MR lymphography for predicting lymph node involvement in prostate cancer. *Int J Radiat Oncol Biol Phys,* 2010.

[32] Heesakkers, R., et al., Prostate cancer: detection of lymph node metastases outside the routine surgical area with ferumoxtran-10-enhanced MR imaging. *Radiology,* 2009. 251(2): p. 408-14.

[33] Bayens, Y., et al., Orchidectomy followed by radiotherapy in 176 stage I and II testicular seminoma patients: benefits of a 10-year follow-up study. *Radiother Oncol,* 1992. 25(2): p. 97-102.

[34] Coleman, J., et al., The management and clinical course of testicular seminoma: 15 years' experience at a single institution. *Clin Oncol,* 1998. 10(4): p. 237-41.

[35] Fossa, S., et al., Optimal planning target volume for stage I testicular seminoma: A Medical Research Council randomized trial. Medical Research Council Testicular Tumor Working Group. *J Clin Oncol,* 1999. 17(4): p. 1146-54.

[36] Santoni, R., et al., Stage I seminoma of the testis: a bi-institutional retrospective analysis of patients treated with radiation therapy only. *BJU Int,* 2003. 92(1): p. 47-52.

[37] Hultenschmidt, B., et al., Results of radiotherapy for 230 patients with stage I-II seminomas. *Strahlenther Onkol,* 1996. 172(4): p. 186-92.

[38] Logue, J., et al., Short course para-aortic radiation for stage I seminoma of the testis. *Int J Radiat Oncol Biol Phys,* 2003. 57(5): p. 1304-9.

[39] Classen, J., et al., Para-aortic irradiation for stage I testicular seminoma: Results of a prospective study in 675 patients. A trial of the German cancer study group (GTCSG). *Br J Cancer,* 2004. 90(12): p. 2305-11.

[40] Jones, W., et al., Randomized trial of 30 versus 20 Gy in the adjuvant treatment of stage I testicular seminoma: A report on Medical Research Council Trial TE18, European Organization for the Research and Treatment of Cancer Trial 20942 (ISRCTN 18525328). *J Clin Oncol,* 2005. 23(6): p. 1200-08.

[41] Mead, G., et al., Relapse patterns in 2, 466 stage 1 seminoma patients entered into Medical Research Council randomised trials. *J Clin Oncol,* 2008. 26: p. A5020.

[42] Mead, G., et al., Randomized trials in 2466 patients with stage I seminoma: Patterns of relapse and follow-up. *JNCI,* 2011. 103: p. 241-9.

[43] Zagars, G., et al., Mortality after cure of testicular seminoma. *J Clin Oncol,* 2004. 22(4): p. 640-7.

[44] Huddart, R., et al., Cardiovascular disease as a long-term complication of treatment for testicular cancer. *J Clin Oncol,* 2003. 21(8): p. 1513-23.

[45] Haugnes, H., et al., Cardiovascular risk factors and morbidity in long-term survivors of testicular cancer: A 20-year follow-up study. *JCO,* 2010. 29: p. 4649-57.

[46] Wethal, T., et al., Treatment-related differences in cardiovascular risk factors in long-term survivors of testicular cancer. *J Cancer Surviv,* 2007. 1(1): p. 8-16.

[47] Bieri, S., M. Rouzaud, and R. Miralbell, Seminoma of the testis: is scrotal shielding necessary when radiotherapy is limited to the para-aortic nodes? *Radiother Oncol,* 1999. 50: p. 349-53.

[48] Jacobsen, K., et al., External beam abdominal radiotherapy in patients with seminoma stage I: Field type, testicular dose, and spermatogenesis. *Int J Radiat Oncol Biol Phys,* 1997. 38(1): p. 95-102.

[49] Travis, L., et al., Second cancers among 40576 testicular cancer patients: focus on long-term survivors. *JNCI*, 2005. 97(18): p. 1354-65.

[50] van den Belt-Dusebout, A., et al., Treatment-specific risks of second malignancies and cardiovascular disease in 5-year survivors of testicular cancer. *J Clin Oncol*, 2007. 25(28): p. 4370-8.

[51] Zwahlen, D., et al., Effect of radiotherapy volume and dose on secondary cancer risk in stage I testicular seminoma. *Int J Radiat Oncol Biol Phys*, 2008. 70(3): p. 853-8.

[52] Sculier, J., et al., A comparison of methods of calculation for estimating carboplatin AUC with a retrospective pharmacokinetic-pharmacodynamic analysis in patients with advanced non-small cell lung cancer. *Eur J Cancer*, 1999. 35(9): p. 1314-19.

[53] Oliver, R., et al., Pilot studies of 2 and 1 course carboplatin as adjuvant for stage I seminoma: should it be tested in a randomized trial against radiotherapy? *Int J Radiat Oncol Biol Phys*, 1994. 29(1): p. 3-8.

[54] Oliver, R., et al., Radiotherapy versus single-dose carboplatin in adjuvant treatment of stage I seminoma: a randomised trial. *Lancet*, 2005. 366(9482): p. 293-300.

[55] Dieckmann, K., et al., Adjuvant treatment of clinical stage I seminoma: is a single course of carboplatin sufficient? *Urology*, 2000. 55(1): p. 102-6.

[56] Krege, S., et al., Phase II study: adjuvant single-agent carboplatin therapy for clinical stage I seminoma. *European Urology*, 1997. 31(4): p. 405-7.

[57] Aparicio, J., et al., Multicenter study evaluating a dual policy of postorchidectomy surveillance and selective adjuvant single-agent carboplatin for patients with clinical stage I seminoma. *Ann Oncol*, 2003. 14(6): p. 867-72.

[58] Agirovic, D., Germ cell testicular tumors in clinical stage A and normal values of serum tumor markers post-orchiectomy: The experience in the management of 300 consecutive patients. . *J BUON*, 2005. 10(2): p. 195-200.

[59] Oliver, R., et al., Randomized trial of carboplatin versus radiotherapy for stage I seminoma: Mature results on relapse and contralateral testis cancer rates in MRC TE19/EORTC 30982 study (ISRCTN27163214). *J Clin Oncol*, 2011.

[60] Oliver, R., et al., Radiotherapy versus carboplatin for stage I seminoma: Updated analysis of the MRC/EORTC randomized trial (ISRCTN27163214). *JCO*, 2008. 26: p. A1.

[61] Powles, T., et al., The long-term risks of adjuvant carboplatin treatment for stage I seminoma of the testis. *Ann Oncol*, 2008. 19: p. 443-7.

[62] Horwich, A. and J. Bell, Mortality and cancer incidence following radiotherapy for seminoma of the testis. *Radiother Oncol*, 1994. 30(3): p. 193-8.

[63] Warde, P., et al., Stage I testicular seminoma: Results of adjuvant radiation and surveillance. *JCO*, 1995. 13: p. 2255-62.

[64] Schmoll, H., et al., Testicular seminoma: ESMO clinical recommendations for diagnosis, treatment and follow-up. *Ann Oncol*, 2009. 20(S4): p. iv83-iv88.

[65] Seminoma, Stage I/II. in International Consultation on Urologic DiseasesInternational *Consultation on Urologic Diseases*. 2009. Shanghai.

[66] Wood, L., et al., Canadian consensus guidelines for the management of testicular germ cell cancer. *Can Urol Assoc J*, 2010. 4(2): p. e19-38.

[67] Chung, P., et al., Stage II testicular seminoma: pattterns of recurrence and outcome of treatment. *Eur Urol*, 2004. 45(6): p. 754-60.

[68] Bayens, Y., et al., Orchidectomy followed by radiotherapy in 176 stage I and II testicular seminoma patients: benefits of a 10-year follow-up study. *Radiother Oncol,* 1992. 25(2): p. 97-102.

[69] Zagars, G. and A. Pollack, Radiotherapy for stage II testicular seminoma. Int *J Radiat Oncol Biol Phys,* 2001. 51(3): p. 643-9.

[70] Classen, J., et al., Radiotherapy for stages IIA/B testicular seminoma: final report of a prospective multicenter clinical trial. *J Clin Oncol,* 2003. 21(6): p. 1101-6.

[71] Vallis, K., et al., Radiotherapy for stages I and II testicular seminoma: results and morbidity in 238 patients. *Br J Radiol,* 1995. 68(808): p. 400-5.

[72] Gilbert, D., et al., Treating IIA/B seminoma with combination carboplatin and radiotherapy. *J Clin Oncol,* 2009. 27(12): p. 2101-2.

[73] Ganjoo, K., et al., Positron emission tomography scans in the evaluation of postchemotherapy residual masses in patients with seminoma. *J Clin Oncol,* 1999. 17(11): p. 3457-60.

[74] Hinz, S., et al., The role of positron emission tomography in the evaluation of residual masses after chemotherapy for advanced stage seminoma. *J Urol,* 2008. 179(3): p. 936-40.

[75] Herr, H., et al., Surgery for a post-chemotherapy residual mass in seminoma. *J Urol,* 1997. 157(3): p. 860-2.

[76] Culine, S. and J. Droz, Optimal management of residual mass after chemotherapy in advanced seminoma: there is time for everything. *J Clin Oncol,* 1996. 14(10): p. 2884-5.

[77] Horwich, A., et al., Residual mass following chemotherapy of seminoma. *Ann Oncol,* 1997. 8(1): p. 37-40.

[78] International Germ Cell Consensus Classification: A prognostic factor-based staging system for metastatic germ cell cancers. *J Clin Oncol,* 1997. 15: p. 594-603.

[79] Kondagunta, G., et al., Etoposide and cisplatin chemotherapy for metastatic good risk germ cell tumors. *J Clin Oncol,* 2005. 23(36): p. 9290-4.

[80] Choo, R., et al., Survey of radiation oncologists: practice patterns of the management of stage I seminoma of testis in Canada and a selected froup in the United States. *Can J Urol,* 2002. 9(2): p. 1479-85.

In: Essentials and Updates in Urologic Oncology
Editor: Philippe E. Spiess

ISBN: 978-1-62081-494-9
© 2013 Nova Science Publishers, Inc.

Chapter XXVII

Non-Seminomatous Germ Cell Testis Tumors

Stephen D. W. Beck and Richard S. Foster

Department of Urologic Oncology, Indiana University,
Indianapolis, Illinois, US

Abstract

The optimal treatment for low stage disease is largely patient driven with surgery, surveillance and chemotherapy considered the primary treatment modalities. In low volume non-seminomatous germ cell cancer, (clinical stage A/B1) retroperitoneal lymph node dissection has maintained its therapeutic benefit while minimizing morbidity with the reduction of the surgical template from a full bilateral dissection to a unilateral nerve-sparring surgery. In the post chemotherapy population, patients with complete radiographic resolution of retroperitoneal disease are typically observed as the relapse rate in this population is ~ 5%. Residual masses after chemotherapy should be resected. A modified post chemotherapy dissection is adequate in carefully selected patients with low volume disease restricted to the primary landing zone of the affected testicle. A full bilateral RPLND remains standard template for larger volume disease. In chemo-refractory disease, aggressive surgery provides a 5-year survival of 31% for patients with active cancer. Excluding chemo-naïve patients, late relapse disease is managed surgically with 50% being cured of disease.

The vast majority (approximately 90 to 95%) of neoplasms of the testis are of germ-cell origin because these cells are mitotically very active and therefore most prone to developing DNA mutations (1). The supporting cells of the testis, Sertoli cell and Leydig cells, have low proliferative rates, and consequently tumors derived from these cells are unusual, comprising fewer than 4% of all testicular tumors (2).

Germ cell tumors are composed of five basic cell types: seminoma, embryonal cell carcinoma, yolk sac tumor, choriocarcinoma, and teratoma. Classic seminoma is the most common tumor of the testis accounting for approximately 35% to 55% of all germ-cell neoplasms. The focus of this chapter is the management of non-seminomatous germ-cell tumors.

Therapeutic Principles in the Management of NSGCT

In general, patients presenting with NSGCT can be broadly divided into two subgroups: those presenting with low volume disease and those presenting with high volume or advanced disease. Management options in low volume disease include surveillance, retroperitoneal lymph node dissection (RPLND) and chemotherapy. The "optimal" treatment modality in low volume disease should individualized based on clinical stage (A/B1/B2), serum tumor marker status, primary tumor histology, and patient comorbidity, fertility status and preference. As cure is typically not a concern in low volume disease, the goal of treating physicians is to decrease treatment related morbidity while maintaining high cure rates. Patients presenting with advanced disease can also be broadly divided into two subgroups: good risk and intermediate/poor risk. Patients with good risk advanced disease have a favorable prognosis, and similar to low volume disease, the goal of the treating physicians is to minimize patient morbidity while preserving treatment efficacy. In poor risk disease, the goal is to improve responses to chemotherapy and cure with acceptable patient morbidity.

Pathology

Embryonal Cell Carcinoma

At the time of clinical presentation, embryonal cell carcinoma usually is seen as a smaller, more asymmetric testicular mass than seminoma. Grossly, on the cut surface, embryonal carcinoma is very heterogeneous. Microscopically, the tumor usually occurs in a solid form and does not have the lobular pattern of seminoma. Embryonal carcinoma cells tend to be larger, demonstrate more pleomorphism, have more mitoses, and have less distinctive cell membranes with nuclear overlapping than seminomatous tumor cells. Most embryonal cell carcinomas are immunoreactive for PLAP, low-molecular weight cytokeratin, CD-30 and POU5F (Oct 3/4). They do not express CD-117, AFP, or HCG. Embryonal cell carcinoma tends to metastasize early and often demonstrates other cell types in these metastatic sites.

Yolk Sac Carcinoma (Endodermal Sinus Tumor)

Yolk sac carcinoma was originally described as a rare tumor of infancy and childhood. Telium thought that the histologic findings in this tumor were similar to the endodermal sinuses present in the rodent. [1] Pierce and co-authors compared the tumor to a mouse yolk sac. [2] Yolk sac elements are found in 38% of adult patients with testis tumors. In 10% of patients, the yolk sac carcinoma is the dominant element of mixed adult testis tumors. Pure adult yolk sac tumors are rare. These tumors are associated with serum elevation of AFP in the overwhelming majority of cases. Shiller-Duval bodies are unique to yolk sac tumors and are perivascular arrangements of cuboidal or low columnar epithelial cell with a labyrinth like network of extracellular spaces. The cytoplasm may contain small, spherical, and densely eosinophilic intracytoplasmic droplets that are PAS positive. These tumors are immunoreactive for AFP and low molecular-weight cytokeratin. PLAP staining is variable. CD117 (c-kit) and CD-30 are usually negative.

Choriocarcinoma

At clinical presentation choriocarcinoma tumors are often extremely small. Despite the small size, wide metastatic spread is common. In its pure form, these tumors are associated with very high levels of serum HCG. On cut surface, the tumor tends to show large areas of hemorrhage with a small rim of viable tumor. Microscopically, two cell elements must be present to qualify as choriocarcinoma: syncytiotrophoblast and cytotrophoblast. Pure choriocarcinoma is extremely rare. It is found more often in association with other tumor elements. Syncytiotrophoblast often form the leading edge of the tumor and allow it to erode in blood vessels, which probably accounts for the large amount of hemorrhage found in the primary and metastatic tumor sites.

Teratoma

By definition, teratoma is composed of two or more embryonic germ cell layers: endoderm, mesoderm and/or ectoderm. Typical endodermal structures seen in teratoma are mucus-secreting glands as in the gastrointestinal, genitourinary, or respiratory tracts. Mesodermal elements often present in teratoma include cartilage, bone, muscle and lymphoid tissue. The ectoderm may be represented by stratified squamous epithelial cell-lined cysts and neural tissue elements. Teratomas may be composed of mature tissues, embryonal type tissue or a mixture of both and historically these tumors were classified as either mature or immature based on the degree of differentiation.

Mixed Histologic Germ Cell Tumors

Excluding seminoma, approximately 70% of germ cell tumor are composed of multiple histologic subtypes. [3] The most common of these mixtures is yolk sac tumor and teratoma. A second frequent pairing is embryonal cell carcinoma and teratoma, and together these elements are frequently referred to as teratocarcinoma.

Management

Clinical Stage A

Despite dramatic advances in cure, controversy remains regarding the optimal management of clinical stage (CS) A nonseminomatous germ cell tumors (NSGCT), defined as disease limited to the testicle with normal abdominal and chest computed tomographic (CT) scans, and normal serum tumor markers post orchiectomy. The presentation of NSGCT confined clinically to the testicle (CS A) is associated with a 30 to 50% incidence of occult retroperitoneal metastases (pathologic stage B) creating the controversy regarding the "best" treatment modality. Currently 3 approaches are considered for treatment in CS A NSGCT: retroperitoneal lymph node dissection (RPLND), surveillance, and primary chemotherapy, all with equal cure rates at 99%.

The primary issue in the adjuvant treatment of patient with CS A NSGCT is tailoring treatment to those 30% of patients who have occult metastatic disease and destined to relapse on a surveillance program. Observation without risk assessment will result in the treatment of recurrence in about one third of patients with the possibility of multiple courses of chemotherapy and potential resection of residual masses. RPLND as well as adjuvant chemotherapy without risk assessment will over treat about 70% of patients. It is therefore essential to identify risk factors identifying patients at high risk of occult metastatic disease.

Risk of Micrometastatic Disease

The Medical Research Council (MRC) in Great Britain has performed the first major study for identifying risk factors for relapse in CSA NSGCT. [4] The multivariate analysis revealed four prognostic factors predictive of recurrence: vascular invasion of the primary tumor, lymphatic invasion, the presence of embryonal carcinoma, and the absence of yolk sac tumor. A prospective MRC trial based on these prognostic variables found the presence of at least three of these four factors to be predictive for relapse in 48% of patients. [5] Vascular invasion was the predominant finding. Conversely, those patients with two or less risk factors were found to recur on surveillance about 20% of the time.

Multiple other studies have identified similar risk factors for relapse with embryonal cell carcinoma dominant tumors and the presence of lymphovascular invasion consistently being the most powerful predictors. Vergouwe et al. performed a review of studies assessing predictors of occult metastases and identified 23 publications reporting on 2,587 patients. [6] Overall 759 (29.3%) patients had occult metastasis. Pooled univariate odds ratios identified that lymphovascular (LVI), embryonal carcinoma (EC) > 50%, pathologic stage pT2-4 versus pT1, and MIB-1 staining > 70% as the strongest predictors. Though somewhat variable, high risk groups, with the presence of either or both lymphovascular invasion and embryonal dominant primary carried an approximate 50% recurrence rate. Low risk groups without either pathologic variable, had a relapse rate of < 20%.

Accurate risk stratification would enable directed therapy: arguably retroperitoneal lymph node dissection (RPLND) or primary chemotherapy for the high-risk group and observation for the low-risk group. Even with this stratification, 50% of so called high-risk patients will still be over treated when otherwise cured with orchiectomy. Likewise, 20% of the low-risk group will be destined to relapse on surveillance and subjected to systemic chemotherapy and possible post chemotherapy RPLND.

Surveillance

The rationale for surveillance includes 1) the low rate of progression/recurrence (overall 30% for all comers and only as high as 50% for the "high risk group") and 2) patients that do relapse remain curable. Irrespective of risk classification, RPLND or immediate chemotherapy, will subject 100% of patients to therapy while benefiting only 30% and up to 50% based on risk classification. That is, even in the high risk group, 50% of patients are unnecessarily treated with RPLND or chemotherapy.

Although estimates of the staging accuracy of currently available technology in CS A nonseminoma patients vary widely, most suggest an immediate false-negative rate of approximately 30%. [7-9] This is confirmed by a large number of clinical trials of surveillance alone in this population, and these have shown a relapse rate of approximately 30% with this strategy, with remarkably few differences between trials regardless of the size of the trial or country of origin (table 1). Table 1 reports a summary of surveillance series involving at least 200 patients. The median time to relapse is 5 to 7 months. The retroperitoneum is the most common site of recurrence observed in up to 60% of relapses [10, 11] while 25% occur in the lung and 10% diagnosed by elevated serum tumor markers. [12]

A pooled analysis recently reported on 59 papers addressing NSGCT surveillance. [13] Of 3613 NSGCT patients on surveillance, 1025 (28%) relapsed. The large majority of patients relapsing did so within 2 years, with up to 85% to 90% occurring in the first 12 months with 90% to 95% of those destined to relapse doing so within 24 months. [14, 15] In the pooled analysis of 1025 relapses, 55 occurred 2 years after orchiectomy accounting for 2% of all surveillance patients from studies that reported late relapse and 6% of all relapses. [13] In this large pooled cohort, only 7 recurrences occurred after five years on surveillance. [16-19]

Table 1. Summary of Surveillance Outcomes for Clinical Stage I NSGCT

Author	N	Median FU (yrs)	# relapse (%)	Med. Time to relapse (months)	DSS
Read [5]	373	5.0	100 (27)	NR	98.7%
Kakiashvili [2]1	371	6.3	104 (28)	7.1	99.2%
Colls [16]	248	4.5	70 (28)	NR	98.4%
Daugard [17]	301	5.0	86 (29)	5.0	100%
Oliver [15]	234	7.0	71 (30)	NR	97.4%

Burden of Therapy

As all treatments in clinical stage A NSGCT have similar cure rates, a key in determining the optimal treatment for the individual is the burden of therapy for each modality. The strategy of surveillance is to reserve therapy for those who relapse and thus avoid therapy in patients otherwise cured with orchiectomy. Most patents that relapse on surveillance present with good risk disease and remain curable with cisplatin-based chemotherapy. In two separate series, 98% (58 of 59) [14] and 96% (70 of 73) [20] of relapses were good risk. Of those relapses receiving chemotherapy approximately a quarter will require surgery. Those patients relapsing in the retroperitoneum with normal serum tumor markers may be candidates for primary RPLND. In the single center series from Toronto, at a median follow up of 6.3 years, 104 of 371 (28%) patients relapsed on surveillance. [21] 57 (55%) received immediate chemotherapy of whom 37 (54%) obtained a complete response, 18 (32%) required RPLND, and 7 underwent thoracotomy. 39 underwent primary RPLND at relapse. Of the 104 patients that recurred, the burden of therapy included: chemotherapy alone in 31, surgery alone in 31, and a combination of chemotherapy, surgery and radiation in the remaining 42 patients. Therefore, for approximately 60% of relapses, burden of therapy is no different than primary RPLND or chemotherapy at initial presentation; however, for the remaining 40% (11% of the initial cohort starting surveillance) the burden of therapy is significant.

Survival

In the pooled analysis of 3424 patients on surveillance in series that reported death, 47 died of disease with a 98.6% disease specific survival. [13] Some investigators noted that patients who died of disease were those who dropped out of surveillance or refused therapy upon relapse. [16, 22-24] Thus, there is little doubt from the existing literature on surveillance that with motivated, compliant patients, that the cure rate with this strategy is similar to that of primary RPLND, that is, patients that relapse on surveillance remain curable.

Compliance has been a concern when placing patients on a surveillance protocol with studies showing up to a third of patients missing at least one clinic visit. [10, 25] The concern of non-compliance is that it may translate into a decrease in disease specific survival. A recent evaluation of compliance of clinical stage A NSGCT at the University of Calgary showed extremely poor compliance with follow up as scheduled. In this study, compliance with clinic visits and tumor markers was only 61% during the first year and 35% in year 2, and with scheduled CT scans only 25% compliance in year 1 and 12% in year 2. The only two deaths in 76 patients were in individuals who were non-compliant with follow up. Nevertheless, the true impact of non-compliance on survival is unknown. A national surveillance study in New Zealand failed to correlate non-compliance with compromise in cure. [16]

Surveillance Follow-up

Table 2. Toronto CSI NSGCT Surveillance Schedule

	Month 2	Month 4	Month 6	Month 8	Month 10	Month 12
Year 1	Markers CXR	Marker CXR CT AandP	Markers CXR	Marker CXR CT AandP	Markers CXR	Marker CXR CT AandP
Year 2	Marker CXR	Marker CXR CT AandP	Markers CXR	Marker CXR CT AandP	Markers CXR	Marker CXR CT AandP
Year 3		Markers CXR		Markers CXR		Markers CXR
Year 4			Markers CXR			Markers CXR
Year 5						Markers CXR

The success of a surveillance strategy seems to depend on the early detection of recurrence. As the relapse rates are higher in the first 2 years more intensive follow-up is required in this time period using a combination of physical exam, CXR, serum TM, and abdominal/pelvic CT scan. Due to recent evidence regarding an increased secondary cancer risk due to diagnostic radiation exposure, controversy remains regarding the optimal frequency of imaging. A randomized trial evaluated CT scans at 3 and 12 months versus 3, 6, 9, 12, and 24 months and found no benefit in more frequent CT scans. This study involved 414 patients with a median follow-up of 40 months though only 10% of patient were considered high risk based on vascular invasion. [20] In the Toronto series, CT scan of the abdomen and pelvis, as a single modality, was most likely to detect recurrences (76.9%). CXR alone never identified relapse and the combination of CT scan and serum tumor makers identified relapse in 30%. The suggested Toronto CSA follow-up schedule is seen in table 2.

Adjuvant Chemotherapy

The rationale for chemotherapy in CSA NSGCT is that it virtually eliminates the risk for relapse at an incidence much lower than observed with either primary RPLND or surveillance. Surveillance protocols leave patients at a 30% to 50% risk of relapse depending on risk classification. Primary RLPND cures 75% of patients with pathologic stage B (PSB) disease, the remaining 25% will relapse and require systemic therapy for cure. If the lymph nodes are negative at RPLND (pathologic stage A) the risk of progression is 10% and as high as 25% in high risk patients. The risk of relapse with adjuvant chemotherapy after chemotherapy is < 2% (table 3) though exposes all patients to chemotherapy including those 50% never destined to relapse.

Table 3. Chemotherapy for High Risk Clinical Stage 1 NSGCT

First Author	Year	Chemotherapy	Risk Factors	No. of patients (evaluable/all)	Relapse Rate	DOD
Oliver [26]	1992	2 BEP	>2 MRC RF	22/22	1 (4.5%)	1 (4.5%)
Cullen [27]	1996	2 BEP	>3 MRC RF	109/114	2 (1.8%)	1 (0.9%)
Pont [107]	1996	2 BEP	VI	29/42	2 (6.9%)	1 (3.4%)
Klepp [108]	1997	3 BEP	VI	32/34	1 (3.0%)	0
Ondrus [109]	1998	2 BEP	VI and/or ECP	18/18	0	0
Bohlen [110]	1999	2 BEP or PVB	VI+and /or LI or >pT2 or EC	58/60	1 (1.7%)	0
Hendry [111]	2000	2 BEP	>3 MRC RF	60/60	1 (1.7%)	1 (1.7%)
Chevreau [29]	2004	2 BEP	VI+ and/or LI+ and or EC+	36/40	0	0
Amato [112]	2004	CEB	1 or more: AFP>80, >80% EC, VI or LI	68/76	1 (1.5%)	0
Maroto [28]	2005	2 BEP	VI and or EC	231/231	2 (0.9%)	0
Dearnaley [31]	2005	2 PVB	VI and /or LI or local invasion	115/115	2 (1.7%)	1 (0.9%)
Westermann [30]	2008	1 BEP	VI and/or LI and/or ECP	37/40	1 (2.7%)	1 (2.7%)
Albers [32]	2008	1 BEP	VI in 41.8% of patients	174/191	2 (1.1%)	0
Total				989/1043	16 (1.6%)	6 (0.6%)

BEP bleomycin, etoposide, cisplatin; *PVB* bleomycin, vincristine, cisplatin; *CEB* carboplatin, etoposide, bleomycin; *PVB* cisplatin, vinblastine, bleomycin; *RF* risk factors; *MRC* medical research council; *DOD* dead of disease

The first study evaluating the efficacy of 2 courses of bleomycin, etoposide and cisplatin (BEP) as adjuvant therapy following orchiectomy included 22 "high risk" patients reported by Oliver in 1992. [26] High risk was defined as the presence of two or more following pathologic features: vascular invasion (VI), lymphatic invasion, presence of undifferentiated cells and absence of yolk sac elements. At a median follow up of 2 years, 21 (95.5%) patients remain free of disease. The single patient that relapsed died of disease.

In a multicenter UK Medical Research Council study reported in 1996, 114 patients with at least 3 of 4 risk factors (VI, lymphatic invasion, presence of undifferentiated cells and absence of yolk sac elements) received 2 cycles of BEP. [27] At a median follow up of 4 years there have been 2 relapses. One patient relapsed at 7 months recurring in the retroperitoneum, liver, and chest and ultimately died of disease and the second patient relapsed at 18 months in the groin, the patient is alive though on review the primary tumor was thought to be rete adenocarcinoma. One patient died of a cerebrovascular accident during treatment.

Similar relapse rates were reported by the Spanish Germ Cell Group involving 231 high risk patients who received two courses of BEP. [28] Two patients (0.9%) relapsed and both are disease free after salvage therapy. Long-term follow extending 10 years has confirmed the low relapse-rates with adjuvant chemotherapy. [29, 30]

In an effort to decrease toxicity of therapy, The Medical Research Council reported a new regimen of adjuvant chemotherapy replacing etoposide with vincristine (BOP). [31] The 5-year disease free survival of 98.3% in the BOP arm was similar to that of BEP, though neurotoxicity was present in 12% at 2 years. The authors concluded no benefit of BOP over BEP.

Investigators have attempted to decrease the exposure to chemotherapy by treating patients with a single cycle of chemotherapy. The Swiss Group for Clinical Cancer Research reported outcomes of high risk stage 1 patients receiving a single course of BEP in the adjuvant setting. [30] Of the 45 patients, 35 showed no evidence of disease during a median follow up of 99 months. One patient developed pulmonary metastases after 13 months and died of pneumonia. Two patients developed contralateral testis cancer and two patients were free of disease at 10 and 31 months when lost to follow-up.

The German Testicular Cancer Study Group randomized 382 patients (42% with VI) to either RPLND or one cycle of BEP. [32] After a median follow up of 4.7 years, 2 recurrences were observed in the intention to treat population with chemotherapy. The 2-year disease free survival after one course of chemotherapy was 99.5%.

There is little doubt on the efficacy of adjuvant chemotherapy in managing CSA NSGCT and of the three treatment modalities it has the lowest relapse rate. As the other treatment modalities decrease the risk of requiring chemotherapy (especially primary RPLND) while maintaining similar cure rates, the primary concern with adjuvant chemotherapy in this young population is the potential serious late toxicity of systemic therapy. The Royal Marsden Hospital reported a 2-fold greater risk of developing cardiovascular disease in testis cancer patients treated with chemotherapy and radiation. [33] Others have reported that cured patients treated with cisplatin-based chemotherapy have significantly higher levels of blood pressure, a higher prevalence of hypertension, and an excessive weight gain compared with patients treated with other modalities and compared to controls. [34] A recent report evaluated the long-term toxicity of cisplatin-based chemotherapy in 1409 men at a median follow-up of 10.7 years. [35] All chemotherapy groups had statically higher odds of toxicity than men who did not receive chemotherapy and included: Raynaud-like phenomena in 39%, paresthesias in the hands or feet in 29%, hearing impairment in 21% and tinnitus in 22%.

Even in the risk assessment of the MRC, only 50% of the high-risk group will relapse. Although this is an improvement on the prediction without histopathologic criteria that 30%

will relapse, by definition one half of the patients treated with chemotherapy in this setting are already cured with orchiectomy. Three cycles of therapy represents standard of care for patients with disseminated, or relapsed disease, [36] and the data with surveillance has shown the same excellent cure rate in relapsing patients who are monitored closely. This means that with adjuvant chemotherapy 1) 50% of patients who are cured with orchiectomy alone will unnecessarily receive chemotherapy and, 2) 50% of patients who would be destined to relapse (if on surveillance) will be cured with two cycles of chemotherapy (instead of the three cycles that would be required at relapse). If a prognostic model that predicts a much higher relapse rate can be developed (lessening the percentage of pathologic stage A patients exposed to immediate therapy), then this strategy may need to be re-examined. To date, immediate chemotherapy in clinical stage A disease has not been readily adopted in the United States though is recommended by the European Consensus as the treatment of choice for high risk patients. [37]

Retroperitoneal Lymph Node Dissection

The rationale for RPLND in the management of clinical stage A NSGCT is easily described. Several benefits to the patient accrue from the performance of this procedure. First, because approximately 30% of patients with clinical stage A disease are pathologic stage B, there exists a benefit in immediate staging. Second, if the patient has retroperitoneal metastasis, surgical removal of such disease is curative in 50% to 90% of patients, depending on the volume of disease resected. [38-40] Hence, the procedure is not simply a staging procedure but is therapeutic in the majority of patients. A third benefit relates to the ease of follow-up. Because retroperitoneal recurrence is exceedingly rare with a properly performed procedure, follow-up examination after RPLND includes only chest x-ray, serum tumor marker evaluation, and physical examination. Because recurrence beyond 2 years of follow-up is rare, intensive follow-up in necessary for only 2 years. Fourth, patients managed by surveillance strategy are known to have significant problems with anxiety regarding recurrence in the follow-up period. By effectively staging and treating the testis cancer early in the course of management, such anxiety is understandably decreased. Fifth, RPLND decreases the overall risk of requiring systemic chemotherapy, a benefit which may have growing importance as data emerges regarding the long-term toxicity of chemotherapy. Sixth, with nerve-sparing RPLND and nearly universal preservation of antegrade emission, surgery arguably has the lowest impact on fertility. Finally, although late recurrence is a rare phenomenon in NSGCT, performance of RPLND early in the course of therapy likely decreases the chance of such late recurrence. [41] Based on these factors, RPLND remains an effective and reasonable method of management.

History and Template Modification

The traditional full bilateral suprahilar RPLND involved removal of all lymphatic tissue from the suprahilar areas to the bifurcation of the common iliac arteries, from ureter to ureter. This was, by intent, a radical procedure because chemotherapeutic rescue was not available when full bilateral RPLND was developed. All sympathetic efferent fibers were sacrificed and lymphatic tissue was removed en bloc. Therefore, these patients suffered from anejaculation post-operatively.

With the advent of CT scanning, it became apparent that the pathway of lymphatic channels from the abdomen to the chest was posterior through the crus of the diaphragm and not anterior to the suprahilar zones. In addition, it was noted that suprahilar metastasis was exceedingly uncommon in the situation of low-volume retroperitoneal metastasis. Therefore, the suprahilar aspect of the full bilateral RPLND was eliminated. Because no modification of template below the renal vessels occurred during the full bilateral dissection, anejaculation again was the rule post-operatively.

The next development in the evolution of RPLND involved the use of anatomic mapping studies to modify the surgical resection templates. These mapping studies were performed in patients undergoing full bilateral RPLND for both low- and moderate-volume retroperitoneal metastasis. These studies clearly showed that patients with minimal volume retroperitoneal disease characteristically had involvement of the retroperitoneum unilaterally. Specifically, patients with low-volume retroperitoneal tumor from a left sided primary characteristically had metastases localized to the upper left periaortic zone, and patients with low-volume disease from a right-sided primary were found to have metastases to the interaortocaval or precaval zones. These facts led investigators to modify the traditional full bilateral RPLND further and limit the dissection to the templates depicted in figs 1 and 2. With these templates, right and left sided dissection would remove lymphatic tissue at high risk of harboring metastatic disease but preserve other retroperitoneal lymphatic tissue at low risk for containing metastasis. The advantages of limiting the dissection in this group of patients were shorter operative times, and shorter postoperative ileus. Additionally, and most importantly, these templates saved some retroperitoneal efferent sympathetic fibers as the dissections were basically unilateral and these fibers exist bilaterally. Hence, modified dissection were capable of preserving emission and ejaculation in roughly 50% to 70% of the time.

The most recent modification in technique for RPLND for low-stage disease is the nerve-sparing dissection. This dissection was developed by experienced retroperitoneal surgeons who realized that efferent sympathetic fibers, though quite small, were able to be identified. In the nerve-sparing procedure these fibers are dissected prospectively after which the modified lymphadenectomy is performed (fig 3-6). The intent of the modified nerve-sparing dissection is to preserve the staging aspect of the procedure, preserve the therapeutic aspect of lymphadenectomy and to eliminate the major source of morbidity in traditional lymphadenectomy for low-stage disease, the loss of emission/ejaculation.

Efficacy of RPLND

Pathologic Stage A

RPLND remains the most accurate means of staging patients presenting with CS A NSGCT. Depending on risk classification roughly 50% to 70% will be pathologic stage A. Despite no evidence of lymphatic spread, approximately 10% pathologic Stage A patients will relapse with the cure rate approaching 100%. Indiana University reported on the outcome of 464 patients with clinical stage A NSGCT from 1965-1989 with a mean follow-up of 96.2

months. [42] In this analysis, 323 (70%) patients had pathologic stage A disease with 37 (11%) relapsing, with an overall survival of 99.4%. Though the overall relapse rate in PSA is 10%, patients with high risk features in the orchiectomy specimen (lymphovascular invasion and/or embryonal dominant histology) relapse at a rate of 20% to 25%. [43] Without high risk features the relapse rate is less than 5%. Relapses typically occur in the chest or serologically and treated with systemic chemotherapy.

Pathologic Stage B

Approximately 30% to 50% of CSA patients undergoing primary RPLND will harbor micrometastatic disease (PSB). Though the cure rate in this population is nearly 100%, the pathway to obtain this high rate of cure varies from patient to patient. Management of PSB disease after RPLND is either observation or 2 courses of adjuvant chemotherapy. In a randomized trial comparing adjuvant chemotherapy to close observation with chemotherapy reserved for those patients who relapse, there was no difference in the survival rates (95%) at a median follow up of 4 years. [44]

Relapse after primary RPLND in PSB disease is roughly 30%. These patients remain curable at relapse with 3 courses of standard cisplatin-based chemotherapy.

In the Indiana series of 464 patients with CS A disease undergoing primary RPLND from 1965 to 1989, pathologic stage B disease was identified in 112 (30%) patients. Of these, 64 did not receive adjuvant chemotherapy of whom 22 (34%) relapsed with one death. Memorial Sloan Kettering reported a 81% four-year progression free probability (PFP) for PB1 patients not receiving adjuvant chemotherapy. [45] Interestingly, the 4-year PFP prior to 1999 was 79% and increased to 90% after 1999 though this later cohort consisted of only 11 patients.

Low volume retroperitoneal lymphatic disease does not preclude surgery as a primary treatment modality in NSGCT, and the extent of nodal cancer, at least in the population with pB1 disease, does not appear to be predictive of outcome. In an effort to identify clinical and pathologic parameters predictive of relapse, Rabbani and Sheinfeld reported outcome in 45 patients with pB1 disease and were unable to detect variables predictive of relapse including vascular invasion in the primary tumor, and primary and retroperitoneal lymph node histology. [46] Richie et al. evaluated risk factors for relapse for 39 patients with B1 disease of whom 3 (8%) recurred. [40] Once again, pathologic features of the primary tumor including predominant embryonal histology, vascular invasion and T stage failed to predict relapse. Recently the results of RPLND in patients with high risk, clinical stage A disease treated at Indiana University were reviewed. [47] High risk was defined by the 2 criteria of embryonal predominance and vascular invasion in the orchiectomy specimen. Embryonal predominance was defined as embryonal carcinoma present at a level greater than any other histologic subtype in the orchiectomy specimen. The presence of each risk factor predicted pathologic stage B disease at the 46.5% level. Of patients with pathologic stage B disease who elected not to receive adjuvant chemotherapy only a third had recurrence after RPLND, indicating that two-thirds of these high risk patients were cured with retroperitoneal lymph node dissection only.

A series reported from Indiana University included 118 patients with PB1 disease not receiving adjuvant chemotherapy with a minimum follow up of 2 years. The 5 year disease free survival was 68% and neither the histology of the retroperitoneal nodes, number of nodes involved nor the presence of extra nodal extension predicted for relapse. [48-50] To date, no predictive variable has been identified to accurately stratify patients as high risk for relapse. These series clearly demonstrate that a properly performed RPLND is not simply a staging procedure but therapeutic curing 70% of patients with PB1 disease. The remaining third that relapse remain curable with systemic chemotherapy.

In an attempt to decrease this relapse rate some investigators recommend adjuvant chemotherapy. Eight studies involving 653 patients receiving adjuvant chemotherapy reported a relapse rate of 1.8% (table 4). While adjuvant therapy does virtually eliminate the risk of relapse for those 30% destined to relapse after RPLND it negates any therapeutic benefit of surgery subjecting the 70% of patients (otherwise cured with surgery) unnecessarily to chemotherapy.

Table 4. Adjuvant chemotherapy after primary RPLND in pathologic stage B NGCGT

Author	Number of patients	Chemotherapy (number of cycles)	Number of relapses	Median follow up (mos)
Vugrin [113]	42	VAB-6 (2)	1	24
Williams [44]	92	PVB (2)	1	48
Weissbach [114]	221	PVB (2-4)	7	43
Gerl [115]	85	PVB or BEP (2-4)	1	72
Kennedy [116]	37	PVB (4)	0	125
Culine [117]	44	VAB-6 or EP (4)	0	72
Behnia [51]	82	BEP (2)	1	85
Kondagunta [118]	87	EP (2)	1	96
Total	653		12 (1.8%)	

Important in the philosophy of treating low stage germ-cell cancer is the goal of achieving cure by a single treatment modality. As demonstrated in the studies referenced above, primary RPLND cures 50% to 70% of patients with pathologic stage B disease. Two courses of adjuvant chemotherapy administered to patients with pathologic stage B disease does eliminate the risk of recurrence but potentially adds to patient morbidity. [51, 52] If the rationale is to administer post operative chemotherapy in patients with pathologic B disease in order to avoid recurrence and not rely on surgery for cure, most testis cancer physicians feel that the surveillance is better suited. If this is the case, those patients on surveillance who do relapse would avoid surgery and still be cured with 3 courses chemotherapy.

Toxicity of RPLND

With the introduction of nerve sparing technique, the morbidity from retroperitoneal lymph node dissection is in essence that of a laparotomy. [53-55] A review of the experience at Indiana University showed that the only significant long-term morbidity is an approximate 1% chance of postoperative small bowel obstruction due to adhesions. [56] The same institution reviewed the last 75 primary retroperitoneal lymph node dissections. [57] In this population the mean operative time was 132 minutes, mean blood loss was 207 cc. Nasogastric tubes are not routinely used in either primary or post chemotherapy surgery, and in this series only 2 patients had NG tubes. The mean hospital stay was 2.8 days (range: 2-4).

Fertility

The major impetus behind the development of the surveillance strategy was the loss of emission or ejaculation after standard full bilateral RPLND. With the development of the nerve-sparing technique antegrade emission is preserved in 99% of patients; therefore, surgery itself should have no negative impact on fertility. [55, 58, 59] Furthermore, with decreasing the risk of receiving systemic chemotherapy, RPLND may have the lowest impact on fertility for stage A NSGCT compared to surveillance or immediate chemotherapy. Fertility rates for surveillance approach 65% though decreases to 20% for patients that relapse. [60] After primary RPLND fertility is observed in 75% of men. [53, 58]

Laparoscopic RPLND

The morbidity of open (O) RPLND has continued to decline over the last 30 years and nerve-sparing can preserve antegrade emission in nearly all patients. The impetus behind the introduction of laparoscopic (L) RPLND was to further decrease patient morbidity while maintaining similar oncologic efficacy to that of O-RPLND.

The decline in patient morbidity with L-RPLND is debatable with some series demonstrating a decline in hospital stay, blood loss and overall complication rates[61, 62] while others have shown a longer hospital stays, blood loss and operative time though attribute some of this is attritbuted to the "learning curve". [63, 64]

Before L-RPLND becomes widely accepted the therapeutic efficacy must be defined. One major concern physicians have with current L-RLPND is that often if metastatic disease is found in the retroperitoneal lymph nodes, the procedure is either aborted and adjuvant chemotherapy is administered or it is completed and adjuvant chemotherapy is administered. [63, 65]

Results of > 800 patients treated by L-RPLND reported in 34 articles was recently published. [66] Five publications with a follow-up of 63 months included 557 patients. 126 of 140 (90%) patients with positive nodes received adjuvant chemotherapy with relapse rate of 1.4%. Because adjuvant chemotherapy in this setting is so curative (with or without surgery), the oncologic efficacy of L-RPLND is unknown.

Follow-up

In PS A NSGCT, follow up includes physical exam, serum tumor marker evaluation, and chest x-ray every other month the first year and every 4 months the second year. It is rare for PS A patients to relapse beyond 2 years and further imaging studies can be dramatically reduced after this time period. Follow up in PB1 includes physical exam, serum tumor marker evaluation, and chest x-ray every month the first year, every 2 months the second year and slowly increasing the interval between visits over the next 3years. Neither group requires routine abdominal/pelvic CT imaging as it is rare to have a local relapse after RPLND. There is; however, no universally accepted guidelines for following these patients.

Special Considerations

Clinical Stage1s

A special subset of clinical stage A patients are those with persistently increased serum tumor markers that do not decrease at a rate consistent with their know half-lives after orchiectomy. By virtue of the increased markers, these patients are know to have persistent disease, unlike clinical stage A patients with negative markers who have only a 30% risk of having persistent disease. Although some would argue for RPLND in these patients, disease might not be confined to the retroperitoneum and a post-RPLND increased marker would then require chemotherapy. Even if the marker normalizes with RPLND, some would advocate two cycles of adjuvant chemotherapy. Thus, most investigators have concluded that primary chemotherapy for a persistent maker increase after orchiectomy represents the most reasonable treatment option for these patients. [67, 68]

Chemotherapy Resistant Histologies

Surveillance is a reasonable management option is stage A NSGCT because the disease at relapse remains chemosensitive and the cure rate is similar to RPLND. Unusual histologies including adenocarcinoma, primitive neuroectodermal tumor, and teratoma with malignant transformation may be present in the orchiectomy specimen. These histologies are chemo-resistant and thus if on surveillance these histologies are present at relapse salvage therapy (surgery or chemotherapy) is by in large ineffective. Thus, even if a component of these histologies is present in the primary tumor, most physicians would recommend primary RPLND en lieu to surveillance.

Clinical Stage B/C

Clinical stage B NSGCT includes patients with evidence of retroperitoneal metastases based on clinical staging (CT scan). Patients with serum TM normalization post orchiectomy with small volume (< 5 cm) retroperitoneal disease may be treated with either chemotherapy or primary RPLND. Clinical stage B patients with persistently elevated serum TM post orchiectomy and all stage C disease are treated with cisplatin-based chemotherapy.

Primary RPLND

The rationale to proceed with primary RPLND in clinical stage B NSGCT with normal serum TM is multifactorial. Not all retroperitoneal tumors (clincal stage B) represent metastatic disease and therefore would not respond to systemic chemotherapy. These patients would therefore require PC surgery due to this "persistent mass". Donohue reported on 174 clincal stage B patients undergoing primary RPLND form 1965 to 1989, 41 patients (23%) were in fact pathologic stage A. [69] Further more, patients with teratoma in the orchiectomy specimen may have teratoma in the retroperitoneum and more likely to have a persistent mass post chemotherapy and require RPLND. Therefore this subset may have a higher likelihood of dual therapy (chemotherapy and surgery) for cure. Alternatively, primary RPLND would irradiate retroperitoneal teratoma and potentially cure the patient while avoiding systemic therapy. If retroperitoneal pathology reveals active cancer (with or without teratoma), surgery remains curative in 50% to 70% of patients. Surgery should be a consideration for all patients presenting with clinical stage B disease with normal serum TM especially those with teratoma in the primary.

Chemotherapy

Systemic therapy for metastatic germ cell tumors consists of cisplatin-based chemotherapy. For good risk disease, the accepted standard is 3 courses of Bleomycin, Etoposide, and Cisplatin (BEP). [36, 70] Due to concerns of pulmonary toxicity, patients with a strong smoking history or older than 50 years of age can be alternatively managed with 4 courses of EP. Standard therapy for intermediate and poor risk disease remains 4 courses of BEP. Randomized trials evaluating high dose chemotherapy (HDCT) versus BEP x 4 in poor risk patients as initial therapy failed to show an improved outcome in the HDCT arm. [71]

Depending upon the patient population selected, roughly 70% of patients treated with first line chemotherapy will obtain a complete clinical response with normalization of serum tumor markers and complete resolution of all metastatic disease. The policy at Indiana University, in agreement with the European Germ Cell Cancer Consensus Group [72], is to observe these patients as only 3 to 5% will relapse. [73, 74] Patients not achieving a complete clinical response, with residual radiographic tumor and serum tumor marker normalization routinely undergo PC RPLND. Pathology of the residual mass at PC surgery consists of necrosis in 45%, teratoma in 45% and cancer in 10%.

Patients with tumors that relapse or with tumors that progress despite first line chemotherapy are candidates for salvage therapy. A minority of patients will have anatomically confined disease that is amenable to surgical resection. [75, 76] For the remaining majority of patients treatment options include salvage chemotherapy with cisplatin plus ifosfamide plus vinblastine, [77] or paclitaxel [78] for four courses or high-dose chemotherapy with autologous hematopoietic stem-cell transplantation to rescue the bone marrow from the myeloablative effect of chemotherapy. [79-81]

Management after a Complete Radiographic Response

At most centers, the management of patients achieving a complete radiographic response (CR) to systemic chemotherapy is observation. Historically, the rationale to this was 1) the low incidence of teratoma or active cancer at surgery [44], 2) the relapse rate in this population is 5% and 3) those patients that relapse remain curable.

Recent studies; however, have documented the incidence of microscopic teratoma to be 20 to 25%. [82, 83] As such, some centers have recommend PCRPLND for all patients. The question arises as to why the discrepancy between the pathologic finding of microscopic teratoma in 25% though a clinical relapse rate of 5%. Would the relapse rate increase with longer follow up (10 to 20 years) or in fact is microscopic teratoma by in large biologically inert?

Two recent large studies attempted to address this question. Nichols and others reported outcome of 161 patients with a CR to induction chemotherapy after a median follow up of 52 months. Ten patients relapsed (6%), nine in the retroperitoneum. All but 2 patients relapsed within 24 months. Eight of the 10 relapses were teratoma and rendered NED with delayed PC

RPLND. Two patients recurred with marker positive, viable cancer and rendered NED with chemotherapy alone (one patient) or chemotherapy plus surgery for residual teratoma. All 10 patients remain NED at a median follow up of 64 months. Indiana University reported relapse rates for 141 patients achieving a CR to first-line chemotherapy after a median follow up of 15.5 years. Six patients (4%) experienced recurrence in the retroperitoneum of whom 2 patients died of disease. Five patients had late relapse (range 3 to 13 years), including 2 patients in the retroperitoneum. All five patients are currently NED.

The data suggest that those 5% of patients that relapse on observation remain curable and there is no evidence that immediate PC surgery on all CR's would improve the overall survival on the 5% that will relapse nor that immediate surgery would prevent those relapses though does subject all patients to the morbidity of PC RPLND.

The current recommendations from The European and Canadian Testicular Cancer Consensus Conference and Indiana University is observation for patients achieving complete radiographic remission or minimal residual disease (< 1.0 cm). [37]

Post Chemotherapy RPLND for Residual Mass

The surgical resection of necrotic tissue after chemotherapy offers no therapeutic benefit to the patient. Therefore, post chemotherapy surgery with the finding of necrosis is a staging procedure alone. The recurrence rate in this population is less than 5% and typically most centers would not re-image the retroperitoneum and follow the patient only with physical exam, chest imaging and serum tumor markers. [84] Ideally patients with known residual fibrosis would be excluded from surgery though presently we are unable to accurately predict necrosis with the use of clinical parameters. The EORTC/MRC recently assessed the external validity of a prediction rule developed to predict the probability of retroperitoneal metastases being only necrosis after chemotherapy. [6] Patients with a high probability of necrosis might be offered surveillance as opposed to surgery. Criteria used to calculate the probability of benign histology included: the absence/presence of teratoma in the primary tumor, pre-chemotherapy serum tumor marker levels, and maximal transversal mass size measured on CT before and after chemotherapy. In the validation set, only 4% of residual masses were classified as benign and would have received surveillance en lieu of surgery. Though the prediction rule accurately identified benign histology, so few patients met the classification criteria that the clinical usefulness of this tool remains limited.

Surgical resection of residual cancer or teratoma is rational and well accepted as both entities may grow and metastasize and lead to significant patient morbidity and even death. Teratoma is not sensitive to chemotherapy and therefore surgical resection is the only therapeutic option. Recurrence rate for resected teratoma is 10 to 20% with a greater chance of local (retroperitoneal) recurrence the larger the volume of disease. [85-87] Donohue and Foster reported a 89% progression free survival for 273 patients harboring residual teratoma at surgery. [84] Stenning et al reported similar results in a cohort of 153 patients undergoing PCRPLND. [88] The 2-year progression free survival for resected mature and immature teratoma was 86% and 89%, respectively. With a median post chemotherapy mass size of 3.0 cm, Memorial Sloan Kettering reported disease free survival of 83% at 5-years for resected teratoma. [86] In this study, patients with residual mass size less than 2 cm, 2 to 5 cm and > 5 cm had 5-year probabilities of freedom from recurrence of 94%, 91% and 59%, respectively (p < 0.0005). Investigators from Indiana University recently reported recurrence rates after resection of large volume (> 10 cm) teratoma. [89] The 2 and 5-year recurrence free survival for the 99 patients was 86% and 75% with a mean follow up of 42 months.

Typically in the post chemotherapy setting after resecting residual teratoma most would recommend CT scans of the abdomen and pelvis periodically in addition to serial chest imaging, physical exam and serum tumor markers due to the risk of retroperitoneal recurrence of teratoma.

Active cancer is identified in 10% of patients after standard PC surgery with a reported relapse free rate of 70% for those who received adjuvant chemotherapy. [90, 91] Fizazi et al reported on 238 patients with viable residual disease after first-line chemotherapy. [92] The 5-year progression free survival was 64%. Three variables significant on multivariate analysis were used to risk stratify this population and included: incomplete surgery, viable malignant cells > 10%, and poor or intermediate IGCCC. Patients with no adverse factors experienced a 5-year progression free survival of 90% compared to 41% for 2 or more risk factors. This International Study Group further compared progression free survival and overall survival in patients receiving and not receiving adjuvant chemotherapy following PC RPLND. The 5-year relapse free rate for 166 patients receiving adjuvant chemotherapy was 69% compared to 52% for the 65 patients not receiving post operative chemotherapy (p < 0.001). On multivariate analysis post operative chemotherapy was associated with a significantly better progression free survival (p < 0.001), but overall survival was not improved (p = 0.26). While adjuvant chemotherapy does not improve overall survival it does decrease the risk of recurrence and thus avoiding the morbidity of second line chemotherapy (high dose therapy). It seems that the presence of viable NSGCT portends a poor prognosis and as such, it has been standard practice to give two courses of adjuvant chemotherapy in this population.

Extent of Surgery

Retroperitoneal mapping studies have accurately documented the predictable lymphatic spread of testicular cancer allowing for the use of more limited surgical templates in low volume metastatic disease. [93] In the surgical management of clinical stage A disease, surgical boundaries over the last 3 decades have been down-sized from a full bilateral suprahilar dissection to a unilateral nerve sparing template without compromising cure. [59] In the management of post chemotherapy masses, there has been no such consistent reduction in the retroperitoneal surgical boundaries with a full bilateral dissection considered standard therapy.

In the 1970's and 1980's lower stage metastatic disease was more often treated with surgery in an attempt to avoid additional courses of chemotherapy. With improvement of antiemetics, growth factors, and supportive care, the toxicity of cisplatin based chemotherapy has decreased. Subsequently a greater number of low stage patients have been treated with primary chemotherapy. Many patients from the 1970's and 1980's undergoing post chemotherapy surgery had high volume residual disease and the decision to perform a full bilateral RLND was therefore rational and appropriate. Since chemotherapy is now being administered for relatively low volume retroperitoneal disease, and since these tumors are typically restricted to the primary landing zone of the affected testicle, the question has arisen as to the appropriateness of full bilateral RPLND in this population. Concern of modified dissections; however, is the risk of unresected microscopic disease outside the template of dissection. In an unselected population undergoing full bilateral surgery the incidence of extra template disease was 7 to 32% and is highly dependent on patient selection and template boundaries. [94]

Proponents of modified dissections feel that with appropriate patient selection, the risk of extra-template disease and its clinical significance is low. In 1992, investigators from Memorial Sloan-Kettering published a series of 113 patients undergoing full bilateral PCRPLND, with an 8% incidence of disease (cancer/teratoma) identified in the contralateral landing zone. [95] This cohort all presented with "bulky disease" and treated with cisplatin or carboplatin-based chemotherapy protocols. This group concluded that a modified dissection should be considered in patients with 1) no palpable residual tumor mass, 2) left primary tumors, and 3) right primary tumors that have no evidence of cancer/teratoma on frozen section analysis of the residual mass. Fossa et al. reported the results of 87 patients undergoing modified post chemotherapy RPLND in a group of patients with residual masses less than 20 mm. [83] Pathology revealed necrosis in 67%, teratoma in 26%, and cancer in 7%. Five relapses occurred in this study with no in field recurrences, indicating that the template of dissection was adequate. Indiana University recently reported outcomes of 100 patients undergoing a modified post chemotherapy dissection. [96] The selection criteria included low-volume retroperitoneal disease (< 5 cm), both pre- and post chemotherapy, restricted to the primary landing zone of the affected testicle. Pathology revealed cancer in 2%, teratoma in 62% and necrosis in 36%. Three patients relapsed all outside the boundaries of a full bilateral dissection and the 2-year progression free survival of 95%. Others have also demonstrated the safety of a modified PCRPLND in select patients. [97, 98]

The advantages of a modified dissection in the post chemotherapy setting are the same as those at primary RPLND, mainly preservation of the contralateral efferent sympathetic fibers to maintain antegrade seminal emission. It appears that a modified dissection is rational is select patients with small volume disease limited to the primary landing zone after chemotherapy.

Complicated Post Chemotherapy Surgery

The term "complicated" RPLND applies to patients who have received more than induction chemotherapy only (salvage), have experienced a retroperitoneal recurrence after initial RPLND (redo), or have progression of disease during or immediately after chemotherapy (desperation). In this group there is a higher incidence of nephrectomy, aortic replacement and caval resection. This aggressive approach is justified as ensuring a complete resection with additional procedures provides a therapeutic benefit.

Donohue et al analyzed 860 patients who underwent PCRPLND . [90] Relapse rates for patients with any one of the complicated factors mentioned above was 45% compared to 12% for patients without these factors. In the salvage population, the incidence of active cancer was 50% with an overall survival of 50% to 60% with no apparent benefit from adjuvant chemotherapy. In this same review, Donohue analyzed the effect of "redo" RPLND on patient outcome. That is, the significance of incomplete resection at initial surgery. An overall survival of 63% was observed in 188 patients undergoing redo RPLND versus 86% for 613 patients undergoing primary PCRPLND. Likewise, in a contemporary series, Memorial Sloan-Kettering reported a 67% 5-year disease specific survival for 57 patients undergoing redo surgery. [99] Redo RPLND, probably the only prognostic variable not absolutely dictated by the biological aggressiveness of the disease, largely reflects prior inadequate retroperitoneal technique, underscoring the importance of complete surgical resection at initial RPLND.

Persistent serum tumor marker elevation after chemotherapy has historically been considered a relative contraindication to surgery due to supposed systemic disease and low chance of cure with local therapy alone. These patients have typically been treated with subsequent salvage chemotherapy. Over the last 15 years, however, several centers have experienced surgical cures in this population. [75, 76, 100, 101] Approximately 50% of patients undergoing post chemotherapy surgery with elevated serum tumor markers are alive at 5-years. Half these patients are found to harbor viable non-teratomatous germ cell tumor with a third alive at 5-years with no observed benefit from adjuvant chemotherapy. These studies demonstrate that a subset of patients with elevated serum tumor markers after chemotherapy are curable with surgery. The decision to proceed with surgery en lieu of second or third line chemotherapy includes identifying both patients felt unlikely to obtain a complete response with systemic therapy (and thus require surgery), and patients with resectable tumors that are potentially curable with surgery.

Late Relapse

Late relapse of testis cancer is defined as recurrence of disease later than 2 years after initial successful treatment. This entity is very important because it behaves differently compared with *de novo* testis cancer. [41, 102] Late relapse disease is predominately a surgical disease as late relapse tumors are not likely to be cured with chemotherapy alone. In a pooled analysis of 5880 patients with testis cancer revealed late relapse in 119 of 3704 (3.2%) and in 31 of 2176 (1.4%) patients with non-seminoma and seminoma, respectively. The retroperitoneum space is the predominant site of relapse followed by the lung.

Teratoma is the most common histology followed by yolk sac tumor. Though yolk sac tumor at late relapse histologically appears similar to *de novo* yolk sac tumor, it is not chemosensitive, and therefore, late relapse is treated surgically. Because yolk sac elements are common at relapse, an elevated alpha feto protein is sometimes the initiating event that provokes a radiographic evaluation. Around 40% to 50% of patients with late relapse are cured, and the vast majority are cured surgically because the lack of chemosensitive late relapse.

Management of Extra Retroperitoneal Disease

Of patients presenting with supradiaphragmatic disease, approximately 10% will undergo pulmonary resection for residual disease after platinum based chemotherapy. Hematogenous spread from the testicle to the lung occurs directly from the testicle or indirectly through lymphatic spread into the thoracic duct, draining into the subclavian vein and then to the lung.

Predictors of Pulmonary Pathology

Selection of patients for pulmonary resection typically includes patients with residual lung nodules and normal serum tumor markers after chemotherapy. Resection of residual teratoma or active cancer can be therapeutic and therefore the morbidity of thoracotomy is justified. Conversely, resection of residual necrosis is a staging procedure only. Efforts have been made to predict pulmonary histology based on retroperitoneal pathology, testicular pathology and serum tumor levels in an attempt to avoid the morbidity of thoracotomy in patients predictived to harbor necrosis only.

Excluding series with less than 100 patients, there are only 2 retrospective studies identifying variables predictive of pulmonary histology. Tognini et al reviewed 143 post chemotherapy patients who underwent resection of residual retroperitoneal and chest disease under the same anesthetic. [103] Concordance existed in 77.5% of patients with necrosis, 70% with teratoma, and 69% with cancer of the abdomen. Categorizing patients as uncomplicated (first line chemotherapy, normalization of serum tumor markers and no previous RPLND) revealed a concordance of 86% for patients with necrosis in the retroperitoneum and in the chest.

An international, multicenter, retrospective review evaluated the concordance of retroperitoneal and pulmonary histology in 215 patients. [104] The pulmonary mass histology was necrosis in 116 (54%), mature teratoma in 70 (33%), and cancer in 29 (13%). The strongest predictor of pulmonary histology was the histology found at RPLND. If RPLND histology revealed necrosis, the probability of necrosis at thoracotomy was 89%. When the RPLND histology was necrosis and the primary tumor was teratoma negative, the predictive probability of necrosis at thoracotomy was as high as 93%. For patients with a teratoma positive tumor, the probability was slightly lower at 87%.

With the above data as well as other studies, a cogent argument can be made to observe pulmonary nodules in order to avoid the morbidity of thoracotomy in a subgroup of patients. In subgroups with necrosis in the retroperitoneum, observation of pulmonary nodules would spare more than 90% of patients from surgery. Arguably, with observation strategies with chest imaging every 2 months for the first year and every 4 months for the second year, the small portion of patients with residual teratoma (5%) or active cancer (1% to 4%) will be identified and treated early with no detriment in cancer survival. Proponents of surgery state the risk of growing teratoma syndrome or malignant transformation for residual teratoma and the risk of disease progression in the small population with active cancer. There is no data comparing immediate resection of residual pulmonary nodules/masses versus delayed resection upon progression. Decision-making with regard to residual mass resection must take into account technical feasibility, patient morbidity and potential benefit, access to heath care, and patient preference.

Residual post chemotherapy mediastinal or neck masses are typically removed either at time of RPLND or at staged procedure. Approximately 70% of resected liver lesions are necrosis and the histologic concordance between retroperitoneal histology and liver histology was 94.4% for necrosis, 25.9% for teratoma and 38.5% for active cancer. [105] Observation of liver metastases should be considered when retroperitoneal histology reveals necrosis or when the volume and/or location of the hepatic involvement necessitates a significant surgical undertaking. If on follow up, the mass enlarges then surgery or second-line chemotherapy should be considered. Brain metastasis is rare (1%) and Cisplatin-based chemotherapy is recommended as initial therapy in patients with brain metastases at initial presentation. Balmaceda et al reported a 57% complete response rate in 68 patients with brain involvement with chemotherapy alone. [106] Surgical resection should be considered for residual disease. Radiotherapy does not appear to influence survival in this select population.

References

[1]   Teilum G. Endodermal sinus tumors of the ovary and testis. Comparative morphogenesis of the so-called mesoephroma ovarii (Schiller) and extraembryonic (yolk sac-allantoic) structures of the rat's placenta. *Cancer* 1959;12:1092-105.

[2]   Pierce GB, Bullock WK, Huntington RW, Jr. Yolk sac tumors of the testis. *Cancer* 1970;25(3):644-58.

[3]   Mosharafa AA, Foster RS, Leibovich BC, et al. Histology in mixed germ cell tumors. Is there a favorite pairing? *J Urol* 2004;171(4):1471-3.

[4]   Freedman LS, Parkinson MC, Jones WG, et al. Histopathology in the prediction of relapse of patients with stage I testicular teratoma treated by orchidectomy alone. *Lancet* 1987;2(8554):294-8.

[5]   Read G, Stenning SP, Cullen MH, et al. Medical Research Council prospective study of surveillance for stage I testicular teratoma. Medical Research Council Testicular Tumors Working Party. *J Clin Oncol* 1992;10(11):1762-8.

[6]   Vergouwe Y, Steyerberg EW, de Wit R, et al. External validity of a prediction rule for residual mass histology in testicular cancer: an evaluation for good prognosis patients. *Br J Cancer* 2003;88(6):843-7.

[7]   Bradey N, Johnson RJ, Read G. Abdominal computed tomography in teratoma of the testis: its accuracy in stage I disease and an assessment of the distribution of retroperitoneal lymph-node metastases in other stages of the disease. *Br J Radiol* 1987;60(713):487-91.

[8]   Rowland RG, Weisman D, Williams SD, Einhorn LH, Klatte EC, Donohue JP. Accuracy of preoperative staging in stages A and B nonseminomatous germ cell testis tumors. *J Urol* 1982;127(4):718-20.

[9]   Tesoro-Tess JD, Pizzocaro G, Zanoni F, Musumeci R. Lymphangiography and computerized tomography in testicular carcinoma: how accurate in early stage disease? *J Urol* 1985;133(6):967-70.

[10]   Divrik RT, Akdogan B, Ozen H, Zorlu F. Outcomes of surveillance protocol of clinical stage I nonseminomatous germ cell tumors-is shift to risk adapted policy justified? *J Urol* 2006;176(4 Pt 1):1424-29; discussion 9-30.

[11]   Sturgeon JF, Jewett MA, Alison RE, et al. Surveillance after orchidectomy for patients with clinical stage I nonseminomatous testis tumors. *J Clin Oncol* 1992;10(4):564-8.

[12]   Albers P. Management of stage I testis cancer. *Eur Urol* 2007;51(1):34-43; discussion - 4.

[13]   Groll RJ, Warde P, Jewett MA. A comprehensive systematic review of testicular germ cell tumor surveillance. *Crit Rev Oncol Hematol* 2007;64(3):182-97.

[14]   Kollmannsberger C, Moore C, Chi KN, et al. Non-risk-adapted surveillance for patients with stage I nonseminomatous testicular germ-cell tumors: diminishing treatment-related morbidity while maintaining efficacy. *Ann Oncol* 2009.

[15]   Oliver RT, Ong J, Shamash J, et al. Long-term follow-up of Anglian Germ Cell Cancer Group surveillance versus patients with Stage 1 nonseminoma treated with adjuvant chemotherapy. *Urology* 2004;63(3):556-61.

[16] Colls BM, Harvey VJ, Skelton L, et al. Late results of surveillance of clinical stage I nonseminoma germ cell testicular tumours: 17 years' experience in a national study in New Zealand. *BJU Int* 1999;83(1):76-82.

[17] Daugaard G, Petersen PM, Rorth M. Surveillance in stage I testicular cancer. *Apmis* 2003;111(1):76-83; discussion -5.

[18] Nicolai N, Pizzocaro G. A surveillance study of clinical stage I nonseminomatous germ cell tumors of the testis: 10-year followup. *J Urol* 1995;154(3):1045-9.

[19] Rorth M, Jacobsen GK, von der Maase H, et al. Surveillance alone versus radiotherapy after orchiectomy for clinical stage I nonseminomatous testicular cancer. Danish Testicular Cancer Study Group. *J Clin Oncol* 1991;9(9):1543-8.

[20] Rustin GJ, Mead GM, Stenning SP, et al. Randomized trial of two or five computed tomography scans in the surveillance of patients with stage I nonseminomatous germ cell tumors of the testis: Medical Research Council Trial TE08, ISRCTN56475197--the National Cancer Research Institute Testis Cancer Clinical Studies Group. *J Clin Oncol* 2007;25(11):1310-5.

[21] Kakiashvili DM, Zuniga A, Jewett MA. High risk NSGCT: case for surveillance. *World J Urol* 2009;27(4):441-7.

[22] Gels ME, Hoekstra HJ, Sleijfer DT, et al. Detection of recurrence in patients with clinical stage I nonseminomatous testicular germ cell tumors and consequences for further follow-up: a single-center 10-year experience. *J Clin Oncol* 1995;13(5):1188-94.

[23] Kakehi Y, Kamoto T, Kawakita M, Ogawa O. Follow-up of clinical stage I testicular cancer patients: cost and risk benefit considerations. *Int J Urol* 2002;9(3):154-60; discussion 60-1.

[24] Raghavan D, Colls B, Levi J, et al. Surveillance for stage I non-seminomatous germ cell tumours of the testis: the optimal protocol has not yet been defined. *Br J Urol* 1988;61(6):522-6.

[25] Meinke AH, 3rd, Estes NC, Ernst CB. Chylous ascites following abdominal aortic aneurysmectomy. Management with total parenteral hyperalimentation. *Ann Surg* 1979;190(5):631-3.

[26] Oliver RT, Raja MA, Ong J, Gallagher CJ. Pilot study to evaluate impact of a policy of adjuvant chemotherapy for high risk stage 1 malignant teratoma on overall relapse rate of stage 1 cancer patients. *J Urol* 1992;148(5):1453-5; discussion 5-6.

[27] Cullen MH, Stenning SP, Parkinson MC, et al. Short-course adjuvant chemotherapy in high-risk stage I nonseminomatous germ cell tumors of the testis: a Medical Research Council report. *J Clin Oncol* 1996;14(4):1106-13.

[28] Maroto P, Garcia del Muro X, Aparicio J, et al. Multicentre risk-adapted management for stage I non-seminomatous germ cell tumours. *Ann Oncol* 2005;16(12):1915-20.

[29] Chevreau C, Mazerolles C, Soulie M, et al. Long-term efficacy of two cycles of BEP regimen in high-risk stage I nonseminomatous testicular germ cell tumors with embryonal carcinoma and/or vascular invasion. *Eur Urol* 2004;46(2):209-14; discussion 14-5.

[30] Westermann DH, Schefer H, Thalmann GN, Karamitopoulou-Diamantis E, Fey MF, Studer UE. Long-term followup results of 1 cycle of adjuvant bleomycin, etoposide and cisplatin chemotherapy for high risk clinical stage I nonseminomatous germ cell tumors of the testis. *J Urol* 2008;179(1):163-6.

[31] Dearnaley DP, Fossa SD, Kaye SB, et al. Adjuvant bleomycin, vincristine and cisplatin (BOP) for high-risk stage I non-seminomatous germ cell tumours: a prospective trial (MRC TE17). *Br J Cancer* 2005;92(12):2107-13.

[32] Albers P, Siener R, Krege S, et al. Randomized phase III trial comparing retroperitoneal lymph node dissection with one course of bleomycin and etoposide plus cisplatin chemotherapy in the adjuvant treatment of clinical stage I Nonseminomatous testicular germ cell tumors: AUO trial AH 01/94 by the German Testicular Cancer Study Group. *J Clin Oncol* 2008;26(18):2966-72.

[33] Huddart RA, Norman A, Shahidi M, et al. Cardiovascular disease as a long-term complication of treatment for testicular cancer. *J Clin Oncol* 2003;21(8):1513-23.

[34] Sagstuen H, Aass N, Fossa SD, et al. Blood pressure and body mass index in long-term survivors of testicular cancer. *J Clin Oncol* 2005;23(22):4980-90.

[35] Brydoy M, Oldenburg J, Klepp O, et al. Observational study of prevalence of long-term Raynaud-like phenomena and neurological side effects in testicular cancer survivors. *J Natl Cancer Inst* 2009;101(24):1682-95.

[36] Einhorn LH, Williams SD, Loehrer PJ, et al. Evaluation of optimal duration of chemotherapy in favorable-prognosis disseminated germ cell tumors: a Southeastern Cancer Study Group protocol. *J Clin Oncol* 1989;7(3):387-91.

[37] Krege S, Beyer J, Souchon R, et al. European consensus conference on diagnosis and treatment of germ cell cancer: a report of the second meeting of the European Germ Cell Cancer Consensus group (EGCCCG): part I. *Eur Urol* 2008;53(3):478-96.

[38] Donohue JP, Thornhill JA, Foster RS, Rowland RG, Bihrle R. Primary retroperitoneal lymph node dissection in clinical stage A non-seminomatous germ cell testis cancer. Review of the Indiana University experience 1965-1989. *Br J Urol* 1993;71(3):326-35.

[39] Donohue JP, Thornhill JA, Foster RS, Rowland RG, Bihrle R. Clinical stage B non-seminomatous germ cell testis cancer: the Indiana University experience (1965-1989) using routine primary retroperitoneal lymph node dissection. *Eur J Cancer* 1995;31A(10):1599-604.

[40] Richie JP, Kantoff PW. Is adjuvant chemotherapy necessary for patients with stage B1 testicular cancer? *J Clin Oncol* 1991;9(8):1393-6.

[41] Baniel J, Foster RS, Gonin R, Messemer JE, Donohue JP, Einhorn LH. Late relapse of testicular cancer. *J Clin Oncol* 1995;13(5):1170-6.

[42] Donohue JP, Thornhill JA, Foster RS, Rowland RG, Bihrle R. Retroperitoneal lymphadenectomy for clinical stage A testis cancer (1965 to 1989): modifications of technique and impact on ejaculation. *J Urol* 1993;149(2):237-43.

[43] Hermans BP, Sweeney CJ, Foster RS, Einhorn LE, Donohue JP. Risk of systemic metastases in clinical stage I nonseminoma germ cell testis tumor managed by retroperitoneal lymph node dissection. *J Urol* 2000;163(6):1721-4.

[44] Williams SD, Stablein DM, Einhorn LH, et al. Immediate adjuvant chemotherapy versus observation with treatment at relapse in pathological stage II testicular cancer. *N Engl J Med* 1987;317(23):1433-8.

[45] Stephenson AJ, Bosl GJ, Motzer RJ, et al. Retroperitoneal lymph node dissection for nonseminomatous germ cell testicular cancer: impact of patient selection factors on outcome. *J Clin Oncol* 2005;23(12):2781-8.

[46] Rabbani F, Sheinfeld J, Farivar-Mohseni H, et al. Low-volume nodal metastases detected at retroperitoneal lymphadenectomy for testicular cancer: pattern and prognostic factors for relapse. *J Clin Oncol* 2001;19(7):2020-5.

[47] Sweeney CJ, Hermans BP, Heilman DK, Foster RS, Donohue JP, Einhorn LH. Results and outcome of retroperitoneal lymph node dissection for clinical stage I embryonal carcinoma--predominant testis cancer. *J Clin Oncol* 2000;18(2):358-62.

[48] Beck SD, Cheng L, Bihrle R, Donohue JP, Foster RS. Does the presence of extranodal extension in pathological stage B1 nonseminomatous germ cell tumor necessitate adjuvant chemotherapy? *J Urol* 2007;177(3):944-6.

[49] Beck SD, Foster RS, Bihrle R, Cheng L, Donohue JP. Does the histology of nodal metastasis predict systemic relapse after retroperitoneal lymph node dissection in pathological stage B1 germ cell tumors? *J Urol* 2005;174(4 Pt 1):1287-90; discussion 90.

[50] Beck SD, Foster RS, Bihrle R, Cheng L, Ulbright TM, Donohue JP. Impact of the number of positive lymph nodes on disease-free survival in patients with pathological stage B1 nonseminomatous germ cell tumor. *J Urol* 2005;174(1):143-5.

[51] Behnia M, Foster R, Einhorn LH, Donohue J, Nichols CR. Adjuvant bleomycin, etoposide and cisplatin in pathological stage II non-seminomatous testicular cancer. the Indiana University experience. *Eur J Cancer* 2000;36(4):472-5.

[52] Motzer RJ, Sheinfeld J, Mazumdar M, et al. Etoposide and cisplatin adjuvant therapy for patients with pathologic stage II germ cell tumors. *J Clin Oncol* 1995;13(11):2700-4.

[53] Foster RS, McNulty A, Rubin LR, et al. Fertility considerations in nerve-sparing retroperitoneal lymph-node dissection. *World J Urol* 1994;12(3):136-8.

[54] Heidenreich A, Albers P, Hartmann M, et al. Complications of primary nerve sparing retroperitoneal lymph node dissection for clinical stage I nonseminomatous germ cell tumors of the testis: experience of the German Testicular Cancer Study Group. *J Urol* 2003;169(5):1710-4.

[55] Jewett MA. Nerve-sparing technique for retroperitoneal lymphadenectomy in testis cancer. *Urol Clin North Am* 1990;17(2):449-56.

[56] Baniel J, Foster RS, Rowland RG, Bihrle R, Donohue JP. Complications of primary retroperitoneal lymph node dissection. *J Urol* 1994;152(2 Pt 1):424-7.

[57] Beck SDW, Peterson MD, Foster RS, Bihrle R, Donohue JP. What is the short-term morbidity of primary retroperitoneal lymph node dissection in a contemporary group of patients? *American Urologic Association* 2006(Abstract): .

[58] Beck SD, Bey AL, Bihrle R, Foster RS. Ejaculatory status and fertility rates after primary retroperitoneal lymph node dissection. *J Urol* 2010;184(5):2078-80.

[59] Foster RS, Donohue JP, Bihrle R. Stage A nonseminomatous testis carcinoma: rationale and results of nerve-sparing retroperitoneal lymphadenectomy. *Urol Int* 1991;46(3):294-7.

[60] Herr HW, Bar-Chama N, O'Sullivan M, Sogani PC. Paternity in men with stage I testis tumors on surveillance. *J Clin Oncol* 1998;16(2):733-4.

[61] Abdel-Aziz KF, Anderson JK, Svatek R, Margulis V, Sagalowsky AI, Cadeddu JA. Laparoscopic and open retroperitoneal lymph-node dissection for clinical stage I nonseminomatous germ-cell testis tumors. *J Endourol* 2006;20(9):627-31.

[62] Janetschek G, Hobisch A, Holtl L, Bartsch G. Retroperitoneal lymphadenectomy for clinical stage I nonseminomatous testicular tumor: laparoscopy versus open surgery and impact of learning curve. *J Urol* 1996;156(1):89-93; discussion 4.

[63] Albqami N, Janetschek G. Laparoscopic retroperitoneal lymph-node dissection in the management of clinical stage I and II testicular cancer. *J Endourol* 2005;19(6):683-92; discussion 92.

[64] Kenney PA, Tuerk IA. Complications of laparoscopic retroperitoneal lymph node dissection in testicular cancer. *World J Urol* 2008;26(6):561-9.

[65] Cresswell J, Scheitlin W, Gozen A, Lenz E, Teber D, Rassweiler J. Laparoscopic retroperitoneal lymph node dissection combined with adjuvant chemotherapy for pathological stage II disease in nonseminomatous germ cell tumours: a 15-year experience. *BJU Int* 2008;102(7):844-8.

[66] Rassweiler JJ, Scheitlin W, Heidenreich A, Laguna MP, Janetschek G. Laparoscopic retroperitoneal lymph node dissection: does it still have a role in the management of clinical stage I nonseminomatous testis cancer? A European perspective. *Eur Urol* 2008;54(5):1004-15.

[67] Davis BE, Herr HW, Fair WR, Bosl GJ. The management of patients with nonseminomatous germ cell tumors of the testis with serologic disease only after orchiectomy. *J Urol* 1994;152(1):111-3; discussion 4.

[68] Saxman SB, Nichols CR, Foster RS, et al. The management of patients with clinical stage I nonseminomatous testicular tumors and persistently elevated serologic markers. *J Urol* 1996;155(2):587-9.

[69] Donohue JP, Thornhill JA, Foster RS, Rowland RG, Bihrle R. Clinical stage B nonseminomatous germ cell testis cancer: the Indiana University experience (1965-1989) using routine primary retroperitoneal lymph node dissection. *Eur J Cancer* 1995;31A(10):1599-604.

[70] Culine S, Kerbrat P, Kramar A, et al. Refining the optimal chemotherapy regimen for good-risk metastatic nonseminomatous germ-cell tumors: a randomized trial of the Genito-Urinary Group of the French Federation of Cancer Centers (GETUG T93BP). *Ann Oncol* 2007;18(5):917-24.

[71] Motzer RJ, Nichols CJ, Margolin KA, et al. Phase III randomized trial of conventional-dose chemotherapy with or without high-dose chemotherapy and autologous hematopoietic stem-cell rescue as first-line treatment for patients with poor-prognosis metastatic germ cell tumors. *J Clin Oncol* 2007;25(3):247-56.

[72] Krege S, Beyer J, Souchon R, et al. European consensus conference on diagnosis and treatment of germ cell cancer: a report of the second meeting of the European Germ Cell Cancer Consensus Group (EGCCCG): part II. *Eur Urol* 2008;53(3):497-513.

[73] Ehrlich Y, Brames MJ, Beck SD, Foster RS, Einhorn LH. Long-Term Follow-Up of Cisplatin Combination Chemotherapy in Patients With Disseminated Nonseminomatous Germ Cell Tumors: Is a Postchemotherapy Retroperitoneal Lymph Node Dissection Needed After Complete Remission? *J Clin Oncol* 2009.

[74] Debono DJ, Heilman DK, Einhorn LH, Donohue JP. Decision analysis for avoiding postchemotherapy surgery in patients with disseminated nonseminomatous germ cell tumors. *J Clin Oncol* 1997;15(4):1455-64.

[75] Beck SD, Foster RS, Bihrle R, Einhorn LH, Donohue JP. Outcome analysis for patients with elevated serum tumor markers at postchemotherapy retroperitoneal lymph node dissection. *J Clin Oncol* 2005;23(25):6149-56.

[76] Murphy BR, Breeden ES, Donohue JP, et al. Surgical salvage of chemorefractory germ cell tumors. *J Clin Oncol* 1993;11(2):324-9.

[77] Loehrer PJ, Sr., Gonin R, Nichols CR, Weathers T, Einhorn LH. Vinblastine plus ifosfamide plus cisplatin as initial salvage therapy in recurrent germ cell tumor. *J Clin Oncol* 1998;16(7):2500-4.

[78] Motzer RJ, Sheinfeld J, Mazumdar M, et al. Paclitaxel, ifosfamide, and cisplatin second-line therapy for patients with relapsed testicular germ cell cancer. *J Clin Oncol* 2000;18(12):2413-8.

[79] Einhorn LH, Williams SD, Chamness A, Brames MJ, Perkins SM, Abonour R. High-dose chemotherapy and stem-cell rescue for metastatic germ-cell tumors. *N Engl J Med* 2007;357(4):340-8.

[80] Motzer RJ, Mazumdar M, Sheinfeld J, et al. Sequential dose-intensive paclitaxel, ifosfamide, carboplatin, and etoposide salvage therapy for germ cell tumor patients. *J Clin Oncol* 2000;18(6):1173-80.

[81] Rick O, Beyer J, Kingreen D, et al. High-dose chemotherapy in germ cell tumours: a large single centre experience. *Eur J Cancer* 1998;34(12):1883-8.

[82] Karellas M, Carver BS, Stasi J, Motzer RJ, Bosl GJ, Sheinfeld J. Clinical outcome following post-chemotherapy retroperitoneal lymph node dissection for the with CII non-seminomatous germ cell tumors and a radiographically normal retroperitoneum. *J Urol* 2007;177(4):277.

[83] Oldenburg J, Alfsen GC, Lien HH, Aass N, Waehre H, Fossa SD. Postchemotherapy retroperitoneal surgery remains necessary in patients with nonseminomatous testicular cancer and minimal residual tumor masses. *J Clin Oncol* 2003;21(17):3310-7.

[84] Donohue JP, Foster RS. Management of retroperitoneal recurrences: Seminoma and Nonseminoma. In: *Urologic Clinics of North America*; 1994:761-72.

[85] Loehrer PJ, Sr., Hui S, Clark S, et al. Teratoma following cisplatin-based combination chemotherapy for nonseminomatous germ cell tumors: a clinicopathological correlation. *J Urol* 1986;135(6):1183-9.

[86] Carver BS, Shayegan B, Serio A, Motzer RJ, Bosl GJ, Sheinfeld J. Long-term clinical outcome after postchemotherapy retroperitoneal lymph node dissection in men with residual teratoma. *J Clin Oncol* 2007;25(9):1033-7.

[87] Svatek RS, Spiess PE, Sundi D, et al. Long-term outcome for men with teratoma found at postchemotherapy retroperitoneal lymph node dissection. *Cancer* 2009;115(6):1310-7.

[88] Stenning SP, Parkinson MC, Fisher C, et al. Postchemotherapy residual masses in germ cell tumor patients: content, clinical features, and prognosis. Medical Research Council Testicular Tumour Working Party. *Cancer* 1998;83(7):1409-19.

[89] Beck SDW, Foster RS, Bihrle R, Donohue JP, Einhorn LH. Long term outcomes for patients with high volume retroperitoneal teratoma undergoing post chemotherpay surgery. *Journal of Urology*, Abstract 2007;177:331.

[90] Donohue JP, Leviovitch I, Foster RS, Baniel J, Tognoni P. Integration of surgery and systemic therapy: results and principles of integration. *Semin Urol Oncol* 1998;16(2):65-71.

[91] Spiess PE, Tannir NM, Tu SM, et al. Viable germ cell tumor at postchemotherapy retroperitoneal lymph node dissection: can we predict patients at risk of disease progression? *Cancer* 2007;110(12):2700-8.

[92] Fizazi K, Tjulandin S, Salvioni R, et al. Viable malignant cells after primary chemotherapy for disseminated nonseminomatous germ cell tumors: prognostic factors and role of postsurgery chemotherapy--results from an international study group. *J Clin Oncol* 2001;19(10):2647-57.

[93] Donohue JP, Zachary JM, Maynard BR. Distribution of nodal metastases in nonseminomatous testis cancer. *J Urol* 1982;128(2):315-20.

[94] Carver BS, Shayegan B, Eggener S, et al. Incidence of metastatic nonseminomatous germ cell tumor outside the boundaries of a modified postchemotherapy retroperitoneal lymph node dissection. *J Clin Oncol* 2007;25(28):4365-9.

[95] Wood DP, Jr., Herr HW, Heller G, et al. Distribution of retroperitoneal metastases after chemotherapy in patients with nonseminomatous germ cell tumors. *J Urol* 1992;148(6):1812-5; discussion 5-6.

[96] Beck SDW, Foster RS, Bihrle R, Donohue JP. Is full bilateral retroperitoneal lymph node dissection always necessary for post chemotherapy resdual tumor? *AUA,* San Antonia Texas 2005;Abstract.

[97] Ehrlich Y, Yossepowitch O, Kedar D, Baniel J. Distribution of nodal metastases after chemotherapy in nonseminomatous testis cancer: a possible indication for limited dissection. *BJU Int* 2006;97(6):1221-4.

[98] Rabbani F, Goldenberg SL, Gleave ME, Paterson RF, Murray N, Sullivan LD. Retroperitoneal lymphadenectomy for post-chemotherapy residual masses: is a modified dissection and resection of residual masses sufficient? *Br J Urol* 1998;81(2):295-300.

[99] McKiernan JM, Motzer RJ, Bajorin DF, Bacik J, Bosl GJ, Sheinfeld J. Reoperative retroperitoneal surgery for nonseminomatous germ cell tumor: clinical presentation, patterns of recurrence, and outcome. *Urology* 2003;62(4):732-6.

[100] Eastham JA, Wilson TG, Russell C, Ahlering TE, Skinner DG. Surgical resection in patients with nonseminomatous germ cell tumor who fail to normalize serum tumor markers after chemotherapy. *Urology* 1994;43(1):74-80.

[101] Wood DP, Jr., Herr HW, Motzer RJ, et al. Surgical resection of solitary metastases after chemotherapy in patients with nonseminomatous germ cell tumors and elevated serum tumor markers. *Cancer* 1992;70(9):2354-7.

[102] George DW, Foster RS, Hromas RA, et al. Update on late relapse of germ cell tumor: a clinical and molecular analysis. *J Clin Oncol* 2003;21(1):113-22.

[103] Tognoni PG, Foster RS, McGraw P, et al. Combined post-chemotherapy retroperitoneal lymph node dissection and resection of chest tumor under the same anesthetic is appropriate based on morbidity and tumor pathology. *J Urol* 1998;159(6):1833-5.

[104] Steyerberg EW, Donohue JP, Gerl A, et al. Residual masses after chemotherapy for metastatic testicular cancer: the clinical implications of the association between retroperitoneal and pulmonary histology. Re-analysis of Histology in Testicular Cancer (ReHiT) Study Group. *J Urol* 1997;158(2):474-8.

[105] Jacobsen NE, Beck SD, Jacobson LE, Bihrle R, Einhorn LH, Foster RS. Is retroperitoneal histology predictive of liver histology at concurrent post-chemotherapy retroperitoneal lymph node dissection and hepatic resection? *J Urol*;184(3):949-53.

[106] Balmaceda C, Heller G, Rosenblum M, et al. Chemotherapy without irradiation--a novel approach for newly diagnosed CNS germ cell tumors: results of an international cooperative trial. The First International Central Nervous System Germ Cell Tumor Study. *J Clin Oncol* 1996;14(11):2908-15.

[107] Pont J, Albrecht W, Postner G, et al. Adjuvant chemotherapy for high-risk clinical stage I nonseminomatous testicular germ cell cancer: long-term results of a prospective trial. *J Clin Oncol* 1996;14(2):441-8.

[108] Klepp O, Dahl O, Flodgren P, et al. Risk-adapted treatment of clinical stage 1 non-seminoma testis cancer. *Eur J Cancer* 1997;33(7):1038-44.

[109] Ondrus D, Matoska J, Belan V, Kausitz J, Goncalves F, Hornak M. Prognostic factors in clinical stage I nonseminomatous germ cell testicular tumors: rationale for different risk-adapted treatment. *Eur Urol* 1998;33(6):562-6.

[110] Bohlen D, Borner M, Sonntag RW, Fey MF, Studer UE. Long-term results following adjuvant chemotherapy in patients with clinical stage I testicular nonseminomatous malignant germ cell tumors with high risk factors. *J Urol* 1999;161(4):1148-52.

[111] Hendry WF, Norman A, Nicholls J, Dearnaley DP, Peckham MJ, Horwich A. Abdominal relapse in stage 1 nonseminomatous germ cell tumours of the testis managed by surveillance or with adjuvant chemotherapy. *BJU Int* 2000;86(1):89-93.

[112] Amato RJ, Ro JY, Ayala AG, Swanson DA. Risk-adapted treatment for patients with clinical stage I nonseminomatous germ cell tumor of the testis. *Urology* 2004;63(1):144-8; discussion 8-9.

[113] Vugrin D, Whitmore WF, Jr., Herr H, Sogani P, Golbey RB. Adjuvant vinblastine, actinomycin D, bleomycin, cyclophosphamide and cis-platinum chemotherapy regimen with and without maintenance in patients with resected stage IIB testis cancer. *J Urol* 1982;128(4):715-7.

[114] Weissbach L, Hartlapp JH. Adjuvant chemotherapy of metastatic stage II nonsemino-matous testis tumor. *J Urol* 1991;146(5):1295-8.

[115] Gerl A, Clemm C, Kohl P, al. e. Adjuvant chemotherapy of stage II non-seminomatous germ cell tumors. *Oncol Rep* 1994(1):209-12.

[116] Kennedy BJ, Torkelson JL, Fraley EE. Adjuvant chemotherapy for stage II nonseminomatous germ cell cancer of the testis. *Cancer* 1994;73(5):1485-9.

[117] Culine S, Theodore C, Farhat F, Bekradda M, Terrier-Lacombe MJ, Droz JP. Cisplatin-based chemotherapy after retroperitoneal lymph node dissection in patients with pathological stage II nonseminomatous germ cell tumors. *J Surg Oncol* 1996;61(3):195-8.

[118] Kondagunta GV, Sheinfeld J, Mazumdar M, et al. Relapse-free and overall survival in patients with pathologic stage II nonseminomatous germ cell cancer treated with etoposide and cisplatin adjuvant chemotherapy. *J Clin Oncol* 2004;22(3):464-7.

In: Essentials and Updates in Urologic Oncology
Editor: Philippe E. Spiess

ISBN: 978-1-62081-494-9
© 2013 Nova Science Publishers, Inc.

Chapter XXVIII

Systemic Chemotherapy for Testicular Cancer

Brian P. Mulherin, Noah M. Hahn and Lawrence H. Einhorn
Department of Genitourinary Oncology, University of Indiana,
Indianapolis, Indiana, US

Abstract

Testicular cancer is an uncommon malignancy, accounting for about 1% of all cancers in men. However, it represents the most common solid neoplasm in young adult males. Germ cell tumors are one of the most curable of all neoplasms, even in the metastatic setting. They are extremely sensitive to cisplatin-based combination chemotherapy, and surgical resection of residual disease has been shown to improve outcomes further. By combining chemotherapy, surgery, and sometimes radiotherapy, the vast majority of patients can now be cured. Testicular cancer has become a model for a curable neoplasm.

Epidemiology

Testicular cancer is an uncommon malignancy, representing about 1% of all cancers in men [1]. Despite its rarity, it represents the most common solid neoplasm in adult males between the ages of 15 and 35, and thus has disproportionate effects on quality of life and economic activity. Germ cell tumors (GCT) account for 95% of testicular cancer, and will be the focus of the remainder of this chapter; the term "testicular cancer" as used in this chapter (and in common parlance) pertains to GCT exclusively. Other testicular malignancies include sex cord-stromal tumors (e.g. Sertoli cell tumors, Leydig cell tumors), gonadoblastoma, lymphoma, metastatic carcinoma, and others.

Testicular cancer represents one of the most curable of all neoplasms, even in the metastatic setting. Its incidence has been rising for the past several decades; although the causes behind this rise remain uncertain, several risk factors for developing testicular cancer have been identified. Patients with cryptorchidism have a relative risk of 2.5 to 14 times that of control subjects, both in the undescended and descended testis. Orchiopexy appears not to alter the risk for further development of testicular cancer. Of note is that only 10% of patients with testicular cancer have a history of maldescent [2]. An emerging number with familial germ cell tumors have been reported, representing between 1 and 3% of all new patients [3-4]. An international consortium study found similar clinicopathologic manifestations of GCT in identified kindreds vs. nonfamilial cases in 461 families with 985 cases [5]. Other risk factors include hypospadias (relative risk 2.13) [6], HIV infection (e.g. rate of seminoma 21-fold higher in HIV-positive patients vs. general population in Pennsylvania) [7], and race. Ethnicity plays an important part in GCT, with the highest rates observed in Caucasians and much lower rates in African Americans and Asians. Carcinoma in situ appears to be a premalignant condition; in two sample reports in infertile men and unilateral GCT undergoing contralateral testicular biopsies, 50% of men developed invasive tumors by 5 years and 70% by 7 years [8,9]. Klinefelter's syndrome is associated with small, atrophic testes and an increased risk for developing testicular and primary mediastinal GCT [10-12]. Down's syndrome has also been associated with an elevated risk of GCT [13].

Primary Sites of Germ Cell Neoplasms

Germ cell neoplasms may develop in midline structures. Primordial germ cell precursors migrate during embryogenesis before traveling to the gonads; thus, midline structures such as the pineal gland, anterior mediastinum, retroperitoneum, and testis (in men) and ovaries (in women) are at risk.

Isochromosome 12p

Patients with GCT have almost routinely been found to have an abnormality (an isochromosome) in the short arm of chromosome 12, abbreviated i(12p). One or more copies of i(12p) can be detected in 85% of patients with GCTs using fluorescence in situ hybridization (FISH) [14]. Virtually all patients with GCTs demonstrate multiple copies of 12p. This finding is particularly useful diagnostically in patients who present with extragonadal tumors or carcinomas of unknown primaries, in which the histologic or serologic diagnosis of germ cell tumor is in doubt.

Pathology

Seminoma

Pure seminoma accounts for 40-50% of all testis cancer (50% of patients with cryptorchidism have seminoma) [15]. The "classic" subtype accounts for more than 90% of pure seminomas. Individuals with classic seminomas typically present in the fourth or fifth decade of life, and approximately 75% have stage I disease at diagnosis. Pathologically, seminomas have a uniform distribution of rounded cells with large, centralized nuclei. The cytoplasm stains positively for glycogen. Approximately 10% of pure seminomas have syncytiotrophoblast proliferation; such patients may have modest elevations of serum β-human chorionic gonadotropin (b-HCG). Of note, any elevation of alpha-fetoprotein (AFP) connotes the presence of a nonseminomatous germ cell tumor (NSGCT). For example, an individual with pure seminoma on pathologic examination and AFP elevation should be treated as a NSGCT.

Spermatocytic seminoma accounts for 1-5% of all seminomas. They differ from classic seminomas in several respects. They present later in life (typically 60s and 70s), do not contain i(12p), and metastasize at an extremely low rate in the absence of sarcomatous differentiation. Thus, orchiectomy is often the only required treatment [16-17].

Nonseminomatous Germ Cell Tumors (NSGCT)

Embryonal carcinoma. Embryonal carcinoma accounts for about 20% of all patients with germ cell tumors, although it frequently represents a component of mixed germ cell tumors. AFP, hCG, or both may be elevated. Embryonal cell carcinoma has a variable pathologic appearance, often with large polygonal cells with indistinct cytoplasmic borders. The cytoplasm is usually pale with large nuclei and centrally located nucleoli. As in chorio-carcinoma (see below), this tumor may undergo widespread hematogeneous dissemination (potentially skipping retroperitoneal lymph nodes), and can undergo hemorrhagic necrosis in response to chemotherapy.

Yolk sac carcinoma. As a pure entity, yolk sac carcinoma is relatively uncommon. However, up to 50% of patients with primary mediastinal tumors will have some component of yolk sac carcinoma. This tumor type is associated with an elevated AFP or hCG.

Choriocarcinoma. Pure choriocarcinoma is rare; when present, it is often associated with a small primary tumor and widespread metastases. These tumors are variably associated with focal hemorrhage within the tumor. They may be quite vascular, leading to intra-tumoral bleeding in metastatic sites (e.g., lung or central nervous system), which may be the presenting local symptom. They can also undergo hemorrhagic necrosis after exposure to cytotoxic chemotherapy, leading to persistent radiographic abnormalities. This tumor type is associated with extremely high elevation of hCG, and thus, serologic remission is extremely important.

Teratoma. Teratoma is a GCT that contains differentiated tissues from at least one, and often all, of the three germ layers (endoderm, mesoderm, and ectoderm). Teratoma is a frequent component of mixed germ cell tumors. Resection is important, as it can not only grow locally and expand, but also undergo malignant transformation months to years after the original diagnosis. Teratomas are not chemosensitive, and require surgical excision for cure. They are not PET-avid, and do not produce elevations in serum tumor markers (see below). Teratomas with malignant transformation may resemble a variety of different tumors and are seen in primary and postchemotherapy specimens of germ cell tumor. Histologic findings include small cell carcinoma, adenocarcinoma, peripheral neuroectodermal tumor (PNET), rhabdomyosarcoma, and Wilms' tumor [18].

The only curable option for these patients is complete surgical resection of their disease, although chemotherapy tailored to the specific histology has been employed [19-20].

Clinical Presentation

Presenting Signs of Testicular Cancer

Retroperitoneal lymphadenopathy may cause back pain, typically in the lumbar region. Further lymphatic spread to supraclavicular lymph nodes (Virchow's node) may also be seen. Pulmonary metastases may produce cough, shortness of breath, and hemoptysis. A large mediastinal mass may cause superior vena cava syndrome. Disease spread to the central nervous system and bone is rare; thus, routine radiographic or radionuclide screening is not warranted in the absence of symptoms. Some patients present with gynecomastia. Although common in adolescents, new onset of gynecomastia in young adults should suggest germ cell malignancy or other endocrine abnormalities. Marked production of hCG can produce paraneoplastic hyperthyroidism. hCG and thyroid stimulating hormone (TSH) share a common alpha- and beta-subunit with considerable homology, and so hCG may mimic activity of TSH [21].

Testicular Physical Examination and Ultrasound Findings

Most patients with testicular cancer present with a painless scrotal mass. This may be confused with epididymitis, particularly when pain is present. Carefully separating the testis from the epididymis or spermatic cord should generally be sufficient to differentiate a testicular mass from epididymitis. Testicular ultrasound will confirm the findings. Translumination of the testis may determine if the patient has a hydrocele, which can be seen in about 20% of patients. Findings on ultrasound include solitary or multiple hyperechoic lesions. Small areas of speckled calcifications suggest carcinoma in situ. Over 95% of patients with a testicular mass will have malignant pathology.

Further Imaging and Initial Surgery

Diagnosis and treatment are closely tied. The preferred approach in a patient with a testicular mass is a radical orchiectomy using the inguinal approach. Fine-needle aspiration (FNA) or trans-scrotal biopsy may lead to aberrant spread of tumor to inguinal and iliac lymph nodes, and are, therefore, contraindicated. Chest radiography or chest CT should be performed to rule out the possibility of pulmonary disease. An abdominal CT scan should be done to evaluate for retroperitoneal lymphadenopathy. Right-sided testicular tumors typically spread to interaortocaval lymph nodes, while left-sided tumors typically spread to paraaortic nodes. Routine CNS imaging and bone scans are not indicated, as discussed above. PET scans can be useful for follow-up in advanced seminomas (see below), but have no role in initial staging.

Tumor Markers

hCG and AFP are elevated in about 85% of the patients with disseminated GCTs. These markers are useful diagnostically and therapeutically. In a patient with pathologic stage I testicular cancer, an orchiectomy should result in the reduction of serum HCG and AFP levels according to their half-lives (18-36 hours and 5 days, respectively). During treatment with chemotherapy, at least a one log reduction of serum HCG should occur every 3 weeks (although this may be more delayed with marked elevations, e.g. greater than 60,000). Patients with elevated AFP have a less predictable decline. Persistent elevation of tumor markers after orchiectomy in presumed stage I disease requires chemotherapy for cure (see below).

False-positive markers. hCG and AFP may not always decline, despite chemotherapy. Reasons for "false"-positive markers may include a tumor sanctuary site (central nervous system or contralateral testicle) that chemotherapy does not adequately penetrate. In addition, false elevation of b-HCG can be observed with cross-reactivity with luteinizing hormone in patients with relative hypogonadotropism.

This can be easily diagnosed by treating the patient with a depot form of testosterone and repeating the b-HCG 2 weeks later. Marijuana usage can result in modest elevation of b-HCG through elevation of LH, which cross-reacts with b-HCG in the assay. Patients with hepatocellular damage, such as hepatitis or cirrhosis, may have AFP elevation falsely attributed to germ cell malignancy. Finally, there are reported familial cases of persistent mildly elevated AFP levels [22].

Staging

Several staging systems for germ cell neoplasms have evolved from the original staging system proposed by Boden and Gibb [23]. In general, testicular cancer can be separated into three stages: stage I (or A), confined to the testis alone; stage II (or B), regional lymphadenopathy; and stage III (or C), distant metastatic disease. Stage II disease can be subcategorized by size or number of lymph nodes (see Table 1).

For patients with disseminated disease, the International Germ Cell Cancer Collaborative Group staging system is useful to determine prognosis and for defining those patients with good- or poor-risk disease [24]. This system uses the clinical and serologic data from both of these prior systems to separate patients into good-, intermediate-, and poor-risk disease categories. Of note, the tumor markers utilized are post-orchiectomy (see Table 2).

Clinical Stage I Disease

Radical inguinal orchiectomy is the mainstay of therapy. Normal serum markers and normal chest and abdominal CT scans following orchiectomy defines a patient with a clinical stage I disease. Below follows a discussion of several possible adjuvant treatments.

Table 1. Testicular cancer staging (GCT only) [101]

Primary tumor (T)

pTX: Primary tumor cannot be assessed
pT0: No evidence of primary tumor
pTis: Intratubular germ cell neoplasia (carcinoma in situ)
pT1: Tumor limited to the testis and epididymis without vascular/lymphatic invasion; tumor may invade into the tunica albuginea but not the tunica vaginalis
pT2: Tumor limited to the testis and epididymis with vascular/lymphatic invasion, or tumor extending through the tunica albuginea with involvement of the tunica vaginalis
pT3: Tumor invades the spermatic cord with or without vascular/lymphatic invasion
pT4: Tumor invades the scrotum with or without vascular/lymphatic invasion

Regional lymph nodes (N)

Clinical
NX: Regional lymph nodes cannot be assessed
N0: No regional lymph node metastasis
N1: Metastasis with a lymph node mass 2 cm or less in greatest dimension; or multiple lymph nodes, none more than 2 cm in greatest dimension
N2: Metastasis with a lymph node mass more than 2 cm but not more than 5 cm in greatest dimension; or multiple lymph nodes, any one mass greater than 2 cm but not more than 5 cm in greatest dimension
N3: Metastasis with a lymph node mass more than 5 cm in greatest dimension
Pathologic (pN)
pNX: Regional lymph nodes cannot be assessed
pN0: No regional lymph node metastasis
pN1: Metastasis with a lymph node mass 2 cm or less in greatest dimension and less than or equal to five nodes positive, none more than 2 cm in greatest dimension
pN2: Metastasis with a lymph node mass more than 2 cm but not more than 5 cm in greatest dimension; or more than five nodes positive, none more than 5 cm; or evidence of extranodal extension of tumor
pN3: Metastasis with a lymph node mass more than 5 cm in greatest dimension

Distant metastasis (M)

M0: No distant metastasis
M1: Distant metastasis
• M1a: Nonregional nodal or pulmonary metastasis
• M1b: Distant metastasis other than to nonregional lymph nodes and lung

Serum tumor markers (S)

SX: Marker studies not available or not performed
S0: Marker study levels within normal limits
S1: LDH <1.5 x Nand hCG (mIu/ml) <5000 and AFP (ng/ml) <1000
S2: LDH 1.5-10 x N or hCG (mIu/ml) 5000-50,000 or AFP (ng/ml) 1000-10,000
S3: LDH >10 x N or hCG (mIu/ml) >50,000 or AFP (ng/ml) >10,000

Note: "N" above = upper limit of normal

Stage groupings

Stage	Primary tumor (T)	Regional lymph nodes (N)	Distant metastasis (M)	Serum tumor markers (S)
0	pTis	N0	M0	S0
I	pT1-4	N0	M0	SX
IA	pT1	N0	M0	S0
IB	pT2	N0	M0	S0
	pT3	N0	M0	S0
	pT4	N0	M0	S0
IS	Any pT/Tx	N0	M0	S1-3
II	Any pT/Tx	N1-3	M0	SX
IIA	Any pT/Tx	N1	M0	S0
	Any pT/Tx	N1	M0	S1
IIB	Any pT/Tx	N2	M0	S0
	Any pT/Tx	N2	M0	S1
IIC	Any pT/Tx	N3	M0	S0
	Any pT/Tx	N3	M0	S1
III	Any pT/Tx	Any N	M1	SX
IIIA	Any pT/Tx	Any N	M1a	S0
	Any pT/Tx	Any N	M1a	S1
IIIB	Any pT/Tx	N1-3	M0	S2
	Any pT/Tx	Any N	M1a	S2
IIIC	Any pT/Tx	N1-3	M0	S3
	Any pT/Tx	Any N	M1a	S3
	Any pT/Tx	Any N	M1b	Any S

Table 2. IGCCCG Risk-Group Classification [24]

Poor-risk disease (NSGCT only), any ONE of the following:
LDH > 10 times upper limit of normal, OR hCG > 50,000 IU/mL, OR AFP >10,000 ng/mL
PMNSGCT
Non-pulmonary visceral metastases (bone, liver, brain, etc.)
Intermediate-risk disease:
Seminoma: any primary site, AND non-pulmonary visceral metastases, AND normal markers
NSGCT: any testis/retroperitoneal site, NO non-pulmonary visceral metastases, AND intermediate markers (AFP 1000-10,000 ng/mL, OR hCG 5000-50,000 IU/mL)
Good-risk disease: all others

Radiation Therapy

Radiation therapy is typically utilized in patients with pure seminoma who have stage I or early stage II disease (i.e. <3 cm, see below). Following radical orchiectomy, patients with clinical stage I seminoma may be prophylactically irradiated to 2000 cGy to a target area (including the periaortic region from approximately the 11th thoracic vertebrae to the lumbar region and extending to the ipsilateral renal hilum). Routine radiation of the iliac lymph nodes is no longer required. Relapse rates are reduced to 3% with prophylactic radiation [25]. Pelvis irradiation does confer a higher risk for secondary malignancies; in the aforementioned trial, six new non-GCT diagnoses were confirmed on follow-up, all in patients treated with 30 Gy vs. 20 Gy (one scalp melanoma, one scalp basal cell carcinoma, 2 prostate cancers, one bladder cancer, and one low-grade non-Hodgkin lymphoma [25]. Bulky stage II disease is usually treated with moderately higher dosages of 35 to 40 cGy. Radiotherapy is not useful in treating NSGCT.

Surgery

Retroperitoneal lymphadenectomy. Retroperitoneal surgery for metastatic testis cancer consists of two primary operations. In low-stage disease, a modified template of dissection is used contingent upon the side of the primary tumor. Hence, the field of dissection for a right-sided testicular tumor includes the right paracaval and interaortocaval regions. For a left testicular primary, the field includes the left periaortic and preaortic lymphatics. The ipsilateral sympathetics are preserved to guarantee maintenance of emission and ejaculation postoperatively. RPLND may be utilized as an adjuvant treatment for clinical stage I NSGCT. It may also be employed in early stage II disease (see below). Surgical success is predicated on the predictable pattern of metastatic spread from the testis to the retroperitoenum prior to distant sites (although embryonal cell carcinoma and choriocarcinoma may present with widespread hematogeneous dissemination, even in the absence of retroperitoneal disease). Surgical operations have evolved from a variety of templates to minimize complications of retrograde ejaculation.

Surveillance

Another option for the management of patients with clinical stage I testicular cancer is surveillance. In NSGCT, patients have an approximately 30% chance of developing recurrent disease due to occult metastases to the retroperitoneal lymph nodes. The incidence of relapse varies based on histology and the presence or absence of lymphovascular invasion, with embryonal cell carcinoma coupled with the latter conferring a relapse rate of approximately 50%. Relapse rates for clinical stage I seminoma vary based on tumor size, with tumors less than 3 cm having a 90% cure rate with orchiectomy alone and those greater than 4 cm having a 70% cure rate with orchiectomy alone. Most of these recurrences occur within the first 1 to 2 years, but relapse beyond 2 years can occur. With close follow-up, most patients with recurrent disease will present with low-volume disease and, thus, should be cured with systemic cisplatin-based chemotherapy. Since close follow-up is essential to detect early relapses or new primary sites of disease, this should only be offered to highly motivated patients.

Adjuvant Chemotherapy

Recently, administration of one cycle of BEP (bleomycin, etoposide, cisplatin) chemotherapy has been shown to decrease the recurrence rate of clinical stage I NSGCT to less than 1% after nearly five years of follow-up. This may be an attractive option in a patient with unreliable follow-up who wishes to avoid surgery. Patients randomized to RPLND in the aforementioned trial experienced a recurrence rate of nearly 8%. Therefore, standard post-orchiectomy options for clinical stage I NSGCT include observation, one cycle of BEP, or RPLND [26]. A single cycle of adjuvant carboplatin may also be given for clinical stage I seminoma, reducing the expected recurrence rate to approximately 3%. Standard post-orchiectomy options for clinical stage I seminoma, therefore, include surveillance, a single cycle of carboplatin, or retroperitoneal radiotherapy.

Stage II Disease

For patients with NSGCT with low-volume disease (< 3 cm in cross-sectional diameter) and normal (or within predicted half-life) serum markers, primary retroperitoneal lymph node dissection (RPLND) is the preferred treatment. In such patients, RPLND will result in cures of approximately 70%, without additional therapy. If observed without adjuvant therapy, approximately 30% of patients have recurrence, but three cycles of BEP should produce virtually a 100% cure rate for those with relapsing disease. Thus, the long-term outcome for a surgically resected stage II patient who is compliant with follow-up should be similar with or without adjuvant therapy. In patients with resected seminoma and low-volume retroperitoneal nodes (<3 cm), radiotherapy to the retroperitoneum can also confer a high cure rate.

For patients with rising markers following orchiectomy or with retroperitoneal disease greater than 3 cm in cross-sectional diameter, primary chemotherapy is indicated. In the absence of supradiaphragmatic disease and hCG and AFP below 5000 IU/L and 1000 ng/mL, respectively, three cycles of BEP are standard therapy. Bleomycin should be avoided in patients with significant pulmonary pathology, renal dysfunction (to avoid excessive muco-cutaneous toxicity), patients older than age 50, or in primary mediastinal NSGCT (PMNSGCT, see below). In good-risk patients, a fourth cycle of BEP does not improve long-term outcomes compared to three cycles, and should be avoided [27, 28].

Bleomycin is associated with serious and potentially fatal pulmonary toxicity, and several randomized trials have explored eliminating bleomycin from standard treatment regimens. However, removing bleomycin from BEP results in inferior outcomes, as demonstrated in a phase III Eastern Cooperative Oncology Group (ECOG) trial. This trial compared three cycles of BEP vs. the identical therapy without bleomycin. Out of 173 evaluable patients, 94% receiving BEP attained a no evidence of disease status (NED), compared to 88% for cisplatin and etoposide alone. Failure-free survival (FFS) also favored bleomycin (86% vs. 69%, respectively, p=0.004), as did overall survival (OS; 95% vs. 86%, respectively, p=0.011) [29]. Multiple other randomized trials have also evaluated the role of bleomycin [30-35]; in every trial, the bleomycin arm had fewer deaths overall, while the risk of death was increased in the EP arm in several studies. The overall survival difference in most trials was not statistically significant. Bleomycin thus remains a critical component of most chemotherapy regimens for testicular cancer.

Although carboplatin confers less nephrotoxicity, neurotoxicity, and ototoxicity than cisplatin, trials utilizing carboplatin have demonstrated inferior survival. One trial substituting carboplatin for cisplatin in BEP [36], and another trial evaluating the same substitution with

EP [37], have demonstrated inferior survival rates, relapse rates, and NED rates. We recommend not substituting carboplatin for cisplatin.

Four cycles of etoposide and cisplatin have also been explored as treatment for good-risk disease (cisplatin 20 mg/m2 on days 1-5 and etoposide 100 mg/m2 on days 1-5 every 3 weeks for 4 cycles; EP). In a French study evaluating BEP x 3 vs. EP x 4 for good-risk metastatic NSGCT, response rates, 4-year event-free survival rates (EFS), and four-year overall survival rates (OS) were not statistically significantly different. However, adverse events were numerically more common with EP x 4, PFS was numerically superior with BEP x 3 (91% vs. 86%, respectively), and 4-year OS was numerically superior with BEP x 3 (96% vs. 92%). The trial concluded BEP x 3 remained the treatment of choice for metastatic NSGCT patients [35]. Concerning toxicity, the advantage of the 3 cycles of BEP regimen is the shorter duration of therapy and less cisplatin, while 4 cycles of EP avoids complications associated with bleomycin [38]. We recommend three cycles of BEP as first-line therapy for most patients, with four cycles of EP reserved for those patients unable to tolerate bleomycin (see above).

Postchemotherapy Retroperitoneal Lymph Node Dissection (PC-RPLND)

This procedure is performed for residual retroperitoneal tumor after administration of chemotherapy for metastatic testis cancer, typically defined as nodes measuring more than 1 cm in the transverse dimension. The metastatic tumor can be very adherent to the great vessels and other structures; thus, proper tissue planes are difficult to determine. Specialized vascular techniques are sometimes necessary to completely resect the retroperitoneal tumor, but complete resection of all tumor is essential to ensure a good outcome. Surgeons who attempt PC-RPLND should be experienced with the procedure. It is very difficult to predict the degree of difficulty of the procedure based on preoperative clinical parameters. See below for a discussion of residual masses in seminomas.

In patients with NSGCT with initial large retroperitoneal masses who achieve a complete radiographic and serologic remission after chemotherapy, routine RPLND has been recommended by some authors. In a retrospective analysis of 141 patients observed without a post-chemotherapy RPLND at Indiana University, only 9% relapsed after a median follow-up of 15.5 years; of these, two-thirds now have no evidence of disease (NED), and four patients died of disease [39].

Stage III Disease

Patients with disseminated disease are treated with cisplatin-based combination chemotherapy. Patients with good-risk disease can be treated with three cycles of BEP or four cycles of EP, although BEP x 3 has been numerically superior in several trials (see above). For patients with intermediate and poor-risk disease, cure rates are approximately 75% and 65%, respectively. As such, these patients are candidates for potentially more aggressive therapy. The standard treatment approach is four cycles of BEP or VIP (see below).

Although we typically recommend initial orchiectomy, patients with a heavy metastatic burden are often quite symptomatic at diagnosis. For example, a male with choriocarcinoma and overwhelming pulmonary metastases may have dyspnea, hypoxia, and hemoptysis. In this instance, administering chemotherapy upfront is appropriate. For symptomatic patients requiring immediate systemic treatment, orchiectomy can be delayed until immediately following chemotherapy (e.g. day 6 of BEP). Since chemotherapy has poor penetrance into testes (i.e. they are a sanctuary site), they can serve as potential foci for relapse later, underscoring the need for orchiectomy in all patients.

Neutropenia may occur with cytotoxic chemotherapy. Given the potential for cure, we do not recommend delaying treatment for asymptomatic neutropenia. If patients have neutropenic fevers, we recommend administering the next cycle with granulocyte-colony stimulating factor (G-CSF) support, and typically dose-reduce the etoposide by 25%. The dose of cisplatin should NOT be reduced. Delaying or reducing therapy may compromise long-term cure rates.

Ifosfamide-Based Therapy

Ifosfamide has single-agent activity in NSGCT that relapse following cisplatin-based therapy, and has been combined with cisplatin and either etoposide (VIP) or vinblastine (VeIP) in this population (see below). An intergroup trial evaluated upfront ifosfamide in intermediate- and poor-risk disease. This seminal trial compared four cycles of either BEP or VIP (etoposide 75 mg/m2, ifosfamide 1.2 g/m2, and cisplatin 20 mg/m2, all administered daily for five consecutive days every 21 days; patients randomized to ifosfamide received mesna for uroprotection). Overall complete remission rates (ORR) were comparable (37% vs. 31% for VIP and BEP, respectively), as were FFS rates (64% vs. 60%), and OS (74% vs. 71%). As expected, VIP proved more toxic, with more hematologic and genitourinary side effects in this cohort [40]. With longer follow-up, progression-free survival (PFS) and OS remained comparable with poor-risk disease (PFS, 56% for VIP for 49% for BEP; OS, 62% vs. 57%, respectively) [41]. A third, smaller trial yielded similar results [42].

Based on the above, four cycles of BEP remain the standard of care for intermediate- or poor-risk disease. VIP may be considered in the following circumstances: patients with significant underlying lung disease, who are at increased risk for bleomycin-induced pulmonary toxicity; patients with extensive pulmonary metastases causing hypoxia, who likely require supplemental oxygen and are, therefore, at similarly increased risk for bleomycin-induced pulmonary toxicity; and patients with PMNSGCT, who will require extensive surgical resections and large amounts of time on supplemental oxygen.

Residual Masses

As stated above, patients may have residual radiographic abnormalities following primary chemotherapy. Resection of residual disease in patients with normal tumor markers yields necrotic tissue in 40-50%, teratoma in 30-40%, and residual viable GCTs in 10-20% [43-44]. In the latter case, two additional cycles of cisplatin and etoposide are generally indicated. Post-surgical "adjuvant" therapy may potentially be avoided if a complete resection could be achieved, specimens contain less than 10% viable tumor cells, and if patients had an optimal IGCCCG at presentation [45-47].

For NSGCT, current recommendations are to resect all residual masses following chemotherapy (barring technical infeasibility). This includes residual retroperitoneal lymph nodes measuring more than 1 cm in transverse diameter. In patients with unresectable disease or those in whom complete resection of all residual disease is not possible, close observation is indicated. Generally, we would follow these patients with monthly chest radiographs, serum markers, and periodic CT scans. In many patients with unresectable residual disease and normal serum markers, the tumor may continue to regress, supporting the fact that the patient merely has residual necrotic tumor. Salvage chemotherapy would be reserved for those patients who demonstrate progressive disease radiographically or serologically. Even in patients with chemorefractory disease with persistently elevated tumor markers, resection of residual masses may be followed by markers normalization and long-term survival [48-49]. Indiana University recently reviewed its experience of desperation RPLND to determine the therapeutic benefit of surgery in this population. [50[. This study included 114 patients all with elevated serum tumor markers after either induction chemotherapy alone (50 patients) or salvage chemotherapy (64 patients). The 5-year overall survival was 54%. Sixty-one patients (53.5%) are alive with a median follow-up of 5 years. Fifty-three patients died of disease, with a median time to death of 8.0 months. Retroperitoneal pathology revealed germ-cell cancer in 53.5%, teratoma in 34.2%, and fibrosis in 12.2%, with 5-year survival rates of 31%, 77%, and 86%, respectively.

Salvage Therapy

Salvage therapy is indicated for patients who relapse from complete remission or who have an incomplete partial response to primary chemotherapy. VeIP (vinblastine, ifosfamide, and cisplatin) produces durable complete remissions in about 25% to 30% of patients with recurrent nonseminomatous germ cell tumor (NSGCT) treated with second-line therapy. In patients with recurrent seminoma, VeIP chemotherapy will produce durable complete remissions in approximately 50% of patients [51-56].

Another approach to salvage therapy includes 4 courses of paclitaxel, ifosfamide, and cisplatin (TIP) every 3 weeks with G-CSF support. In a study of 46 patients with progressive metastatic GCTs, TIP as second-line therapy yielded a complete response (CR) rate of 70%, and 29 of 46 were continuously NED at a median follow-up of 69 months. 3 patients (7%) relapsed after an initial CR. The durable CR rate measured 63%, with a 2-year progression-free survival (PFS) of 65%. These patients had more favorable prognostic features, including six or fewer cycles of cisplatin, no PMNSGCT, either a complete response (CR) or partial response (PR) for greater than six months following chemotherapy with normal markers [57].

High-dose chemotherapy with carboplatin and etoposide with peripheral blood stem-cell rescue (HDCT, performed as two tandem transplants) offers a high rate of cure for relapsed or progressive disease after first-line therapy. In the largest series from Indiana University, median follow-up was 48 months. 68% of individuals who received transplant as first-line salvage therapy have no evidence of disease, while 48% of patients have no evidence of disease when transplant was used as third-line or later therapy. Overall survival with seminoma is over 90%. Individuals receiving high-dose therapy as third-line or later therapy had an inferior outcome [58].

A phase I/II single-arm German trial studied standard-dose VIP coupled with up-front high-dose VIP requiring peripheral blood stem cell rescue in advanced GCT with poor prognostic features (performed as one cycle of VIP followed by three to four sequential cycles of high-dose VIP with stem cell support at six consecutive dosage levels every three weeks). Results suggested a favorable outcome with initial high-dose therapy compared to historical controls, albeit at significantly worse toxicity [59]. An intergroup phase III trial randomized patients with intermediate- or poor-risk GCT to first-line BEP x 4 or four cycles of BEP followed by two cycles of high-dose chemotherapy containing carboplatin followed by HDCT. 1-year durable complete response rates were unchanged, and no survival difference could be detected [60].

For patients relapsing after HDCT, several chemotherapeutic options exist. These patients generally can be considered for investigational trials. Drugs such as paclitaxel, gemcitabine, and oral etoposide have produced response rates in the range of 15% to 30% in the salvage setting, with some durable complete remissions observed [61]. In a phase II trial employing paclitaxel and gemcitabine for patients relapsing after HDCT (generally within one year), 31% of patients had an objective response, and four of 32 patients (12.5%) are NED for 36+, 96+, 94+, and 64+ months. These four patients received no subsequent chemotherapy or curative surgery [62].

The German Testicular Cancer Study Group has evaluated single-agent oxaliplatin in this population; in either cisplatin-refractory or HDCT-refractory patients, response rates reached 13%, and 2 additional patients achieved disease stabilization [63]. Oxaliplatin has also been combined with gemcitabine and paclitaxel (GOP), with a 5% complete response rate and overall response rate of 51% [64].

Patients who are candidates for salvage therapy have mixed prognostic factors. Patients with pure seminoma or longer relapse-free intervals (but < 2 years) have better prognosis than those patients whose tumors progress on cisplatin, multiple regimens, or mediastinal primary tumors.

The Indiana series on high-dose chemotherapy also identified the following additional adverse prognostic variables in patients receiving transplant: high-dose therapy received as third-line or later therapy versus second-line therapy, and favorable initial IGCCCG score (International Germ Cell Cancer Collaborative Group) [58]. A European retrospective review identified additional adverse prognostic factors as age <40 at primary diagnosis and multiple sites of metastatic disease at relapse [65]. A scoring system by Beyer et al. utilizes the following prognostic variables to risk-stratify patients at relapse: site of primary tumors, response to first-line treatment, relapse-free survival, level of hCG at relapse, and level of AFP at relapse. Hazard ratios in favor of high-dose therapy for overall survival measured 0.77-0.83, and 0.72-0.84 for progression-free survival (depending on the type of analyses used) [66]. A recent multicenter retrospective study on 1984 patients with relapsed/refractory germ cell tumors identified PMNSGCT, elevated AFP (particularly greater than 1000 ng/mL), hCG above 1000 U/l, non-pulmonary visceral metastases, and progressive disease as adverse prognostic factors [67].

Late Relapse

Approximately 2% of patients will relapse from a complete remission after 2 years, more than 50% of these greater than five years out. This represents a unique subset of patients with recurrent disease, who are not generally curable with systemic therapy. A typical scenario is the patient with elevated serum markers (usually AFP) presenting several years after primary therapy. Radiographic evaluation will generally reveal a mass that may be in the area of prior disease and oftentimes associated with prior histology of teratoma. If the patient has isolated disease, surgical resection is indicated and is capable of curing above 50% of such patients. In instances of pure nodal disease and AFP elevation, the cure rate approaches 50% in series from Indiana University; hematogeneous disease and elevations of hCG have lower cure rates [68]. Survival approaches 100% in case of single site teratoma. Systemic chemotherapy may produce brief responses, but by itself rarely produces durable complete remission except in those patients who are chemotherapy naïve. There are reports of high-dose therapy with autologous stem cell rescue for treating late relapses, with 6-year overall survival <20% [69].

Residual Masses Post-Chemotherapy in Seminomas

Controversy still exists over the optimal management of residual masses after initial therapy in patients with seminomas. Resecting residual masses postchemotherapy can be technically challenging owing to an intense fibrotic reaction. Some series note a correlation between size and probability of viable tumor remaining at surgery; in a series from Memorial Sloan Kettering of 104 patients, for example, only 3% with a residual mass less than 3 cm had GCT histology at surgery or subsequently relapsed at the surgical site, while 27% with residual masses greater than 3 cm had either persistent seminoma or teratoma [70-71] . A smaller series from Indiana University found a similarly low rate of residual disease, but found no correlation with size [72].

Several different techniques including positron-emission tomography (PET) scans have been used to further evaluate residual mass for persistent carcinoma. In the European SEMPET study, PET scans more accurately predicted residual viable seminoma than traditional CT scans [73]. Recent experience at Indiana University has reported a specificity approaching 100% when PET scans are performed at least 6 weeks after chemotherapy is completed, however, the positive predictive value was somewhat disappointing at only 67% [74]. Thus, a negative PET scan can reassure the clinician that surveillance is reasonable. Unfortunately, a positive PET scan does not confirm residual viable seminoma in all cases, potentially requiring confirmation via biopsy.

Extragonadal Tumors

Patients with extragonadal germ cell tumors (primary mediastinal or primary retroperitoneum) present with unique problems. In patients diagnosed with germ cell tumors based on a retroperitoneal biopsy but not orchiectomy, the testicle may also harbor tumor.

Unresected intratesticular tumor is relatively isolated from chemotherapy due to the pampiniform plexus (sanctuary site). We recommend these individuals undergo a testicular ultrasound, and orchiectomy as appropriate.

PMNSGCT confers a dismal prognosis, partly from an often-higher disease burden at diagnosis, and partly from tumor biology. These tumors occur most frequently between the ages of 20 and 40. Presenting clinical symptoms include SVC syndrome, fevers, chills, weight loss, chest pain, cough, and dyspnea. Most have elevations of tumor markers (typically AFP). Due to the extensive surgical resections employed following completion of primary chemotherapy, these patients should not receive bleomycin. Instead, we recommend four cycles of VIP, followed by potential resection of any remaining disease. Resection of all residual masses should be attempted even with rising markers. These operations are often complex, and patients should be referred to surgical oncologists with extensive experience with PMNSGCT if possible. As with retroperitoneal disease, we recommend administering two additional cycles of chemotherapy if viable tumor cells are present on pathology. Unfortunately, salvage chemotherapy has minimal efficacy [75].

PMNSGCT have been associated with several hematologic disorders, including acute megakaryocytic leukemia (FAB-M7) and myelodysplastic syndrome. These hematologic disorders usually develop concurrently or within a few months after diagnosis, and are not, then, thought to be chemotherapy-induced. In one series of 287 patients with PMNSGCT, the relative risk of developing a hematologic disorder was increased 250-fold over an age-matched population, with a median time to onset of six months and a median survival post-diagnosis of five months [76]. These disorders are frequently associated with the same i(12p) mutations seen with the primary tumor [77-78]. These patients also have an elevated risk of sarcomas.

Toxicities of Therapy

Given the unique curative potential of testicular cancer, most men become long-term survivors. The burgeoning field of cancer survivorship has assumed greater importance throughout oncology as more patients enjoy long-term survival. Below follows a brief, selected discussion of treatment-related toxicities unique to testicular cancer.

Bleomycin Toxicity

Bleomycin may cause pneumonitis and pulmonary fibrosis, with toxicity increasing in a dose-dependent fashion. Fatal pulmonary toxicity related to bleomycin is less than 1% with 3 cycles of BEP, although this rises to 1-2% with four cycles of BEP [32-33, 42, 79-81]. In an early trial, approximately 50% of all treatment-related deaths in men receiving chemotherapy for testicular cancer were due to bleomycin-induced pneumotoxicity, which was fatal in 50% [79]. Patients with pneumotoxicity typically present with bibasilar crackles, dyspnea on exertion, and a nonproductive cough. Pulmonary nodules can be seen on chest imaging, which may be confused for metastatic disease. A decline in the diffusing capacity for carbon monoxide (DLCO) may be seen on pulmonary function tests (PFTs), although this is not universal. High concentrations of supplemental oxygen are known to potentiate bleomycin toxicity, particularly relevant for patients with PMNSGCT and symptomatic pulmonary metastases causing hypoxia, or significant underlying lung disease. If patients develop bleomycin-induced pulmonary toxicity, we recommend avoiding further bleomycin, and proceeding either with EP (for good-risk disease) or VIP (for poor-risk disease).

Cisplatin Toxicity (Non-Gonadal)

Cisplatin is the most active single drug for testicular cancer, but has numerous toxicities. In addition to the well-known nephrotoxicity and salt-wasting, cisplatin can cause neuropathy and ototoxicity. The former is typically a cumulative axonal neuropathy affecting the dorsal root ganglia. Patients typically experience dysesthesias, paresthesias, and alterations in proprioception and vibration sense. Given the curative potential for treatment, we recommend not dose-reducing cisplatin. With functional impairment, we recommend physicians discuss the risks and benefits of further cisplatin therapy with patients; however, practitioners must bear in mind that dose reductions may compromise chemotherapeutic efficacy.

Neuropathy eventually improves in most patients, although some have lasting symptoms [82]. 20-30% of patients may have persistent symptomatic neuropathy [82-83], which may be more pronounced after HDCT.

Cisplatin-induced ototoxicity typically presents with tinnitus and higher-frequency hearing loss. Ototoxicity is both schedule- and dose-dependent [83]. With completion of therapy, most patients have complete resolution of ototoxicity, although tinnitus or hearing deficits may persist in approximately 20% [82, 84-85].

Fertility

As discussed early in this chapter, GCT's may be associated with several conditions with impaired fertility (e.g. cryptorchidism, Klinefelter's). Approximately 50% of men with testicular cancer have abnormal sperm motility even prior to therapy [86], and a similarly high proportion of men may have azoospermia or severe oligospermia before undergoing any therapy. Following orchiectomy, spermatogenesis may decline even further [87].

Cisplatin leads to further defects in spermatogenesis in a dose-dependent fashion. Treatment intensity, pretreatment reproductive function, and patient age influence recovery of spermatogenesis [88-90]. Although two courses of BEP as adjuvant therapy for stage I disease has no apparent deleterious effects on long-term fertility [91], transient declines in spermatogenesis occur in most men following three or four cycles of therapy. This nadirs at 10-14 months post-treatment [87-89, 92]. Spermatogenesis recovers in nearly 70% of patients by three years out [88]. Following more prolonged therapy or HDCT (greater than 400 mg/m2 or 850 mg cumulative total dose of cisplatin), approximately 50% of men experience persistent azoospermia [93-96].

Radiotherapy and RPLND may also affect fertility in patients with testicular cancer. Nerve-sparing RPLND's allow higher proportions of patients to preserve ejaculatory function (see other chapters in this book for a full discussion of these techniques).

Given the above, we routinely recommend sperm banking prior to the initiation of chemotherapy (if medically permissible) in patients wishing to preserve fertility.

Leukemia

As above, PMNSGCT may be associated with AML. The incidence of secondary leukemia is typically less than 0.5% after three or four courses of BEP, with a cumulative etoposide dose of less than 2 gm/m2 [97, 98]. Following higher doses of etoposide, however, patients have increased risk for secondary leukemia. This characteristically occurs two to three years after treatment, and involves the typical chromosomal translocation 11q23. This incidence is 2-3% in most studies [99-100].

Conclusion

Although a rare disease, testicular cancer exacts disproportionate effects on life expectancy and quality of life in a predominantly young patient population. Through the combined use of highly effective chemotherapy, radiotherapy, and surgery, the vast majority of patients with GCT can now be cured, even in the metastatic setting. GCT are typically quite chemosensitive, and combination chemotherapy has proven to be highly effective at treating this disease. Uniquely, surgical resection of persistent radiographic disease can help optimize cure rates. Testicular cancer has become a model for a curable neoplasm.

References

[1]   American Cancer Society. *Cancer Facts and Figures* 2010.
[2]   Abratt RP, Reddi VB, Sarembock LA: Testicular cancer and cryptorchidism. *Br J Urol,* 1992:70, 656.
[3]   Dieckmann KP, Pichlmeier U: The prevalence of familial testicular cancer: an analysis of two patient populations and a review of the literature. *Cancer,* 1997:80, 1954.
[4]   Dong C, Lönnstedt I, Hemminki K: Familial testicular cancer and second primary cancers in testicular cancer patients by histological type. *Eur J Cancer,* 2001:37, 1878.
[5]   Mai PL, Friedlander M, Tucker K, et al.: The International Testicular Cancer Linkage Consortium: a clinicopathologic descriptive analysis of 461 familial malignant testicular germ cell tumor kindred. *Urol Oncol,* 2010:28, 492.
[6]   Schnack TH, Poulsen G, Myrup C, et al.: Familial coaggregation of cryptorchidism, hypospadias, and testicular germ cell cancer: a nationwide cohort study. *J Natl Cancer Inst,* 2010:102, 187.
[7]   Lyter DW, Bryant J, Thackeray R, et al.: Incidence of human immunodeficiency virus-related and nonrelated malignancies in a large cohort of homosexual men. *J Clin Oncol,* 1995:13, 2540.
[8]   Skakkebaek NE, Berthelsen JG, Müller J: Carcinoma-in-situ of the undescended testis. *Urol Clin North Am,* 1982: 9, 377.

[9] von der Maase H, Rørth M, Walbom-Jørgensen S, et al.: Carcinoma in situ of contralateral testis in patients with testicular germ cell cancer: study of 27 cases in 500 patients. *Br Med J* (Clin Res Ed), 1986:293, 1398.

[10] Hasle H, Mellemgaard A, Nielsen, et al.: Cancer incidence in men with Klinefelter syndrome. *Br J Cancer*, 1995:71, 416.

[11] Hasle H, Jacobsen BB, Asschenfeldt P, et al.: Mediastinal germ cell tumour associated with Klinefelter syndrome. A report of case and review of the literature. *Eur J Pediatr,* 1992:151, 735.

[12] Dexeus FH, Logothetis CJ, Chong C, et al.: Genetic abnormalities in men with germ cell tumors. *J Urol*, 1988:140, 80.

[13] Dieckmann KP, Rübe C, Henke RP: Association of Down's syndrome and testicular cancer. *J Urol,* 1997:157, 1701.

[14] Houldsworth J, Bosl GJ, Chaganti RSK: Biology and genetics of adult male germ cell tumors. In: Vogelzang NJ, Scardino PT, Shipley WU, et al., eds. *Comprehensive textbook of Genitourinary Oncology.* Baltimore: Williams and Wilkins, 2006:563-571.

[15] Ulbright TM, Amin MB, Young RH: Tumors of the testis, adnexa, spermatic cord, and scrotum. In: *Atlas of Tumor Pathology.* Washington D.C.: Armed Forces Institute of Pathology, 1999:59-102.

[16] Carrière P, Baade P, Fritschi L: Population based incidence and age distribution of spermatocytic seminoma. *J Urol,* 2007:178, 125.

[17] Aggarwal N, Patwani AV: Spermatocytic seminoma. *Arch Pathol Lab Med,* 2009:133, 1985-8.

[18] Motzer RJ, Amsterdam A, Prieto V, et al.: Teratoma with malignant transformation: diverse malignant histologies arising in men with germ cell tumors. *J Urol,* 1998:159, 133.

[19] Donadio AC, Motzer RJ, Bajorin DF, et al.: Chemotherapy for teratoma with malignant transformation. *J Clin Oncol* 2003; 21: 4285.

[20] Ehrlich Y, Beck SD, Ulbright TM, et al.: Outcome analysis of patients with transformed teratoma to primitive neuroectodermal tumor. *Ann Oncol* 2010; 21: 1846.

[21] Oosting SF, de Haas EC, Links TP, et al.: Prevalence of paraneoplastic hyperthyroidism in patients with metastatic non-seminomatous germ-cell tumors. *Ann Oncol,* 2010:21, 104.

[22] Schefer H, Mattman S, Joss RA: Hereditary persistence of alpha-fetoprotein. Case report and review of the literature. *Ann Onc* 1998, 9: 667-672.

[23] Boden G, Gibb R: Radiotherapy and testicular neoplasms. *Lancet* 1951, 2:1195.

[24] International Germ Cell Collaborative Group: International Germ Cell Consensus Classification: a prognostic factor-based staging system for metastatic germ cell cancers. *J Clin Oncol* 1997, 15:594–603.

[25] Jones WG, Fossa SD, Mead GM, et al: Randomized Trial of 30 Versus 20 Gy in the Adjuvant Treatment of Stage I Testicular Seminoma: A Report on Medical Research Council Trial TE18, European Organisation for the Research and Treatment of Cancer Trial 30942. *J Clin Oncol* 2005, 23:1200-1208.

[26] Albers P, Siener R, Krege S, et al.: Randomized Phase III Trial Comparing Retroperitoneal Lymph Node Dissection With One Course of Bleomycin and Etoposide Plus Cisplatin Chemotherapy in the Adjuvant Treatment of Clinical Stage I

Nonseminomatous Testicular Germ Cell Tumors: AUO Trial AH 01/94 by the German Testicular Cancer Study Group. *J Clin Onc*: 2008, 2966-2972.

[27] Einhorn, LH, et al.: Evaluation of optimal duration of chemotherapy in favorable-prognosis disseminated germ cell tumors: a Southeastern Cancer Study Group protocol. *J Clin Oncol*, 1989: 7, 3.

[28] Saxman SB, Finch D, Gonin R, Einhorn LH: Long-term follow-up of a phase III study of three versus four cycles of bleomycin, etoposide, and cisplatin in favorable-prognosis germ-cell tumors: the Indian University experience. *J Clin Oncol* 1998: 16, 2.

[29] Loehrer PJ Sr, et al.: Importance of bleomycin in favorable-prognosis disseminated germ cell tumors: an Eastern Cooperative Oncology Group trial. *J Clin Oncol*, 1995: 13, 2.

[30] Toner GC, et al.: Comparison of two standard chemotherapy regimens for good-prognosis germ-cell tumours: a randomised trial. Australian and New Zealand Germ Cell Trial Group. *Lancet*, 2001: 357, 9258.

[31] Grimison PS, et al.: Comparison of two standard chemotherapy regimens for good-prognosis germ cell tumors: updated analysis of a randomized trial. *J Natl Cancer Inst*, 2010: 102, 16.

[32] Levi JA, et al.: The importance of bleomycin in combination chemotherapy for good-prognosis germ cell carcinoma. Australasian Germ Cell Trial Group. *J Clin Oncol*, 1993: 11, 7.

[33] De Wit R, et al.: Importance of bleomycin in combination chemotherapy for good-prognosis testicular nonseminoma: a randomized study of the European Organization for Research and Treatment of Cancer Genitourinary Tract Cancer Cooperative Group. *J Clin Oncol*, 1997: 15, 5.

[34] Bosl GJ, et al.: A randomized trial of etoposide + cisplatin versus vinblastine + bleomycin + cisplatin + cyclophosphamide + dactinomycin in patients with good-prognosis germ cell tumors. *J Clin Oncol*, 1988: 6, 8.

[35] Culine S, et al.: Refining the optimal chemotherapy regimen for good-risk metastatic nonseminomatous germ-cell tumors: a randomized trial of the Genito-Urinary Group of the French Federation of Cancer Centers (GETUG T93BP). *Annals of Oncology* 2007, 18: 917-924.

[36] Horwich A, et al.: Randomized trial of bleomycin, etoposide, and cisplatin compared with bleomycin, etoposide, and carboplatin in good-prognosis metastatic nonseminomatous germ cell cancer: a Multiinstitutional Medical Research Council/European Organization for Research and Treatment of Cancer Trial. *J Clin Oncol*, 1997: 15, 5.

[37] Bajorin D, Sarosdy MF, Pfister DG, et al.: Randomized trial of etoposide and cisplatin versus etoposide and carboplatin in patients with good-risk germ cell tumors. *J Clin Oncol*, 1993: 11, 598-608.

[38] Feldman DR, Bosl GJ, Sheinfield J, et al.: Medical treatment of advanced testicular cancer. *Journ Amer Med Assoc* 2008, 299: 672-684.

[39] Ehrlich Y, et al: Long-term follow-up of cisplatin combination chemotherapy in patients with disseminated nonseminomatous germ cell tumors: is a postchemotherapy retroperitoneal lymph node dissection needed after complete remission? *J Clin Oncol* 2010, 28: 531-6.

[40] Nichols CR, et al.: Randomized comparison of cisplatin and etoposide and either bleomycin or ifosfamide in treatment of advanced disseminated germ cell tumors: an Eastern Cooperative Oncology Group, Southwest Oncology Group, and Cancer and Leukemia Group B Study. *J Clin Oncol*, 1998: 16, 4.

[41] Hinton S, et al.: Cisplatin, etoposide and either bleomycin or ifosfamide in the treatment of disseminated germ cell tumors: final analysis of an intergroup trial. *Cancer*, 2003: 97, 8.

[42] De Wit R, et al.: Four cycles of BEP vs four cycles of VIP in patients with intermediate-prognosis metastatic testicular non-seminoma: a randomized study of the EORTC Genitourinary Tract Cancer Cooperative Group. European Organization for Research and Treatment of Cancer. *Br J Cancer*, 1998: 78, 6.

[43] Steyerberg EW, Keizer HJ, Fosså SD, et al.: Prediction of residual retroperitoneal mass histology after chemotherapy for metastatic nonseminomatous germ cell tumor: multivariate analysis of individual patient data from six study groups. *J Clin Oncol*, 1995: 13, 1177.

[44] Carver BS, Bianco FJ Jr, Shayegan B, et al.: Predicting teratoma in the retroperitoneum in men undergoing post-chemotherapy retroperitoneal lymph node dissection. *J Urol*, 2006:176, 100.

[45] Fizazi K, Tjulandin S, Salvioni R, et al.: Viable malignant cells after primary chemotherapy for disseminated nonseminomatous germ cell tumors: prognostic factors and role of postsurgery chemotherapy--results from an international study group. *J Clin Oncol*, 2001:19, 2647.

[46] Fizazi K, Oldenburg J, Dunant A, et al.: Assessing prognosis and optimizing treatment in patients with postchemotherapy viable nonseminomatous germ-cell tumors (NSGCT): results of the sCR2 international study. *Ann Oncol*, 2008: 19, 259.

[47] Coogan CL, Foster RS, Rowland RG, et al.: Postchemotherapy retroperitoneal lymph node dissection is effective therapy in selected patients with elevated tumor markers after primary chemotherapy alone. *Urology*, 1997: 50, 957.

[48] Beck SD, Patel MI, Sheinfeld J: Tumor marker levels in post-chemotherapy cystic masses: clinical implications for patients with germ cell tumors. J Urol, 2004: 171, 168.

[49] Murphy BP, Breeden ES, Donohue JP, et al.: Surgical Salvage of Chemorefractory Germ Cell Tumors. *Journ Clin Oncol* 1993, 11: 324-329.

[50] Beck SD, Foster RS, Bihrle R, et al.: Outcome analysis for patients with elevated serum tumor markers at postchemotherapy retroperitoneal lymph node dissection. *J Clin Oncol*, 2005: 23, 6149.

[51] Loehrer PJ, Lauer R, Roth BJ, et al.: Salvage therapy in recurrent germ cell cancer: ifosfamide and cisplatin plus either vinblastine or etoposide. *Ann Intern Med* 1988, 7:540–546.

[52] Motzer RJ, Cooper K, Geller NC, et al.: The role of ifosfamide plus cisplatin-based chemotherapy as salvage therapy for patients with refractory germ cell tumors. *Cancer* 1990, 66:2476–2481.

[53] Ghosn M, Droz JP, Theodore C, et al.: Salvage chemotherapy in refractory germ cell tumors with etoposide plus ifosfamide plus high-dose cisplatin. *Cancer* 1988, 61:24–27.

[54] Pizzocaro G, Salvioni R, Piva L: Modified cisplatin, etoposide (or vinblastine) and ifosfamide salvage therapy for male germ-cell tumors: long-term results. *Ann Oncol* 1992, 3:211–216.

[55] Harstrick A, Schmoll HJ, Wilke H, et al.: Cisplatin, etoposide and ifosfamide salvage therapy for refractory or relapsing germ cell carcinoma. *J Clin Oncol* 1991, 9:1549–1555.

[56] Loehrer PJ, Gonin R, Nichols CR, et al.: Vinblastine plus ifosfamide plus cisplatin as initial salvage therapy in recurrent germ cell tumor. *J Clin Oncol* 1998, 16:2500–2504.

[57] Kondagunta GV, Bacik J, Donadio A, et al.: Combination of paclitaxel, ifosfamide, and cisplatin is an effective second-line therapy for patients with relapsed testicular germ cell tumors. *J Clin Oncol* 2005; 23: 6549-6555.

[58] Einhorn LH, Williams SD, Chamness A, et al.: High-dose chemotherapy and stem-cell rescue for metastatic germ-cell tumors. *NEJM* 2007: 357: 3340-3348

[59] Schmoll HJ, et al. Long-term results of first-line sequential high-dose etoposide, ifosfamide, and cisplatin chemotherapy plus autologous stem cell support for patients with advanced metastatic germ cell cancer: an extended phase I/II study of the German Testicular Cancer Study Group. *Journ Clin Onc* 2003, 21: 4083-4091.

[60] Motzer RJ, Nichols CJ, Margolin KA, et al.: Phase III Randomized Trial of Conventional-Dose Chemotherapy With or Without High-Dose Chemotherapy and Autologous Hematopoietic Stem-Cell Rescue As First-Line Treatment for Patients With Poor-Prognosis Metastatic Germ Cell Tumors. *Journ Clin Onc* 2007, 25: 247-256.

[61] Einhorn LH, Brames MJ, Juliar B, Williams SD. Phase II study of paclitaxel plus gemcitabine salvage chemotherapy for germ cell tumors after progression following high-dose chemotherapy with tandem transplant. *J Clin Oncol* 2007, 25: 513-6.

[62] Mulherin BP, Brames MJ, Einhorn LH: Long-term survival with paclitaxel and gemcitabine for germ cell tumors after progression following high-dose chemotherapy with tandem transplants. *ASCO* 2011 abstract.

[63] Kollmannsberger C, et al.: Activity of oxaliplatin in patients with relapsed or cisplatin-refractory germ cell cancer: study of the German Testicular Cancer Study Group. *Journ Clin Onc* 2002, 20: 2031-2037.

[64] Bokemeyer C, et al.: Combination chemotherapy with gemcitabine, oxaliplatin, and paclitaxel in patients with cisplatin-refractory or multiply relapsed germ-cell tumors: a study of the German Testicular Cancer Study Group. *Ann Onc* 2008, 19: 448-453.

[65] Reilekova K, Mego M, Svcova-Mila Z, et al.: Prognostic factors in patients with relapsed or primary refractory germ cell tumors. *Neoplasma* 2009, 56: 215-223.

[66] Beyer J, Stenning S, Gerl A, et al.: High-dose versus conventional-dose chemotherapy as first-line salvage treatment in patients with non-seminomatous germ-cell tumors: a matched-pair analysis. *Ann Onc* 2002, 13:599-605.

[67] Lorch A, et al.: Prognostic factors in relapsed or refractory male germ cell tumors: results from an international study of 1593 patients. *J Clin Oncol* 27:15s, 2009 (suppl; abstr 5030).

[68] Murphy BP, Breeden ES, Donohue JP, et al.: Surgical Salvage of Chemorefractory Germ Cell Tumors. *Journ Clin Oncol* 1993, 11: 324-329.

[69] Lorch A, Rick O, Wündisch, et al.: High Dose Chemotherapy as Salvage Treatment for Unresectable Late Relapse Germ Cell Tumors. *Journ Urol* 2010, 184: 168-173.

[70] Motzer R, Bosl G, Heelan R, et al: Residual Mass: An Indication for Further Therapy in Patients With Advanced Seminoma Following Systemic Chemotherapy. *J Clin Oncol* 1987, 5:1064-1070.

[71] Bosl GJ, Mencel P, and Motzer RJ: Management of residual mass in advanced seminoma: results and recommendations from the Memorial Sloan-Kettering Cancer Center. *Journ Clin Oncol* 1996, 14: 454-460.

[72] Schultz SM, et al.: Management of postchemotherapy residual mass in patients with advanced seminoma: Indiana University experience. *Journ Clin Onc* 1989, 7: 1497-1503.

[73] Becherer A, DeSantis M, Karanikas G, et al: FDG PET is superior to CT in the prediction of viable tumour in post-chemotherapy seminoma residuals. *European Journal of Radiology* 2005, 54:284-8.

[74] Lewis DA, Tann M, Kesler K, et al: Positron Emission Tomography Scans in Postchemotherapy Seminoma Patients With Residual Masses: A Retrospective Review From Indiana University Hospital. *J Clin Oncol* 2006, 24:e54-55.

[75] Kesler KA, Einhorn LH: Multimodality Treatment of Germ Cell Tumors of the Mediastinum. *Thorac Surg Clin*, 2009: 19, 63-69.

[76] Hartmann JT, Nichols CR, Droz JP, et al.: Hematologic disorders associated with primary mediastinal nonseminomatous germ cell tumors. *J Natl Cancer Inst*, 2000: 92, 54.

[77] Nichols CR, Roth BJ, Heerema N, et al.: Hematologic neoplasia associated with primary mediastinal germ-cell tumors. *NEJM*, 1990: 322, 1425.

[78] Ladanyi M, Samaniego F, Reuter VE, et al.: Cytogenetic and immunohistochemical evidence for the germ cell origin of a subset of acute leukemias associated with mediastinal germ cell tumors. *J Natl Cancer Inst*, 1990: 82, 221.

[79] Williams SD, et al.: Treatment of disseminated germ-cell tumors with cisplatin, bleomycin, and either vinblastine or etoposide. *NEJM*, 1987: 316, 23.

[80] Jules-Elysee K, White DA: Bleomycin-induced pulmonary toxicity. *Clin Chest Med.*, 1990: 11, 1.

[81] Loehrer PJ Sr, et al.: Importance of bleomycin in favorable-prognosis disseminated germ cell tumors: an Eastern Cooperative Oncology Group trial. *J Clin Oncol*, 1995: 13, 2.

[82] Brydøy M, et al.: Observational study of prevalence of long-term Raynaud-like phenomena and neurological side effects in testicular cancer survivors. *J Natl Cancer Inst*, 2009: 101, 24.

[83] Glendenning JL et al.: Long-term neurologic and peripheral vascular toxicity after chemotherapy treatment of testicular cancer. *Cancer*, 2010: 116, 10.

[84] Bokemeyer C, et al.: Analysis of risk factors for cisplatin-induced ototoxicity in patients with testicular cancer. *Br J Cancer*, 1998: 77, 8.

[85] Strumberg D, et al.: Evaluation of long-term toxicity in patients after cisplatin-based chemotherapy for non-seminomatous testicular cancer. *Ann Oncol*, 2002: 13, 2.

[86] Fosså SD, Abyholm T, Aakvaag A: Spermatogenesis and hormonal status after orchiectomy for cancer and before supplementary treatment. *Eur Urol,* 1984: 10, 3.

[87] Petersen PM, Skakkebaek NE, Rørth M, Giwercman A: Semen quality and reproductive hormones before and after orchiectomy in men with testicular cancer. *J Urol*, 1999: 161, 3.

[88] Lampe H, et al.: Fertility after chemotherapy for testicular germ cell cancers. *J Clin Oncol,* 1997: 15, 1.

[89] Aass N, Fosså SD, Theodorsen L, Norman N: Prediction of long-term gonadal toxicity after standard treatment for testicular cancer. *Eur J Cancer*, 1991: 27, 9.

[90] Brydøy M, et al.: Paternity following treatment for testicular cancer. *J Natl Cancer Inst,* 2005: 97, 21.

[91] Cullen MH, et al.: Short-course adjuvant chemotherapy in high-risk stage I nonseminomatous germ cell tumors of the testis: a Medical Research Council report. *J Clin Oncol*, 1996: 14, 4.

[92] Fosså SD, Theodorsen L, Norman N, Aabyholm T: Recovery of impaired pretreatment spermatogenesis in testicular cancer. *Fertil Steril*, 1990: 54, 3.

[93] Petersen PM, et al.: Dose-dependent impairment of testicular function in patients treated with cisplatin-based chemotherapy for germ cell cancer. *Ann Oncol*, 1994: 5, 4.

[94] Brydøy M , et al.: Paternity following treatment for testicular cancer. *J Natl Cancer* Inst, 2005: 97, 21.

[95] Ishikawa T, Kamidono S, Fujisawa M: Fertility after high-dose chemotherapy for testicular cancer. *Urology*, 2004: 63, 1.

[96] Gerl A, et al.: The impact of chemotherapy on Leydig cell function in long term survivors of germ cell tumors. *Cancer*, 2001: 91, 7.

[97] Travis LB, et al.: Second cancers among 40,576 testicular cancer patients: focus on long-term survivors. *J Natl Cancer Inst*, 2005: 97, 18.

[98] Kollmannsberger C, Hartmann JT, Kanz L, Bokemeyer C: Therapy-related malignancies following treatment of germ cell cancer. *Int J Cancer*, 1999: 83, 6.

[99] Nichols CR, et al.: Secondary leukemia associated with a conventional dose of etoposide: review of serial germ cell tumor protocols. *J Natl Cancer Inst*, 1993: 85, 1.

[100] Houck W, Abonour R, Vance G, Einhorn LH: Secondary leukemias in refractory germ cell tumor patients undergoing autologous stem-cell transplantation using high-dose etoposide. *J Clin Oncol*, 2004: 22, 11.

[101] Testicular cancer staging. *AJCC Cancer Staging Manual*, Seventh Edition, 2010. Published by Springer New York, Inc.

Section 7. Penile Cancer

Simon Horenblas and Philippe E. Spiess
Section Editors

In: Essentials and Updates in Urologic Oncology
Editor: Philippe E. Spiess

ISBN: 978-1-62081-494-9
© 2013 Nova Science Publishers, Inc.

Chapter XXIX

Surgical Management of the Primary Penile Lesion

Majid Shabbir[*][1], *Nicholas Watkin*[2] *and David Ralph*[3]

[1]Department of Andrology, Institute of Urology,
University College Hospital, London, UK
[2]Penile Cancer and Reconstructive Andrology Unit, St. George's Hospital, London, UK
[3]Department of Andrology, Institute of Urology,
University College London Hospital, London, UK

Abstract

The surgical management of penile cancer has changed significantly over the last decade. Progression in the understanding of this rare malignancy, by pooling of expertise and resources in specialist centres, has challenged the conventional radical surgical approach to penile cancer. While such surgery was effective, the emasculating nature of this treatment had serious psychological and sexual morbidity. Challenges to the traditional belief that a 2 cm margin was required for adequate clearance have paved the way to the concept of new surgical techniques that aim to minimize the impact of the disease and its treatment on the quality of life by preserving as much penile tissue and function as possible, without compromising oncological control. A range of different techniques can be used to effectively treat the primary lesion, and are tailored according to the stage, grade, and extent of the disease. In this chapter we review the current range of different penile preserving surgical techniques used in the modern day management of penile cancer, primarily categorised by stage and location, and critically evaluate their role and efficacy compared to alternative non surgical treatment modalities. In cases where penile preservation is not possible, a range of phallic reconstructive techniques can be used, and the various options are also explored in this chapter.

* Author for Correspondence: Majid Shabbir, Department of Andrology, Institute of Urology, University College London Hospital, 235 Euston Road, London, e-mail: majidshabbir@hotmail.com

Introduction

Penile cancer is a rare malignancy, accounting for <1% of all malignancies in men in Western Europe and the US, with a reported incidence of approximately 1 per 100,000 men per year in England and Wales [1]. Although it is considerably more common in developing countries, where it can account for up to 10% of all male malignancies [2], the low number of cases worldwide have delayed progression and understanding of this disease. There are no randomized control trials comparing different treatment modalities, and most recommendations for treatment are based on small retrospective case series, with relatively short follow up.

The classical approach to treating the primary lesion is radical surgery, either with partial or total penectomy, excising the lesion with a clear margin of 2cm. While this provides excellent oncological control (recurrence rates 0.7% and 4.6% for total and partial penectomy respectively in pooled analysis [3]), the emasculating nature of this procedure is associated with significant psychological and sexual morbidity [4]. This is especially relevant when planning treatment in the cohort of men who develop the disease at a younger age (approximately 20% <40yrs at presentation [1]).

Studies over the last 10 years have challenged the need for such extensive margins. Agrawal et al. reviewed 64 partial and total penectomy specimens, to determine the microscopic spread of tumour beyond the visible tumour margin [5]. They found only 19% of cases had microscopic extension beyond the gross tumour margin. Of these, 75% were < 5mm form the margin. Hoffman et al. reported on their experience of 14 patients who underwent conventional surgery for penile cancer [6]. Half the group had excision margins of < 10mm, although this had no bearing on recurrence as no patient in their series developed recurrence after 33 months follow up. In a series looking at penile preserving techniques, approximately half the 51 patients in the series had clear surgical margins of < 10mm, including 33% with margins < 5mm. Despite this, the local recurrence rate was only 4% after a mean follow up of 26 months, confirming that comparable oncological control to conventional radical surgery could be achieved with excision margins of only a few millimetres [7].

The result of these studies has been a paradigm shift in the surgical management of the primary penile lesion, moving away from more radical surgery to a variety of penile preserving techniques. The use of these techniques has been more prevalent in Western countries such as the UK, where approximately 80% of malignant lesions present on the glans penis and prepuce and are more amenable to an organ conserving approach [8, 9]. Selection of the most appropriate technique is dependent on the stage and location of the primary tumour and the various options are discussed further below. Treatment is best tailored to the individual, taking into account the lesion, the effect of surgery on penile length, the patient's age and co-morbidity. Few would challenge the role of more radical surgery in the treatment of stage T4, high-grade stage T3 or proximal stage T2 disease, which would not suitable for a penile preserving approach. Knowledge and expertise with the different surgical techniques is vital to ensure the best cosmetic, functional, psychological and oncological outcome in patients who present with this potentially devastating disease.

Treatment Options for Primary Penile Lesions at Stage and Location

Carcinoma in Situ (Tis) and Non Invasive Verrucous Carcinoma (Ta)

While surgery has an important role in the treatment of penile carcinoma in situ and Ta disease, the non-invasive nature of these lesions makes them amenable to a number of different non-surgical treatment modalities of which topical chemotherapy, topical immunotherapy, and laser ablation are the most commonly used. Selection of the best therapy depends on the size, site and type of lesion.

Topical Therapies

Topical chemotherapy with 5% 5-Fluorouracil (5-FU) is the most commonly used first line treatment. It is best suited to immunocompetent patients with well defined solitary lesions, and has poor efficacy in the immunosuppressed or those with widespread 'field changes' [10]. It is usually applied topically for between 4-6 weeks on alternate days, and is safe, with low morbidity and minimal systemic absorption. Early studies reported sustained response rates approaching 100% at 5 years, although the numbers of patients treated in these studies is small (<10) [11].

Non or partial responders can be treated with immunotherapy using topical 5% Imiquimod cream for a similar length of time as second line treatment [12]. Although the exact mechanism of action of this novel immunomodulatory therapy is unclear, it is believed to activate the patients own immune system via toll-like receptors leading to secretion of cytokines such as interferon-α, tumour necrosis factor and various interleukins (IFNα, IL-1,6,12, TNFα). Imiquimod can be applied for 5 days a week for a period of 4 to 6 weeks, although the frequency can be reduced provided that the inflammatory response is maintained [13]. While success has been reported in a number of case reports and small case series, no large scale long term efficacy data is currently available [10,12].

Laser Therapy

Carbon dioxide (CO_2) and Neodymium: yttrium aluminium garnet (Nd:YAG) lasers have been used as first line therapy with reasonable response rates and good cosmetic and functional results. The CO_2 laser has a tissue penetration of 2-2.5mm and has the advantage of also being able to be used as a scalpel to excise tissue for histological analysis by direct focussing of the beam. Ablations sites generally heal in 3-4 weeks. The Nd:YAG laser has a tissue penetration of 3-5mm, but causes tissue coagulation preventing histological diagnosis, and a risk of understaging the disease. Larger lesions can be treated using this laser, but ablation sites can take up to 2-3 months to heal. Treatment with either of these lasers is usually well tolerated, with minor complications ranging from minor pain and bleeding at treatment sites, to preputial lymphoedema in those patients who have retained their foreskin [14]. In one study of 19 patients treated with laser therapy, 26% required successful re-treatment for histologically confirmed Tis recurrence after a mean follow up of 32 months, while 1 patient (5%) progressed to invasive disease [15]. In a more recent study assessing the combined use of both lasers, 13/67 (19%) patients had disease recurrence, with upgrading from the original tumour in 3/13 (23%) cases [16]. Higher recurrence rates after laser treatment may reflect a tendency to tackle larger tumours with this minimally invasive approach compared to those treated by other topical therapies. Lasers have been used to treat lesions up to stage T2, but this approach has been shown to be associated with higher overall recurrence (48%), and evidence of nodal progression in 23% [17], highlighting the need for careful case selection.

Surgical Excision

Surgery has an important and emerging role in the treatment of penile carcinoma in situ. Circumcision forms an essential part of the management of premalignant conditions, not only to remove the lesion if confined solely to the prepuce, but also to prevent persistence of an environment suited to HPV infection, chronic inflammation and progression to invasive disease. It facilitates follow up and clinical examination, which is essential with any minimally invasive approach, and can prevent the development of preputial oedema associated with laser therapy. When performing the circumcision, an adequate clearance margin much be achieved. In difficult cases, a swab soaked in 5% acetic acid applied to the penis for up to 5 minutes has been used to help detect occult areas of CIS, staining the abnormal areas white ('acetowhite' reaction), to help guide the extent of excision [9]. However, the use of visual inspection after acetic acid staining has been discredited by many due to its poor sensitivity for detecting the HPV component of CIS (50%), and high false positive staining[18, 19,20,]. As a consequence its use is not advocated by all

Surgical excision of CIS affecting the glans penis has been advocated for patients who have extensive field change, in those unlikely or unwilling to adhere to strict treatment and surveillance protocols, and those with recurrent disease following other conservative therapies. Repeated topical therapies can result in an unsightly scarred and denuded glans that can make clinical monitoring difficult. A total glans resurfacing procedure (TGR) provides the best surgical approach to treatment, excising the diseased area with an adequate margin followed by split thickness skin graft. This technique was first described by Bracka for the management of severe BXO, but has been adapted for Tis/Ta disease [21,22].

Technique of Glans Resurfacing

The procedure is performed under a general anaesthetic with preoperative antibiotic cover and with the use of a tourniquet. The glans epithelium is marked in quadrants from the meatus to the coronal sulcus. A perimeatal and circumcoronal incision is performed, and the glans epithelium and sub-epithelial tissue is then excised from the underlying spongiosum, starting from the meatus to the coronal sulcus for each quadrant (see figure 1). Deep spongiosal biopsies are taken from each quadrant for separate analysis to ensure no invasion. A split thickness skin graft, harvested from the thigh with an air dermatome, is used to cover the 'exposed' glans. Graft thickness can range from 0.008 to 0.016 inch. The graft is sutured and quilted using multiple 5-0 interrupted vicryl rapide sutures. The patient is then catheterised (14F silicone catheter) and the glans penis is dressed with a soft silicone coated dressing (Mepitel) and gauze followed by a foam dressing to help immobilise the graft. The dressing is left in place for 5 days with the patient remaining on strict bed rest for the first 48 hours. On the 5th day the dressing and catheter are removed, and the patient is discharged with wound care advice for review in clinic the following week. This approach allows preservation of maximal penile length, form and function and combines good oncological control with a good cosmetic appearance (see figure 2). In a series of 10 patients treated with total glans resurfacing for recurrent, refractory or extensive disease, no patient had evidence of disease recurrence after a mean follow up of 30 months. In addition, over 80% were sexually active within 3 months of surgery [22].

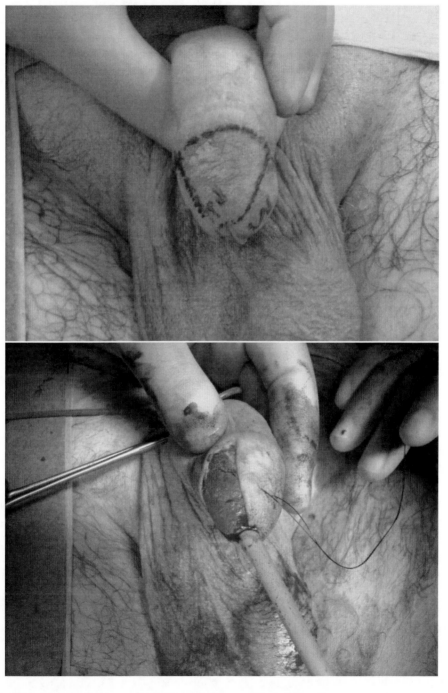

Figure 1. Glans penis marked in quadrants for total glans resurfacing dissection.

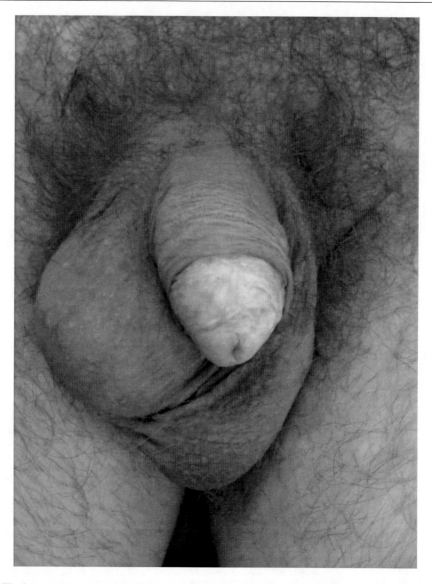

Figure 2. Final post op appearance total glans resurfacing.

One of the main advantages of a surgical approach is its combined diagnostic and therapeutic ability. Whilst completely removing the diseased epithelium, total surgical excision also allows more accurate histopathological staging and diagnosis than the smaller incisional biopsies used with less invasive topical therapies. In a recent series assessing the use of glans resurfacing for CIS as a primary therapy, 10/25 patients (40%) had evidence of invasive carcinoma on the final pathological specimens despite all 25 patients having had pre-operative incisional biopsies confirming evidence of CIS only [23]. This is alarming, given the fact that most patients diagnosed with CIS of the glans are primarily treated on the basis of incisional biopsies only, and are usually treated with topical chemotherapy or laser first line, which would not tackle any invasive element adequately. It may also go some way to explaining the higher recurrence rate with laser therapy (26%), compared to the low recurrence rates of surgical series (0-4%) [15,22,23]. These findings would favour the primary use of surgery to avoid the risk of understaging, inadequate treatment and subsequent progression and may lead to a shift in our approach to managing glanular CIS in the future.

Alternative Surgical Approaches

Partial Glans Resurfacing

In addition to total glans resurfacing, partial glans resurfacing (PGR) has also been used as a primary surgical approach for glanular CIS. This technique involves the same principles as TGR, but is used in cases of solitary, localised foci of CIS affecting <50% of the glans. This approach has the advantage of conserving normal glans skin, allowing better preservation of glanular sensation, and achieving a final appearance closer to the original glans. This approach would be more attractive to younger, sexually active men (see figure 3). In a reported series of primary partial and total glans resurfacing, PGR was associated with a very high risk of positive surgical margins (67%). 40% of this group required further surgical intervention, of which 13% was for positive CIS at the margin and 26% was due to unexpected invasive disease in the final specimen. Patients were still amenable to further penile preserving techniques, including TGR and glansectomy.

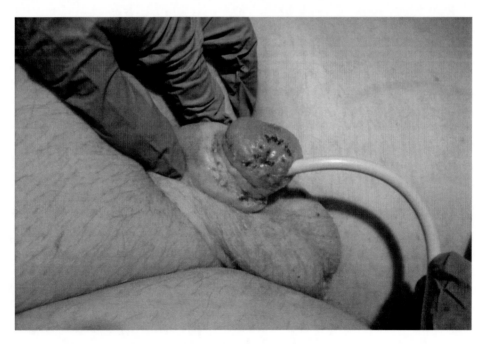

Figure 3. Immediate post op appearance partial glans resurfacing.

Despite the higher positive margin rate, and need for further surgery, the PGR sub-group still had no cases of recurrence or progression after a mean follow up of 29 months [23]. While the exact role and position of PGR in the management of CIS remains unclear, this technique may have a limited role in the management of glanular CIS in carefully selected cases.

Mohs' Micrographic Surgery

An alternative surgical approach is excision using Mohs' micrographic surgery. This techniques involves removing the entire lesion in thin sections, with concurrent histological examination to ensure clear margins microscopically [24]. This technique allows maximal preservation of normal penile tissue, but is difficult and time consuming, requiring both a surgeon and pathologist trained in the technique to ensure adequate oncological clearance. A recent review of outcome from this technique reported a high (32%) recurrence rate [25], and the uptake and use of the technique worldwide has been very limited.

T1 Lesions Invading the Sub-Epithelial Connective Tissue of the Foreskin and Glans Penis

T1 lesions of the foreskin are effectively treated by wide local excision with circumcision. Care must be taken to ensure adequate clearance margins are achieved and exclude concurrent glanular disease.

Small, discrete T1 lesions are the glans can be treated by wide local excision, or partial glansectomy. If the defect after excision is small, and not too close to the urethral meatus, primary closure can be achieved with only minimal glans deformity. Larger defects may be difficult to close without tilting the glans and causing problems directing micturition. In such cases a split skin graft may be required to cover the defect and improve the final cosmetic appearance and functional outcome.

In cases of more extensive glanular invovlement, a total glans resurfacing (TGR) can be used. The procedure is no different to that used for non invasive lesions, and is effective for T1 disease as this technique involves complete removal of the glans epithelium and sub epithelial layers. In a series assessing outcome of TGR for glanular CIS, 7 patients were found to have unexpected foci of G2pT1 disease which was fully excised. No recurrences have been seen in this subset after mean follow up of 29 months (23).

Partial glansectomy and TGR are best suited to those patients with 'low risk' T1a disease (well −moderately differentiated G1/G2 disease, with no evidence of lymphovascular invasion). Close surveillance and follow up is essential to ensure early detection of any recurrences. Careful patient selection is vital, and these techniques should only be offered to those well motivated and compliant enough to ensure close surveillance and success form this surgical approach. Local recurrence, or positive surgical margins, should be treated by total glansectomy, and early detection and 'salvage' surgery has a high success rate, and no adverse effect on disease specific survival [26,27]. Patients with 'high risk' T1b disease (poorly or undifferentiated G3 disease, or evidence of lymphovascular invasion) are better managed by glansectomy at the outset and this technique is described in detail below.

T2 Disease – Tumour Invading the Corpus Spongiosum

The management of T2 lesions confined to the glans has benefitted greatly from developments in penile preserving techniques. Glansectomy is the best surgical approach for T2 disease affecting the corpus spongiosum, and high risk T1b disease. This procedure utilises knowledge of the anatomical plains between the corpora cavernosa and corpus spongiosum first described by Austoni et al [28]. In this procedure, the glans penis is dissected from the corpora cavernosa, with the subsequent formation of a new urethral meatus at the tip of the shaft. The procedure can be combined with a split skin graft to create a 'neo-glans' with excellent cosmesis and a near normal appearance, or can utilise advancement flaps of shaft skin to cover the corporal tips to maintain a functional penis, albeit with a less satisfactory cosmetic appearance.

Technique of Glansectomy and Reconstruction

The procedure is performed under a general anaesthetic with preoperative antibiotic cover and with the use of a tourniquet. A circumferential incision is made a centimetre below the corona on the distal shaft down towards Buck's fascia. A plane of dissection is then created either above the dartos fascia, or below Buck fascia, dependent on the depth and extent of the glanular lesion. The glans 'cap' is dissected free of the corporal heads, taking care not to stray into the spongiosum (see figure 4). Frozen sections from the corporal tips and distal urethral are taken intra-operatively to ensure adequate clearance margins. In cases where the frozen section yields a positive margin, further 'shaving' of the coporal tips or urethra can be performed prior to any planned reconstruction.

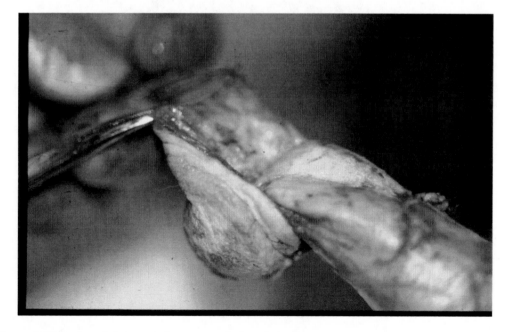

Figure 4. Dissection of glans penis from copora during glansectomy.

As part of the reconstruction, the urethra is spatulated and can also be mobilised, if its position is too ventral, to a more centred location at the tip of the penis. The shaft skin is then secured 2-3 cm from the tip of the penis using multiple 4-0 interrupted vicryl rapide sutures. A split thickness skin graft, harvested from the thigh with an air dermatome, is used to cover the 'exposed' glans. Graft thickness can range from 0.008 to 0.016 inch. The graft is sutured and quilted using multiple 5-0 interrupted vicryl rapide sutures. The patient is then catheterised (14F silicone catheter) and the glans penis is dressed with a soft silicone coated dressing (Mepitel) and gauze followed by a foam dressing to help immobilise the graft. The dressing is left in place for 5 days with the patient remaining on strict bed rest for the first 48 hours. On the 5th day the dressing and catheter may be removed if the graft has taken well, and the patient is discharged with wound care advice for review in clinic the following week. This approach allows maximal preservation of penile length, form and function and combines good oncological control with a good cosmetic appearance (see figure 5).

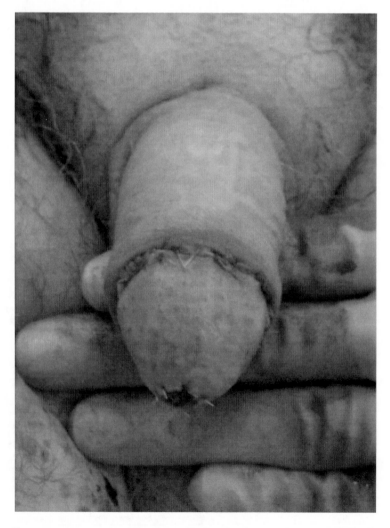

Figure 5. Immediate post op appearance after glansectomy with reconstruction using split skin graft.

Outcome

Hatzichritou et al. reported seven cases of verrucous carcinomas treated by glansectomy without reconstruction [29]. Only one patient required further surgery due to local recurrence at three months. All patients returned to normal sexual function 1 month post operatively and all were alive and disease free after 18–65 months follow up. Morelli et al reported their experience of glansectomy and reconstruction in 15 patients with glans confined SCC. After a mean follow up of 36 months, all patients were disease free, with no cases of local recurrence. All were fully sexually active 2-6 months post operatively, and while all had reduced neo-glans sensitivity, all had preserved orgasm and ejaculatory function highlighting the excellent functional preservation seen with this surgical approach [30]. In the largest reported series to date, only 3 local recurrences were seen in 72 patients treated by glansectomy and reconstruction after a mean follow up of 27 months [31]. The reccurence rate of 4% is similar to that reported from more radical partial penectomy series, highlighting the comparable oncological outcome using a more penile preserving approach.

Role of Radiotherapy

Radiotherapy can be used as an alternative penile preserving treatment for selected small T1-T2 lesions affecting the glans and distal corpora. Ideal candidates should have exophytic lesions <4cm. Treatment can be in the form of external beam radiotherapy, or brachytherapy, although the latter has better results. Treatment is usually combined with circumcision to improve exposure and assessment, and prevent secondary phimosis. Although radiotherapy allows penile preservation, the resultant penis never looks or functions the same again. Local recurrences after treatment are high and have been reported to be up to 40% after external beam radiotherapy, and approximately 20% after brachytherapy [32,33]. It may take several years for recurrence to become apparent because of the difficulty distinguishing active tumour from extensive chronic skin changes seen after radiotherapy. While most cases require radical surgery to regain local control, many are often amenable to penile preserving surgery. In a study assessing patients referred with chronic or recurrent ulceration post radiotherapy the mean time from initial treatment to referral for surgery was 9 years. 14/17patients were managed with glansectomy and reconstruction. No patient had problems with graft take, and after a mean follow up of 3 years, 16/17 were disease free [34]. The emergence of penile preserving surgical techniques has considerably reduced the role of radiotherapy in the management of penile cancer.

T2 Disease - Tumour Invading
the Corpus Cavernosum and T3 Disease -
Invading the Urethra

Evidence of disease extension into the corporeal bodies or urethra requires more extensive resection. The surgical procedure needs to be tailored to the site and size of the lesion, taking into account the overall penile length. The mainstay of treatment for this tumour type is partial penectomy, although resection margins of 2 cm are not required. Excision is combined with frozen section to ensure clear margins are achieved. Subsequent reconstructive techniques can be used to achieve a good cosmetic appearance (see figure 6). If the resultant phallus post resection is too short, lengthening procedures can be used to allow the patient to stand to void, or have penetrative sex. In certain cases where the disease is very proximal, or the resultant phallus too short, a sub-total or total penectomy and perineal urethrostomy may be more appropriate, and these techniques are discussed below.

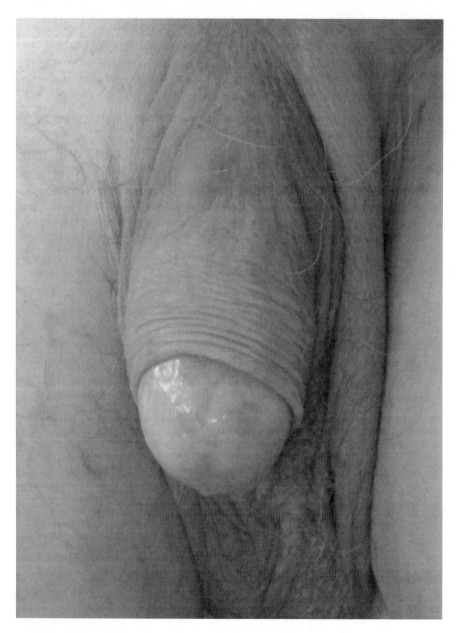

Figure 6. Post op partial penectomy with reconstruction using split skin graft.

Technique of Partial Penectomy and Reconstruction

The procedure is performed under a general anaesthetic with preoperative antibiotic cover and with the use of a tourniquet. A circumferential incision is made a 1-2cm below the proximal limit of the tumour. The shaft skin is degloved to expose the underlying corpora. The corpora are incised to generate a "fish-mouth" appearance that will allow a vertical closure in the midline. A safe margin of 0.5-1cm is considered for partial penectomy (7). The urethra is divided to leave an additional length of approximately 1cm from the end of the corporal dissection to allow for subsequent spatulation and reconstruction. Sections of the distal corporal margins and urethra are sent for frozen section to ensure adequate clearance. The corpora are closed using an absorbable 2/0 PDS suture. The overlying superficial dartos layer can then be reconstructed over the tips of the closed corpora, creating an excellent bed for the subsequent skin graft. As part of the reconstruction, the urethra is spatulated and can also be mobilised, if its position is too ventral, to a more central location at the tip of the penis. The shaft skin is then secured 2-3 cm from the tip of the penis using multiple 4-0 interrupted vicryl rapide sutures. A split thickness skin graft, harvested from the thigh with an air dermatome, is used to cover the 'exposed' glans. Graft thickness can range from 0.008 to 0.016 inch. The graft is sutured and quilted using multiple 5-0 interrupted vicryl rapide sutures. The patient is then catheterised (14F silicone catheter) and the glans penis is dressed with a soft silicone coated dressing (Mepitel) and gauze followed by a foam dressing to help immobilise the graft. The dressing is left in place for 5 days with the patient remaining on strict bed rest for the first 48 hours. On the 5th day the dressing and catheter may be removed if the graft has taken well, and the patient is discharged with wound care advice for review in clinic the following week.

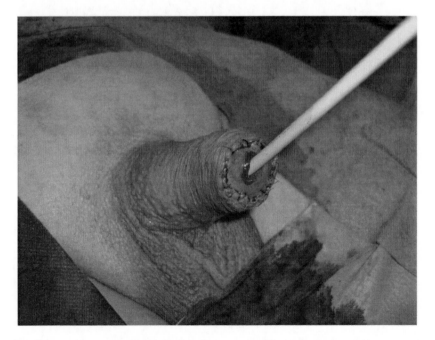

Figure 7. Use of shaft skin advancement flaps for closure instead of reconstruction with split skin graft.

In cases where reconstruction using skin graft is not used or appropriate, shaft skin advancement flaps can be used to cover the corpora and meet the spatulated urethra (see figure 7). This approach often suits older patients who are medically unfit, or unkeen for reconstruction. It may also be more suited to patients where cosmesis or sexual function is less important, although it is still possible to have erections and intercourse after this type of surgery. It has a significantly shorter operative time, and less need for restrictive bed rest, or complex dressings associated with reconstruction and skin graft, and remains a good option in a selected subset of patients.

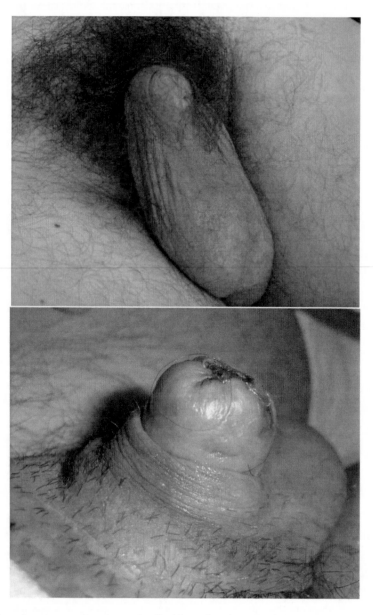

Figure 8. Division of suspensory ligament and split skin graft to increase apparent length of penile stump can be enough to allow a patient to stand and void again.

Penile Lengthening Procedures

In cases where the final penis is too short, subsequent lengthening procedures can allow gain of an additional 2cm of length. This is primarily achieved by dividing the suspensory ligament below the pubic arch, and placing a silicone buffer to preserve the created space and prevent redevelopment of adhesions between the penis and pubic arch. Additional procedures that can be used to improve the apparent penile length include flattening of the suprapubic fat pad to prevent subsequent burying of the penis, and excision of the scrotal web using a VY – plasty to improve the apparent length of the ventral shaft. These additional procedures can provide enough length gain to allow the patient to stand to pass urine comfortably, a major psychological factor for many men undergoing penile cancer surgery (see figure 8).

Outcome

Partial penectomy is a safe oncological procedure, and has a reliably low recurrence rate. Studies over the last decade have confirmed this, with local recurrence rates of between 0 – 7% (mean 4%) reported by different groups worldwide after a follow up of 33- 69 months (mean 50 months) [6, 35-39].

Technique of Total Penectomy and Perineal Urethrostomy

For cases of more proximal T2 or T3 disease, the safest approach is a total penectomy and formation of a perineal urethrostomy. This procedure is performed under a general anaesthetic with the patient's legs up in Lloyd –Davis stirrups. A circumferential incision is made around the base of the phallus after assessment of the scrotal skin to ensure there is adequate tissue to allow for an advancement scrotal flap closure. The incision is deepened through the subcutaneous tissue, taking care to identify and preserve the chordal structures on both sides, and to identify and ligate the vessels of the dorsal venous complex. The urethra is identified, and the dissected free of the corpra cavernosa back as far as the bulbar urethra to allow it to reach the perineal skin tension free for the subsequent urethrostomy. The corpora are dissected back towards their origin under the pubic rami, and divided with a safe 2 cm margin. The cut ends are then closed with a 2/0 PDS suture to ensure haemostasis.

The perineal urethrostomy must be formed with a straight and spatulated urethra, to prevent obstruction due to kinking of the urethra, or stenosis at the new meatus. A midline location should be selected ideally away from the back of the scrotum to prevent soaking during urination. An inverted U- shape incision is made through the perineum to deliver the urethra. The apex of the subsequent U shaped flap is sutured to the apex of the ventrally spatulated urethra (approximately 1cm spatulation) using interrupted 3/0 vicryl suture. The rest of the urethra is then sutured to the U shaped incision to allow wide spatulation, and prevent the most common complication associated of meatal stenosis (up to 9%) [39]. The patient is then catheterised (18F silicone catheter) and Redivac drains are inserted by the penile and perineal wounds. The penile wound is closed using the scrotal skin flap advancement, using a sub-cuticular layer of interrupted 2/0 vicryl, and an interrupted 3/0 vicryl rapide for the skin. The urethrostomy is dressed using a Jelonet (paraffin gauze) and plain gauze dressing, with a padded pressure dressing for the first 24 hours. The drains are removed after 48 hours if the drainage has remained <50mls for 24 hours, and the catheter is removed once the urethrostomy has fully healed (at least one week). While this surgery is more emasculating than a partial penectomy, it provides the best oncological control for proximal high risk disease and avoids leaving the patient with a phallus too short to direct their urinary stream. Patients require careful counselling pre-operatively about their final cosmetic and functional outcome (see figure 9). Selected cases will be suitable for subsequent phalloplasty reconstruction once full oncological control of the primary and regional lymph nodes has been achieved.

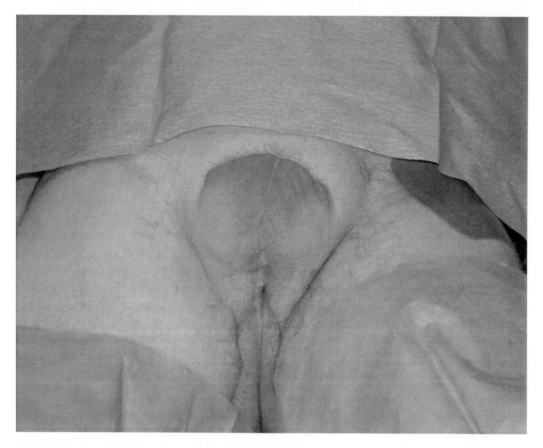

Figure 9. Post op total penectomy with formation of perineal urethrostomy.

Outcome

Total penectomy is a safe oncological procedure and has a very low risk of recurrence. Studies over the last decade have confirmed this, with no local recurrences reported in approximately 100 cases from several series worldwide [6, 35-38].

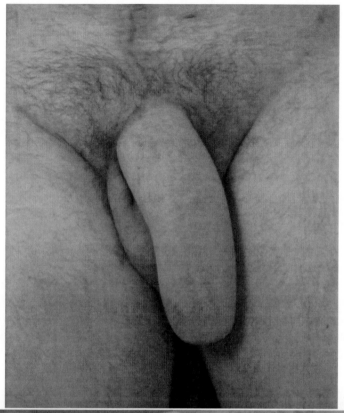

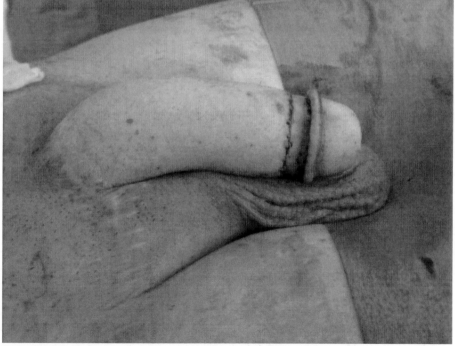

Figure 10. Reconstruction using a radial artery phalloplasty, with subsequent glans resculpting prior to insertion of an inflatable penile prosthesis.

Total Phallic Reconstruction

The more common form of phalloplasty used for penile cancer reconstruction is the Radial Artery Phalloplasty (RAP), made using a radial artery free flap to create a new urethra and phallus using a 'tube-in-a-tube' technique [40]. This procedure allows formation of a phallus, which allows the patient to once again be able to stand to pass urine, and may also have an inflatable penile prosthesis inserted at a later stage to allow return of sexual function. The phalloplasty is not suitable for all, and is best suited to those patients who are healthy, young, well motivated, and non smokers. They should be cancer free, and have stable disease with a favourable prognosis.

The reconstruction is performed in stages, with the first being the creation of the new phallus (see figure 10). For this, one team harvests the forearm flap from the non dominant forearm, while a second surgical team prepares the pubic and groin area to receive the flap, identifying and preparing the urethra, femoral artery, saphenous veins and ilioingiunal nerves for subsequent anastamosis. The defect on the forearm is covered using a full thickness skin graft harvested from the skin-fold between the buttocks and upper thigh. Subsequent stages involve re-sculpting of the phallus to create a neo-glans using further full thickness skin grafts, and insertion of an inflatable penile prosthesis, usually with 3 monthly intervals between each stage (see figure 10). The whole process may take between 6 months and a year to complete.

Outcome

Garaffa et al reported their experience of RAP in 15 patients who had previously undergone subtotal penectomy for T2-T3 tumours [41]. All were disease free after a mean follow up of 7 years (range 2-18 years), and had a mean age of 44 years (range 39-54years). All patients in the series were able to stand to void after reconstruction, with 12/15 (80%) developing full sensation within the phallus. Half the patients had insertion of a penile prosthesis, of whom 5/7 (70%) were using the phallus for intercourse. All were happy with the final cosmetic appearance of the phalloplasty. Complications included urethral strictures in 3/15 (20%), urethral fistulae in 4/15 (26%) cases, and a subsequent explant of the penile prosthesis in 1/7 (14%) patients for infection. Only 1/15 (7%) patients had a subsequent recurrence in the bulbar urethra 2 years after phalloplasty, requiring subsequent urethrectomy formation of a continent catheterisable conduit.

T4 Disease – Tumour Invading Adjacent Structures

Surgery has an important role in the management of locally advanced stage T4 disease, although its role has been redefined by the development of newer chemotherapy regimes. Locally advanced tumours, which have already invaded into adjacent structures, often have metastases at presentation and have a very poor prognosis. In such cases surgery is primarily aimed at palliation and improvement of the patient's quality of life as apposed to cure. The use of neo-adjuvant chemotherapy, usually within the setting of a trial, may allow down-staging of the disease and reduce the extent of surgical excision required. The ideal regime is still unclear, but small studies using neo-adjuvant combinations containing platinum based drugs have shown some promise (42,43).

In more advanced cases, extensive resection may involve excision of part of the anterior abdominal wall or perineum, and even complete excision of the prostate and bladder. Closure will often require more complex reconstruction in conjunction with plastic surgeons using a variety of techniques including the use of rectus abdominus or other local flaps to cover the defect. In cases of cystoprostatectomy, urinary diversion with an ileal conduit may also be required. In patients not suitable for surgical excision, palliative chemotherapy and localised radiotherapy may be more appropriate, dependent on the extent of the disease, the patient's performance status and co-morbidity. As with all patients, case discussion within a multidisciplinary team setting will allow formulation of optimal and individualised treatment plans for such patients.

Follow Up

Careful and close follow forms an essential part of managing penile cancer, especially given the shift towards more penile preserving techniques. Local recurrence after less invasive surgery is more prevalent than after radical surgery, and has been reported to be as high as 32% with techniques such as Moh's micrographic surgery. However, local recurrences do not seem to carry the same impact on survival as regional recurrence, and most patients are still amenable to further penile preserving surgery if the local recurrence is detected early (44,45). Patients should be closely followed up every 3 months for the first 2 years, reducing to 6 monthly thereafter with an aim to complete at least 5 years. After radical surgery the risk of recurrence is very low, and patients need only be seen 6 monthly for the first 2 years, reducing to annual visits up to at least 5 years.

Summary

An increase in the understanding of the nature and natural history of penile cancer has lead to a paradigm shift in how this rare malignancy is treated. In the past, the tendency had been towards over treatment of the primary lesion. While such surgery was effective oncologically, its emasculating nature led to serious psychological and sexual morbidity. The pooling of expertise and resources in specialist centres has improved our knowledge of the necessary clearance margins, and spawned the development of penile preserving techniques, which have limited the impact of the disease and its treatment on patients' quality of life. A range of organ conserving techniques are available, and the selection of the most appropriate one depends on the tumour stage, grade, and location, also taking into account the patient's age, co-morbidity and the expected phallic length that can be preserved (see table1). Close post operative surveillance is essential as the long-term recurrence rates for these techniques are still unknown. Early detection of local recurrence is often still amenable to further penile preserving surgery without any compromise to the oncological outcome. Advances in reconstructive techniques have improved the functional and cosmetic outcome of those treated with radical surgery. The advent of new chemotherapy regimes has improved the options and approach to managing even the most advanced cases, although surgery in this circumstance primarily palliative and aimed at improving the overall quality of life.

Table 1. Treatment Options by Stage

Stage	Tis	Ta-T1a	T1b-T2	T3/T4
Treatment	-Topical chemotherapy / Immunotherapy (Imiquimod, 5-FU) -Laser (CO_2 or Nd:YAG) -Glans resurfacing (partial/ total) -Moh's micrographic surgery	Foreskin -Circumcision Glans -Wide local excision -Glans resurfacing -Glansectomy (partial/ total)	- Total glansectomy and reconstruction if no corpus cavernosum involvement -Partial penectomy if corpus cavernosum invovlved or patient not fit/ suitable for glansectomy/ reconstruction - Radiotherapy (if <4cm)	-Partial penectomy for distal T3 -Radical penectomy and perineal urethrostomy for proximal T2, high grade T3, any T4 -+/- Chemo/ Radiotherapy for advanced T4

References

[1]   Cancer trends in England and Wales, 1950-1999. *www.statistics.gov.uk*. Date accessed 2004.

[2]   Bleeker MC, Heideman DA, Snijders PJ, Horenblas S, Dillner J, Meijer CJ. Penile cancer: epidemiology, pathogenesis and prevention. *World J Urol*. 2009 27(2):141-50.

[3]   Solsona E, Bahl A, Brandes SB, Dickerson D, Puras-Baez A, van Poppel H, Watkin NA. *New developments in the treatment of penile cancer*. Chapter in International Consultation on Penile Cancer PompeoACL, Heyns CF, Abrams P (eds) pp103-127.

[4]   Opjordsmoen S, Fossa SD Quality of life in patients treated for penile cancer. A follow-up study. *Br J Urol* 1994 74(5):652–657

[5]   Agrawal A, Pai D, Ananthakrishnan N et al The histological extent of the local spread of carcinoma of the penis and its therapeutic implications. *BJUI* 2000 85(2):299–301.

[6]   Hoffman M, Renshaw A, Loughlin KR Squamous cell carcinoma of the penis and microscopic pathologic margins. How much margin is needed for local cure? *Cancer* 1999 85(7):1565–1568.

[7]   Minhas S, Kayes O, Hegarty P et al. What surgical resection margins are required to achieve oncological control in men with primary penile cancer? *BJUI* 2005 96:1040–1043.

[8]   Brown, C. T., S. Minhas, and D. J. Ralph, Conservative surgery for penile cancer: subtotal glans excision without grafting: *BJUI* 2005 96(6);911-912.

[9] Pietrzak, P., C. Corbishley, and N. Watkin, , Organ-sparing surgery for invasive penile cancer: early follow-up data: *BJUI* 2004 94(9);1253-1257.

[10] Porter WM, Francis N, Hawkins D, et al. Penile Intraepithelial Neoplasia: Clinical spectrum and treatment of 35 cases. *Br J Dermatol.* 2002; 147(6): 1159-65

[11] Goette DK, Elgart M, DeVillez RL. Erythroplasia of Queyrat treatment with topically applied 5-Fluorouracil. *JAMA* 1975 232(9):934–937

[12] Micali G, Nasca MR, Tedeschi A . Topical treatment of intraepithelial penile carcinoma with imiquimod. *Clin Exp Dermatol* 2003 28(Suppl 1):4–6

[13] Slade HB, Owens ML, Tomai MA, Miller RL. Imiquimod 5% cream (Aldara). *Exp Opin Invest Drugs* 1998; 7: 437–49.

[14] Tietjen DN, Malek RS. Laser therapy of squamous cell dysplasia and carcinoma of the penis. *Urology* 1998 52: 559–565

[15] van Bezooijen BP, Horenblas S, Meinhardt W, Newling DW. Laser therapy for carcinoma in situ of the penis. *J Urol* 2001 166(5):1670–1671.

[16] Windahl T, Andersson SO. Combined laser treatment for penile carcinoma: results after long-term follow up. *J Urol.* 2003 169(6):2118-21.

[17] Meijer RP, Boon TA, van Venrooij GE, Wijburg CJ. Longterm follow-up after laser therapy for penile carcinoma. *Urology* 2007 69(4):759–762.

[18] Ekalaksananan T, Pientong C, Thinkhamrop J, Kongyingyoes B, Evans MF, Chaiwongkot A. Cervical cancer screening in north east Thailand using the visual inspection with acetic acid (VIA) test and its relationship to high-risk human papillomavirus (HR-HPV) status. *J Obstet Gynaecol Res.* 2010 doi: 10.1111/j.1447-0756.2010.01265.x. [Epub ahead of print]

[19] Kellokoski J, Syrjänen S, Kataja V, Yliskoski M, Syrjänen K. Acetowhite staining and its significance in diagnosis of oral mucosal lesions in women with genital HPV infections. *J Oral Pathol Med.* 1990 19(6):278-83.

[20] Frega A, French D, Pace S, Maranghi L, Palazzo A, Iacovelli R, Biamonti A, Moscarini M, Vecchione A. Prevalence of acetowhite areas in male partners of women affected by HPV and squamous intra-epithelial lesions (SIL) and their prognostic significance. A multicenter study. *Anticancer Res.* 2006 26(4B): 3171-4.

[21] Depasquale I, Park AJ, Bracka A. The treatment of balanitis xerotica obliterans. *BJU Int* 2000; 86 : 459–65

[22] Hadway P, Corbishley CM, Watkin NA. Total glans resurfacing for premalignant lesions of the penis: initial outcome data. *BJUI* 2006 98(3):532–536

[23] Shabbir M, Muneer A, Kalsi J, Shukla CJ, Zacharakis E, Garaffa G , Ralph DJ, Minhas S. Glans Resurfacing for the treatment for Carcinoma in situ of the penis: Surgical technique and outcomes. *Eur Urol* 2011 59:1 142-147.

[24] Mohs FE, Snow SN, Larson PO. Mohs micrographic surgery for penile tumors. *Urol Clin North Am.* 1992 19(2):291-304.

[25] Shindel AW, Mann MW, Lev RY, Sengelmann R, Petersen J, Hruza GJ, Brandes SB. Mohs micrographic surgery for penile cancer: management and long-term follow up. *J Urol.* 2007 178(5):1980-5.

[26] Lindegaard JC, Nielsen OS, Lundbeck FA et al. A retrospective analysis of 82 cases of cancer of the penis. *BJUI* 1996 77(6):883–890.

[27] Lont AP, Gallee MPW, Meinhardt W, van Tinteren H, Horenblas S. Penis conserving treatment for T1 and T2 penile carcinoma: clinical implications of a local recurrence. *J Urol.* 2006 176(2):575-80

[28] Austoni E, Fenice O, Kartalas Goumas Y et al. New trends in the surgical treatment of penile carcinoma. *Arch Ital Urol Androl* 1996 68:163–168

[29] Hatzichristou DG, Apostolidis A, Tzortzis V et al. Glansectomy: an alternative surgical treatment for Buschke-Lowenstein tumours of the penis. *Urology* 2001 57:966–969.

[30] Morelli G, Pagni R, Mariani C, Campo G, Menchini-Fabris F, Minervini R, Minervini A. Glansectomy with split-thickness skin graft for the treatment of penile carcinoma. *Int J Impot Res.* 2009 21(5):311-4.

[31] Smith Y, Hadway P, Biedrzycki O et al. Reconstructive surgery for invasive squamous carcinoma of the glans penis. *Eur Urol* 2007 52(4):1179–1185.

[32] Azrif M, Logue JP, Swindell R, et al. External beam radiotherapy in T1-2 N0 penile carcinoma. *Clin. Oncol (R Coll Radiol).* 2006;18(4):320-5.

[33] De Crevoisier R, Slimane K, Sanfilippo N, et al. Long term results of brachytherapy for carcinoma of the penis confined to the glans (N- or Nx). Int *J Radiat Oncol Biol Phys.* 2009;74(4):1150-6.

[34] Shabbir M, Hughes BE, Swallow T, Corbishley C, Perry MJA, Watkin N Management of chronic ulceration after radiotherapy for penile cancer. *J Urol* 2008 179(4):785

[35] Bañón Perez VJ, Nicolás Torralba JA, Valdelvira Nadal P, et al. [Squamous carcinoma of the penis] Carcinoma escamoso de pene. *Arch Esp Urol.* 2000;53(8):693-9.

[36] Ficarra V, Maffei N, Piacentini I, et al. Local treatment of penile squamous cell carcinoma. *Urol Int.* 2002;69(3):169-73.

[37] Chen MF, Chen WC, Wu CT et al. Contemporary management of penile cancer including surgery and adjuvant radiotherapy: an experience in Taiwan. *World J Urol.* 2004;22(1):60-6.

[38] Leijte JA, Kirrander P, Antonini N, et al. Recurrence patterns of squamous cell carcinoma of the penis: recommendations for follow up based on a two-centre analysis of 700 patients. *Eur Urol.* 2008;54(1):161-8.

[39] Korets R, Koppie TM, Snyder ME, et al. Partial penectomy for patients with squamous cell carcinoma of the penis: the Memorial Sloan-Kettering experience. *Ann Surg Oncol.* 2007;14(12):3614-9.

[40] Chang TS, Hwang HY. Forearm flap in one-stage reconstruction of the penis. *Plast Reconstr Surg* 1984 74:251–258

[41] Garaffa G, Raheem AA, Christopher NA, Ralph DJ. Total phallic reconstruction after penile amputation for carcinoma. *BJU Int.* 2009 104(6): 852-6.

[42] Leijte JAP, Kerst JM, Bais E, Antonini N, Horenblas S. Neoadjuvant chemotherapy in advanced penile carcinoma. *Eur Urol* 2007 52(2):488-94.

[43] Barmejo C, Busby JK, Spiess PE, Heller L, Pagliaro LC, Pettaway CA. Neoadjuvant chemotherapy followed by aggressive surgical consolidation for metastatic penile squamous cell carcinoma. *J Urol* 2007 177(4):1335-8.

[44] Horenblas S, Newling DW. Local recurrence tumour after penis-conserving therapy. A plea for longterm follow-up. *Br J Urol* 1993 72(6):976-9.

[45] Leijte JAP, Kirrander P, Antonini N, Windahl T, Horenblas S. Recurrence patterns of squamous cell carcinoma of the penis: recommendations for follow-up based on a two-centre analysis of 700 patients. *Eur Urol* 2008 Jul;54(1):161-8.

In: Essentials and Updates in Urologic Oncology
Editor: Philippe E. Spiess

ISBN: 978-1-62081-494-9
© 2013 Nova Science Publishers, Inc.

Chapter XXX

Management of Pelvic and Inguinal Lymph Nodes

Hussain M. Alnajjar[*][1], *Nicholas A. Watkin*[1]
and Simon Horenblas[2]

[1]St George's Healthcare NHS Trust, Tooting, London, UK
[2]The Netherlands Cancer Institute - Antoni van Leeuwenhoek Hospital,
Amsterdam, The Netherlands

Abstract

In contrast to many cancers squamous cell carcinoma of the penis can be cured despite the presence of lymph node metastases. This characteristic is shared with testicular cancer. But unlike the latter penile carcinoma is not very chemo sensitive and therefore the focus of management has been on surgery. Penile cancer is also characterized by its tendency for prolonged loco regional growth. A characteristic known from other sites like vulvar cancer and head and neck cancers. Another reason for focus on surgery.

As the success of treatment is invariably related to the stage of the disease, the earliest possible detection of lymph node involvement should be strived at.

Unfortunately non invasive detection methods have not been accurate enough with a high probability of false negative findings. This poses a true dilemma for daily practice. With the advent of the dynamic sentinel node procedure a reliable minimal invasive tool has been introduced. As is true in the whole field of surgical oncology, there is mostly only one chance to cure the patient. Considering the tendency for loco regional growth, with hematogenic metastases at a very late stage only and because of the extremely difficult management of locally recurrent disease, local control should be a goal at all costs

---

[*] Hussain M. Alnajjar*, BSc. (MedSci), MBBS, MRCS (Eng.):Clinical Research Fellow in Penile Cancer, Penile Cancer Centre, St George's Healthcare NHS Trust, Tooting, London, SW17 0QT, UK, e-mail: huss@doctors. org.uk, Fax: (0044)2087252915, Tel: (0044)2087252856

This chapter will deal with all aspects of imaging and minimal invasive methods of detecting lymph node involvement. It will focus on the indications of surgical management of the regional nodes, the extent of the surgery and its complications. Also adjuvant therapy is covered.

Introduction

The majority of penile cancers are squamous cell carcinomas (~95%) which typically show a stepwise lymphogenic spread prior to haematogenic dissemination. The primary draining lymph nodes are invariably located within the inguinal lymphatic region. Thereafter, dissemination usually continues to the pelvic nodes and/or distant sites. At initial presentation, distant metastases are present in only 1-2% of the patients and are virtually always associated with clinically evident lymph node metastases.

The presence of nodal involvement is the single most important prognostic factor. [1-7] As the currently available non-invasive staging modalities have a low sensitivity in detecting the regional lymph node status (i.e. missing micro metastatic disease), the optimal management of clinically node-negative (cN0) patients has been the subject of debate. [8] Approximately 20%-25% of these cN0 patients have occult metastasis. Some clinicians manage these patients with close surveillance, while others will perform an inguinal lymphadenectomy.

Other approaches are dynamic sentinel node biopsy, modified lymphadenectomy, and lymphadenectomy in those patients considered to be at risk for occult metastases, so called "risk-adapted approach". [9] While close surveillance may lead to unintentional delay because of outgrowth of occult metastases in 20-25% of cN0 patients, elective as well as risk-adapted inguinal lymphadenectomy is considered unnecessary in 75%-80% of such cases, because of absence of metastases. [10] Furthermore, lymphadenectomy is associated with a high morbidity rate. Up to 35%-70% of patients have short- or long-term complications. [11-14]

Anatomy of the Inguinal Lymph Nodes

The lymph nodes in the inguinal lymphatic region are the first draining nodes for the penis, and the anatomy has been described by various authors. [15, 16] Historically, the inguinal lymphatic region was divided into two groups, the superficial and deep lymph nodes. The superficial inguinal lymph nodes are located beneath Camper's fascia and above the fascia lata covering the muscles of the thigh. The deep inguinal nodes are located deep to the fascia lata and medial to the femoral vein. These nodes intercommunicate with each other and then drain into the pelvic nodes. From a clinical perspective, this anatomic distinction is not very useful as the superficial nodes cannot be distinguished from the deep nodes by physical examination or imaging, Daseler et al. divided the inguinal region into five sections by drawing a horizontal and vertical line through the point where the saphenous vein drains into the femoral vein with one central zone directly overlying the junction. [15]

A recent lymphoscintigraphic study by Leijte *et al.* has shown that the majority of the first draining lymph nodes is located in Daseler's superomedial segment, although there is individual variation. [17]

Assessment of Inguinal Lymph Nodes

The key issue in lymph node staging is the unreliability of the currently available modalities which detect occult nodal involvement. However, given that early resection of the inguinal lymph nodes is associated with a therapeutic benefit, [18-20] it is imperative that those patients with metastatic disease in the inguinal lymph nodes undergo an inguinal lymphadenectomy at the earliest possible time. Unfortunately the high morbidity rate associated with performing an elective inguinal lymphadenectomy makes the operation unsuitable for every penile cancer patient who does not have inguinal nodal involvement. Hence there is uncertainty about the timing of lymphadenectomy as well as identifying those patients who would benefit. However, three clinical groups can be identified: those with clinically node-negative (cN0) groins, those with palpable inguinal lymph nodes (cN+) and those with immobile (fixed) inguinal lymph nodes.

Clinical Examination

The majority of patients diagnosed with penile cancer in Western countries present without any palpable abnormalities in the groins and only 20% present with palpable nodes. [21] Inguinal lymph nodes that become palpable during follow-up are due to metastasis in nearly 100% of cases. [22] Physical examination of the inguinal region is of limited value in accurate detection, especially of small metastases. Approximately 20-25% of cN0-patients will harbour occult metastases. These occult metastases are, by definition, not detected by physical examination. In the cN+ patients approximately 70% will actually have metastatic inguinal nodal involvement. [7] The remainder will have enlarged inguinal nodes secondary to infection of the primary tumour. Traditionally antibiotic treatment was advised for six weeks to treat the inflammation with a further re-assessment of the inguinal lymph nodes thereafter. However, in order to avoid a delay in diagnosis, this is no longer recommended. Patients with lymph node involvement should undergo inguinal lymphadenectomy. [23]

Investigations

The currently available non-invasive staging techniques which can be used to stage the groin besides physical examination, include ultrasonography combined with fine-needle aspiration cytology (FNAC) of morphologically suspicious looking nodes, CT scan, MR imaging and PET/CT-scanning. These modalities are especially useful in the obese patient or those who are difficult to examine as additional imaging may identify metastases not found by physical examination.

Ultrasound with Fine-Needle Aspiration Cytology (FNAC)

Ultrasound is non-invasive, quick and inexpensive and can easily be combined with fine-needle aspiration cytology (FNAC) of morphologically suspicious-looking lymph nodes. In a series of 43 patients with 83 cN0-groins, ultrasound-guided FNAC had a sensitivity and specificity of 39% and 100%, respectively. [24] Ultrasound guided FNAC has been utilised preoperatively to screen the cN0-groin and to further analyze the groins of the patients with palpable inguinal lymph nodes (cN+). In a series of 16 patients staged cN+ and not having antibiotic treatment, FNAC alone (without ultrasonography) showed a sensitivity and specificity of 93% and 91%, respectively. [25] False-negative rates for FNAC have been reported in up to 15%. If the clinician remains suspicious, repeat fine needle aspiration cytology is indicated and if it is still inconclusive, then excisional biopsy can be performed. Care must be taken when performing an open biopsy such that in the event of a malignant node the site of the biopsy can be excised during the subsequent lymphadenectomy.

CT-Imaging

The role of CT in staging the inguinal lymph nodes is poorly understood due to a paucity of studies. One report published in 1991 described a small series of 14 patients that underwent preoperative CT-scan. A sensitivity and specificity of 36% and 100% were found, respectively. None of the occult metastases in cN0-groins were identified. However, these results are a reflection of the CT technology available at the time of the study. Currently with the use of multi-slice CT- scanners and increased spatial resolution results are probably better. Nevertheless, the problem of missing small metastasis still remains. The diagnostic accuracy regarding the pelvic lymph nodes is poor, in accordance with the experience recently reported by other centres. [26] Therefore, CT imaging is not recommended as the initial staging tool for staging in cN0-patients, although it is suitable in those who are difficult to examine (e.g. obese patients). By contrast, CT-scanning can be useful in cN+ patients to determine the extent of disease and this will be discussed later.

MR-Imaging

MR imaging with lymphotrophic nanoparticles (LN-MRI, coated ultra-small particles of iron oxide, USPIOs, ferrumoxtran-10) has shown promising results in identifying occult metastasis in a study of seven patients with penile cancer. [27] MR imaging was performed before and also 24 hours after intravenous ferrumoxtran-10 administration. In this small series, LN-MRI has shown a sensitivity of 100% and a specificity of 97%. This imaging technique has also revealed high diagnostic accuracies in staging lymph nodes in prostate cancer and bladder cancer. [28] However, ferrumoxtran-10 is not FDA-approved, hence it is not commercially available. Furthermore, the manufacturer has withdrawn the application for marketing authorization for lymphotrophic nanoparticles in Europe. In addition, conventional MR imaging is also limited by its spatial resolution. Thus, its use is also limited for staging the cN0-groin.

PET/CT-Scan

Positron emission tomography (PET) instrumentation detects subnanomolar concentrations of radioactive tracer *in vivo*. Following malignant transformation, a range of tumours can be characterized by elevated glucose metabolism and subsequent increased uptake of the intravenously injected radiolabelled glucose analogue [F18]-fluorodeoxyglucose (FDG). PET combined with low-dose CT imaging (PET/CT) in a single scanner fuses the acquired data into one image containing both functional and anatomical information. The accuracy of the combined images is reported to be higher than separate PET and CT images. [29-31]

In 2005, Scher *et al.* published the first results of PET/CT scanning in penile cancer. [32] They found promising results with a sensitivity of 80% and specificity of 100% on a per-patient basis, respectively. However, these results may be a little optimistic. The limitations of MR- imaging with respect to spatial resolution are also true for PET/CT. In a recent prospective study of 42 cN0-groins that underwent preoperative PET/CT scanning without pre treatment antibiotics, PET/CT missed one out of five occult metastases. In addition, three false-positive results were found among the 37 remaining groins leading to a specificity of 92%. [33] The false-positive findings were associated with inflammatory responses within the lymph nodes.

Table 1. Available Management Approaches for cN0-patients.

		Advantages	Disadvantages
1)	Close surveillance	No morbidity in patients without occult metastasis	Survival disadvantage compared with early dissection. Some patients develop inoperable inguinal recurrences
2)	Nomogram/ Risk-adapted lymphadenectomy	Reduction in number of inguinal node dissections and hence decreased overall morbidity	Significant over treatment despite risk adaptation
3)	Minimally invasive staging		
	a) Modified inguinal lymphadenectomy (MIL)	High incidence of detection of micro-metastasis and lower risk of complications than radical surgery	Significant over-treatment (>80% of inguinal specimens will be benign)
	b) Dynamic sentinel node biopsy (DSNB)	Patients are pathological staged with minor morbidity Only pN+ patients suffer from (completion) LND morbidity	In some patients metastases are missed (i.e. false-negative) and develop inguinal recurrences Some patients cannot be salvaged hereafter
4)	Elective bilateral radical lymphadenectomy	No occult metastases are missed	Unnecessary in 80% of patients and severe short and long-term morbidity

Management of the Inguinal Lymph Nodes in Clinically Node-Negative (Cn0) Patients

Several risk-adapted management approaches have been used and advocated during the last decades (Table 1). Basically, these management policies can be divided into non-invasive management (surveillance), minimally-invasive staging (dynamic sentinel node biopsy / modified inguinal lymphadenectomy), or invasive staging techniques (radical lymphadenectomy). The fact that approximately 20% of the cN0-patients have occult metastases, inguinal lymphadenectomy is an unnecessary procedure in approximately 80% of patients. Furthermore, lymphadenectomy is associated with risks and prone to a number of complications which will be discussed later. In general, a lymphadenectomy in all cN0 patients (sometimes described as early, prophylactic or pre-emptive) is not recommended.

1. Close Surveillance

The basis of close surveillance involves a regular clinical examination of the patient proceeding to lymphadenectomy when lymph node metastases become clinically evident. This avoids the morbidity associated with lymphadenectomy and therefore patients with cN0 disease who subsequently are unlikely to develop inguinal lymph node metastases are not over treated. Whilst this has been advocated in the past, with seemingly good results, recent non-randomized retrospective studies indicates that this approach is associated with a negative effect on survival rates. [18-20]

2. Predictive Nomogram for Occult Metastasis/ Risk-Adapted Lymphadenectomy

Another non-invasive approach is the use of a preoperative nomogram predictive of inguinal metastases. [34] In one nomogram the following parameters were used for risk assessment: tumour thickness (≤5 mm. vs. >5mm.), growth pattern (vertical vs. horizontal), grade (well vs. intermediate vs. poor), lymphovascular invasion (absent vs. present), corpora cavernosa infiltration (absent vs. present), corpora spongiosum infiltration (absent vs. present), urethral infiltration (absent vs. present), cN-status (cN0 vs. cN+). In clinical practice this particular nomogram may be a useful tool but still requies validation. It remains to the discretion of the doctor in collaboration with the patient to determine at which cut-off point to embark on a lymphadenectomy.

The basis of risk-adapted approaches is risk assessment of harbouring lymph node metastases based on histopathological factors of the primary tumour, such as tumour stage (T-stage), [35, 36] tumour grade (i.e. grade (G) 1, 2, or 3), [36-38] presence of lymphovascular (LVI), [39-40] perineural invasion (PNI) [37-38] and depth of infiltration. [37] The EAU guidelines have included tumour stage, grade and absence or presence of LVI into a risk-adapted approach for the management of the inguinal regions. Three risk-groups have been identified: low risk tumours (pTis, pTa, pT1G1), intermediate risk tumours (pT1G2, no LVI) and high risk tumours (pT1G3, pT2-3G1-3, or presence of LVI). [9,35] If patients are considered suitable for surveillance, the 2009 EAU guidelines advise follow-up in patients with low risk tumours only, and surgical staging in intermediate and high risk cN0-patients. In a prospective study of 100 patients managed according to these EAU guidelines, none of the patients considered "low-risk" developed lymph node metastases during a mean follow-up of 29 months. On the other hand, elective lymphadenectomy was unnecessary in 82% of the patients with high risk features, because no evidence of metastatic spread was found with histopathology. [10] In another series of 118 patients it was estimated that 63% of high-risk patients will be subjected to unnecessary lymphadenectomy. [41] Both studies indicate that current EAU high-risk stratification is not accurate enough in order to stratify these patients. It appears that the risk of occult nodal involvement in cN0 patients with low-risk (T1G1) is low and these patients can still be subjected to close surveillance with subsequently inguinal lymphadenectomy when metastases become clinically evident.

3. Minimally-Invasive Staging Techniques

To circumvent the abovementioned dilemmas of timing of lymphadenectomy, minimally-invasive staging techniques have been developed. The basis of these techniques is to limit the morbidity in patients with pathological node-negative (pN0) groins, and to identify occult metastases at the earliest moment. Only patients with proven lymphatic spread undergo a completion therapeutic lymphadenectomy. In the last two decades, two approaches have been introduced worldwide: modified inguinal lymphadenectomy (MIL) and dynamic sentinel node biopsy (DSNB).

a.) Modified Inguinal Lymphadenectomy (MIL)

The MIL was proposed by Catalona in 1988 after being performed in 6 patients with invasive carcinoma of the penis or distal urethra. [42] The aim of this approach is to remove all the lymph nodes that are the most probable location of first line lymphatic invasion, and excluding the regions lateral to the femoral artery and caudal to the fossa ovalis. The lymph node packet can be analysed by frozen section and if it confirms metastatic disease then a radical inguinal lymphadenectomy can be performed. The anatomic location of these lymph nodes was based on earlier lymphatic drainage studies. The medial margin of MIL was the adductor longus muscle, the lateral margin was the lateral border of the femoral artery, the superior margin was the external oblique muscle above the spermatic cord and the inferior margin was the fascia lata just distal to the fossa ovalis. The advantage of this MIL is a smaller skin incision and a smaller node dissection resulting in reduced morbidity compared with standard lymphadenectomy. However, limiting the dissection field led to a high number of false-negative findings as reported by several other authors.

b.) Dynamic Sentinel Node Biopsy (DSNB)

Sentinel node biopsy for penile cancer was first reported by Cabañas in 1977. [43] This was based on lymphangiograms of the penis and the lymph node medial to the superficial epigastric vein was identified as being the first echelon lymph node or so called "sentinel node". It was assumed that a negative sentinel node was indicative for absence of further lymphatic spread and therefore no lymphadenectomy was indicated. Sentinel node surgery consisted of identification and removal of this lymph node with completion lymph-adenectomy only in those with a tumour-positive lymph node. However, this initial "static" procedure, based on anatomic landmarks only, did not take into account individual drainage patterns. Several false-negative results were reported, and the technique was largely abandoned. The sentinel node procedure was revived by Morton et al in 1992, by using patent blue-V or isosulfan blue dye as a tracer enabling individual lymphatic mapping. [44] This technique with the addition of a preoperative radioactive tracer (technetium-99m-labelled nanocolloid ^{99m}Tc) forms the basis of the modern sentinel node biopsy era and is also used in, for example, breast cancer and melanoma.

The DSNB procedure for penile cancer was first described by Horenblas *et* al. in 2001 in a report of 55 patients with T2 or greater tumours. [45] With this dynamic approach a sensitivity of 80% was reported. However, the false-negative rates have raised concerns about its diagnostic accuracy. Furthermore, patients with negative sentinel nodes remained on rigid follow-up. During the years, the DSNB protocol has been modified after detailed analysis of the false-negative cases. [46] The initial procedure was extended by pathological examination of the sentinel node by serial sectioning and immunohistochemical staining instead of routine paraffin sections, and addition of preoperative ultrasonography with fine-needle aspiration cytology to detect pathologically enlarged nodes, that fail to pick up radioactivity. Further-more, exploration of groins with nonvisualization on preoperative lymphoscintigram (occurring in approximately 4%-6% of cN0-groins) [47,17,26] and intraoperative palpation of the wound have been introduced. The current modified procedure has evolved into a reliable minimally-invasive staging technique with an associated sensitivity of 93-95% together with a low morbidity, [41,48] and is comparable with the results in breast cancer and melanoma. Recently, in a large prospective series of 323 patients from two tertiary referral hospitals who use essentially the same protocol, DSNB has shown to be a reliable method with a low complication rate. [49] The combined sensitivity of this procedure was 93% with a specificity of 100%. Complications occurred in less than 5% of explored groins and almost all were transient and could be managed conservatively.

Management of the Groin in Clinically Node-Positive (Cn+) Patients

Surgery remains the cornerstone of treatment in patients with metastatic disease in the groins. Cure can be attained in approximately 80% of patients who have one or two involved inguinal nodes without extranodal extension. [1-7] Preoperatively, inguinal nodal involvement can be found with FNAC or excision biopsy. We prefer FNAC as it is easily performed in an out-patient setting, it is relatively non-invasive and it does not interfere with the subsequent lymphadenectomy. Although the reported sensitivity of FNAC is higher in cN+ patients compared to cN0 patients, it is recommended to repeat the ultrasound with FNAC when clinical suspicion remains despite tumour-negative cytological results. If doubt remains an excision biopsy is advised. In removing the suspicious enlarged node the surgeon should pay attention to the anatomical localization of the inguinal incision, as the inguinal scar should be removed at the time of completion inguinal lymphadenectomy.

Patients presenting with fixed inguinal nodes are candidates for neoadjuvant chemotherapy prior to undergoing surgery. [50]

Indications for Therapeutic Lymphadenectomy

Indication for Inguinal Lymphadenectomy

Ipsilateral inguinal lymphadenectomy is indicated when tumour-bearing lymph nodes are found with sentinel node biopsy, FNAC or excision biopsy. Should a bilateral inguinal dissection be undertaken in all patients with unilateral inguinal involvement? At the authors' institutes the timing of detection, the number of palpable nodes and the number of positive nodes found in the resection specimen were considered initially indicative for a contralateral lymphadenectomy. [51] Patients who developed a unilateral inguinal recurrence during follow-up were managed by unilateral dissection assuming that bilateral nodal metastases develop at the same rate and that the absence of clinical nodal involvement of the contralateral side after observation suggested a tumour free groin. Previous studies have suggested that the likelihood of bilateral involvement is related to the number of involved nodes in the unilateral resected inguinal specimen. [1,51] With two or more metastases the probability of occult contralateral involvement is 30% and this may warrant an early contralateral inguinal lymphadenectomy. Currently, ultrasound-guided FNAC and DSNB are used to solve the problem at the authors' institute in those patients presenting initially with unilateral positive nodes. Contralateral groins with tumour-negative sentinel nodes are under close surveillance. Hence, nodal staging and management has emerged from treatment per patient to management per groin.

Indication for Pelvic Lymphadenectomy

In general, 20-30% of patients with positive inguinal nodes have positive pelvic nodes. [1,4,52] Although patients with pelvic lymphadenopathy are considered to have a bleak outcome, pelvic lymphadenectomy can be curative in some patients. Especially, those with occult pelvic metastases may benefit. Several authors have shown that the likelihood of pelvic nodal involvement is related to the number of positive nodes in the inguinal specimen and presence of extranodal extension. [1-7,52] Patients with one intranodal inguinal metastasis have a very low probability of pelvic node involvement (<5%, unpublished data). [4,52] At the authors' institute a pelvic dissection is considered unnecessary in these patients. In all other patients with 2 or more inguinal nodes involved or extranodal extension an ipsilateral pelvic lymphadenectomy of the affected site is performed. There is ample clinical and published evidence that cross over from the groin to the contralateral pelvic area does not occur. [4,52,51] Therefore, contralateral pelvic lymphadenectomy is not recommended in patients with unilateral nodal involvement. Patients with preoperative evidence of pelvic metastases are unlikely to be cured by surgery alone and are candidates for neoadjuvant chemotherapy before undergoing surgery.

Complications of Lymph Node Dissection

Even in the most experienced hands lymphadenectomy is not without complications. This accounts for the reluctance in offering lymphadenectomy to every patient presenting with penile cancer. The reported complication rate varies from 35% to 88%, and appears to be lower when inguinal lymphadenectomy is performed in a prophylactic or therapeutic setting compared with a palliative dissection. [14] Furthermore, pelvic node dissection and radiotherapy have shown to increase the complication rates. [4,12] The most commonly cited complications are wound infection (15±10%), skin necrosis with or without wound dehiscence (14±50%), lymphocele/seroma (10±10%) lymphoedema (27±30%), and other complications including haemorrhage, thrombosis, and even death. A summary of the most frequent complications is listed in Table 2.

Table 2. Complications of Lymphadenectomy (%)

No of dissections	Wound infection	Skin edge necrosis	Seroma formation	Lymph oedema	Death
101 [11]	14	50	16	50	0
405 [12]	17	62	7	27	1
200 [13]	15	45	10	23	-
106 [14]	10	8	10	23	2
102*[4]	22	8	18	56	0

*per-patient

Management of Complications

After removing the suction drains a lymphocele can develop in 10-20% of patients. This can usually be managed by outpatient aspiration with a large needle and a large syringe. After natural resolution of the space in which the lymphocele develops the accumulation of lymphatic fluid stops. Large wound defects can be closed using a Vacuum Assisted Closure (VAC) system. A sponge is inserted in the wound and sealed with plastic and a draining tube is attached to a low vacuum pump. Excellent results have been obtained, increasing the time to secondary healing. If the defect remains large a split skin graft can be laid on top of the granulation tissue.

Despite the use of elastic stockings, lymphedema can still develop in approximately 10% of patients, especially those in whom extensive surgery together with radiation therapy was necessary because of the burden of disease. Supporting therapy includes, lymph massage and compression therapy.

Surgical therapy using lymphatic-venous anastomoses has not been entirely successful. Legs with lymphedema are infection prone, especially with streptococcus A bacteria, leading to erisypelas. At the authors' institutions antibiotic prophylaxis with monthly penicillin depots is strongly advised after two bouts of erisypelas-like infections.

**Table 3. Cancer-specific survival by Pathological Nodal Factors
after Inguinal Lymphadenectomy**

Factors	No of patients with factor	5-yr cancer-specific survival estimates
Pathological node-negative nodes	103^2	95%
	140^7	96%
Pathological node-positive	118^2	53%
	111^7	35%
	102^6	51%
	156^{54}	61%
No of positive nodes		
1	5^1	82%
1-3	58^2	81%
	69^6	76%
≤2	111^{54}	74%
≥3	41^{54}	33%
>3	10^2	50%
4-5	25^6	8%
>5	8^6	0%
Unilateral	43^2	86%
	74^6	63%
	93^{54}	69%
Bilateral	24^1	12%
	25^2	60%
	28^6	21%
	63^{54}	49%
Extranodal extension	22^1	5%
	17^2	0%
	54^6	9%
	79^{54}	42%
Pelvic nodal involvement	22^1	0%
	30^2	0%
	21^6	0%
	13^{55}	30%
	34^{54}	21%

Prognosis and Adjuvant Treatment

The single most important prognostic factor in penile cancer is the presence of nodal involvement. The extent of nodal involvement also has a predictive value for cancer-specific outcome. As mentioned previously, patients with one or two inguinal lymph node metastases have a five-year survival rate of approximately 80%. [1-7] Several studies have indicated that the number of inguinal nodes involved, extranodal extension and pelvic nodal involvement are unfavourable parameters for disease-specific survival (Table 3). [1-7] Hence, the indication for adjuvant treatment is based upon the presence of these adverse prognostic indicators. At the authors' institutions, no adjuvant treatment is indicated when histopathological analysis of the removed inguinal dissected specimen shows one intranodal metastasis as cure alone by surgery can be obtained in these patients. Adjuvant ipsilateral radiotherapy to the inguinal lymphatic region is given when histopathological analysis shows 2 or more inguinal nodes involved or extranodal extension. The rationale for this arises from studies in head and neck squamous cell carcinomas showing an improvement in regional control following adjuvant radiotherapy. [53] Adjuvant radiotherapy to the pelvic region is administrated additionally when pelvic nodes are involved. Prophylactic radiation to the groins in all patients with penile cancer is not advised for the following reasons. Firstly, some patients with nonpalpable nodes will not benefit because they have no occult metastasis as is the case for elective lymphadenectomy. Secondly, all patients will be exposed to the complications of radiation therapy, e.g. short-term complications like epidermolysis, and long-term effects such as lymphoedema and fibrosis. Finally, the follow-up is more complicated because of the fibrotic changes, making physical examination less reliable. Although, Ravi *et al.* have indicated that patients with large (>4 cm.) and/or fixed regional nodes may benefit from preoperative radiotherapy, the above mentioned disadvantages outweigh the preoperative use. There are no studies available that have investigated the efficacy of radiotherapy versus standard lymphadenectomy in terms of local control, (cancer-specific) outcome, or complications.

Despite adjuvant radiotherapy, a previous study at the authors' institution of 102 patients with metastatic penile carcinoma treated between 1956 and 2001 has shown that extranodal extension and pelvic nodal involvement are independent predictors for survival. [4] These results have recently been confirmed in an updated series which has included 156 patients with metastatic penile cancer treated between 1988 and 2008. [54] This data suggest that more effective treatment is needed in this subgroup of patients with high-risk metastatic penile cancer. Whether induction chemotherapy before surgery is of any benefit in this high-risk subgroup warrants further clinical studies.

References

[1]   Srinivas, V., Morse, M. J., Herr, H. W., Sogani, P. C., and Whitmore, W. F., Jr.: Penile cancer: relation of extent of nodal metastasis to survival. *J Urol*, 137: 880, 1987.

[2]   Ravi, R.: Correlation between the extent of nodal involvement and survival following groin dissection for carcinoma of the penis. *Br J Urol*, 72: 817, 1993.

[3]   Horenblas, S. and van Tinteren, H.: Squamous cell carcinoma of the penis. IV. Prognostic factors of survival: analysis of tumor, nodes and metastasis classification system. *J Urol*, 151: 1239, 1994.

[4]   Lont, A. P., Kroon, B. K., Gallee, M. P., van Tinteren, H., Moonen, L. M., and Horenblas, S.: Pelvic lymph node dissection for penile carcinoma: extent of inguinal lymph node involvement as an indicator for pelvic lymph node involvement and survival. *J Urol*, 177: 947, 2007.

[5]   Sanchez-Ortiz, R. F. and Pettaway, C. A.: The role of lymphadenectomy in penile cancer. *Urol Oncol*, 22: 236, 2004.

[6]   Pandey, D., Mahajan, V., and Kannan, R. R.: Prognostic factors in node-positive carcinoma of the penis. *J Surg Oncol*, 93: 133, 2006.

[7] Ornellas, A. A., Kinchin, E. W., Nobrega, B. L., Wisnescky, A., Koifman, N., and Quirino, R.: Surgical treatment of invasive squamous cell carcinoma of the penis: Brazilian National Cancer Institute long-term experience. *J Surg Oncol*, 97: 487, 2008.

[8] Wespes, E.: The management of regional lymph nodes in patients with penile carcinoma and reliability of sentinel node biopsy. *Eur Urol*, 52: 15, 2007.

[9] Solsona, E., Algaba, F., Horenblas, S., Pizzocaro, G., and Windahl, T.: EAU Guidelines on Penile Cancer. *Eur Urol*, 46: 1, 2004.

[10] Hegarty, P. K., Kayes, O., Freeman, A., Christopher, N., Ralph, D. J., and Minhas, S.: A prospective study of 100 cases of penile cancer managed according to European Association of Urology guidelines. *BJU Int*, 98: 526, 2006.

[11] Johnson, D. E. and Lo, R. K.: Complications of groin dissection in penile cancer. Experience with 101 lymphadenectomies. *Urology*, 24: 312, 1984.

[12] Ravi, R.: Morbidity following groin dissection for penile carcinoma. *Br J Urol*, 72: 941, 1993.

[13] Ornellas, A. A., Seixas, A. L., and de Moraes, J. R.: Analyses of 200 lymphadenectomies in patients with penile carcinoma. *J Urol*, 146: 330, 1991.

[14] Bevan-Thomas, R., Slaton, J. W., and Pettaway, C. A.: Contemporary morbidity from lymphadenectomy for penile squamous cell carcinoma: the M.D. Anderson Cancer Center Experience. *J Urol*, 167: 1638, 2002.

[15] DASELER, E. H., ANSON, B. J., and REIMANN, A. F.: Radical excision of the inguinal and iliac lymph glands; a study based upon 450 anatomical dissections and upon supportive clinical observations. *Surg Gynecol Obstet*, 87: 679, 1948.

[16] Dewire, D. and Lepor, H.: Anatomic considerations of the penis and its lymphatic drainage. *Urol Clin North Am*, 19: 211, 1992.

[17] Leijte, J. A., Valdes Olmos, R. A., Nieweg, O. E., and Horenblas, S.: Anatomical mapping of lymphatic drainage in penile carcinoma with SPECT-CT: implications for the extent of inguinal lymph node dissection. *Eur Urol*, 54: 885, 2008.

[18] McDougal, W. S.: Carcinoma of the penis: improved survival by early regional lymphadenectomy based on the histological grade and depth of invasion of the primary lesion. *J Urol*, 154: 1364, 1995.

[19] Lont, A. P., Horenblas, S., Tanis, P. J., Gallee, M. P., van Tinteren, H., and Nieweg, O. E.: Management of clinically node negative penile carcinoma: improved survival after the introduction of dynamic sentinel node biopsy. *J Urol*, 170: 783, 2003.

[20] Kroon, B. K., Horenblas, S., Lont, A. P., Tanis, P. J., Gallee, M. P., and Nieweg, O. E.: Patients with penile carcinoma benefit from immediate resection of clinically occult lymph node metastases. *J Urol*, 173: 816, 2005.

[21] Persson, B., Sjodin, J. G., Holmberg, L., and Windahl, T.: The National Penile Cancer Register in Sweden 2000-2003. *Scand J Urol Nephrol*, 41: 278, 2007.

[22] Ornellas, A. A., Seixas, A. L., Marota, A., Wisnescky, A., Campos, F., and de Moraes, J. R.: Surgical treatment of invasive squamous cell carcinoma of the penis: retrospective analysis of 350 cases. *J Urol*, 151: 1244, 1994.

[23] Pizzocaro, G., Algaba, F., Horenblas, S., Solsona, E., Tana, S., Van Der Poel, H. et al.: EAU Penile Cancer Guidelines 2009. *Eur Urol*, 2010.

[24] Kroon, B. K., Horenblas, S., Deurloo, E. E., Nieweg, O. E., and Teertstra, H. J.: Ultrasonography-guided fine-needle aspiration cytology before sentinel node biopsy in patients with penile carcinoma. *BJU Int*, 95: 517, 2005.

[25] Saisorn, I., Lawrentschuk, N., Leewansangtong, S., and Bolton, D. M.: Fine-needle aspiration cytology predicts inguinal lymph node metastasis without antibiotic pretreatment in penile carcinoma. *BJU Int,* 97: 1225, 2006.

[26] Jensen, J. B., Jensen, K. M., Ulhoi, B. P., Nielsen, S. S., and Lundbeck, F.: Sentinel lymph-node biopsy in patients with squamous cell carcinoma of the penis. *BJU Int,* 103: 1199, 2009.

[27] Tabatabaei, S., Harisinghani, M., and McDougal, W. S.: Regional lymph node staging using lymphotropic nanoparticle enhanced magnetic resonance imaging with ferumoxtran-10 in patients with penile cancer. *J Urol,* 174: 923, 2005.

[28] Thoeny, H. C., Triantafyllou, M., Birkhaeuser, F. D., Froehlich, J. M., Tshering, D. W., Binser, T. et al.: Combined Ultrasmall Superparamagnetic Particles of Iron Oxide-Enhanced and Diffusion-Weighted Magnetic Resonance Imaging Reliably Detect Pelvic Lymph Node Metastases in Normal-Sized Nodes of Bladder and Prostate Cancer Patients. *Eur Urol,* 2009.

[29] Lardinois, D., Weder, W., Hany, T. F., Kamel, E. M., Korom, S., Seifert, B. et al.: Staging of non-small-cell lung cancer with integrated positron-emission tomography and computed tomography. *N Engl J Med,* 348: 2500, 2003.

[30] Antoch, G., Saoudi, N., Kuehl, H., Dahmen, G., Mueller, S. P., Beyer, T. et al.: Accuracy of whole-body dual-modality fluorine-18-2-fluoro-2-deoxy-D-glucose positron emission tomography and computed tomography (FDG-PET/CT) for tumor staging in solid tumors: comparison with CT and PET. *J Clin Oncol,* 22: 4357, 2004.

[31] Ng, S. H., Yen, T. C., Chang, J. T., Chan, S. C., Ko, S. F., Wang, H. M. et al.: Prospective study of [18F]fluorodeoxyglucose positron emission tomography and computed tomography and magnetic resonance imaging in oral cavity squamous cell carcinoma with palpably negative neck. *J Clin Oncol,* 24: 4371, 2006.

[32] Scher, B., Seitz, M., Reiser, M., Hungerhuber, E., Hahn, K., Tiling, R. et al.: 18F-FDG PET/CT for staging of penile cancer. *J Nucl Med,* 46: 1460, 2005.

[33] Leijte, J. A., Graafland, N. M., Valdes Olmos, R. A., van Boven, H. H., Hoefnagel, C. A., and Horenblas, S.: Prospective evaluation of hybrid (18)F-fluorodeoxyglucose positron emission tomography/computed tomography in staging clinically node-negative patients with penile carcinoma. *BJU Int,* 2009.

[34] Ficarra, V., Zattoni, F., Artibani, W., Fandella, A., Martignoni, G., Novara, G. et al.: Nomogram predictive of pathological inguinal lymph node involvement in patients with squamous cell carcinoma of the penis. *J Urol,* 175: 1700, 2006.

[35] Solsona, E., Iborra, I., Rubio, J., Casanova, J. L., Ricos, J. V., and Calabuig, C.: Prospective validation of the association of local tumor stage and grade as a predictive factor for occult lymph node micrometastasis in patients with penile carcinoma and clinically negative inguinal lymph nodes. *J Urol,* 165: 1506, 2001.

[36] Slaton, J. W., Morgenstern, N., Levy, D. A., Santos, M. W., Jr., Tamboli, P., Ro, J. Y. et al.: Tumor stage, vascular invasion and the percentage of poorly differentiated cancer: independent prognosticators for inguinal lymph node metastasis in penile squamous cancer. *J Urol,* 165: 1138, 2001.

[37] Ornellas, A. A., Nobrega, B. L., Wei Kin Chin, E., Wisnescky, A., da Silva, P. C., and Santos Schwindt, A. B.: Prognostic Factors in Invasive Squamous Cell Carcinoma of the Penis: Analysis of 196 Patients Treated at the Brazilian National Cancer Institute. *J Urol,* 2008.

[38] Velazquez, E. F., Ayala, G., Liu, H., Chaux, A., Zanotti, M., Torres, J. et al.: Histologic grade and perineural invasion are more important than tumor thickness as predictor of nodal metastasis in penile squamous cell carcinoma invading 5 to 10 mm. *Am J Surg Pathol*, 32: 974, 2008.

[39] Lopes, A., Hidalgo, G. S., Kowalski, L. P., Torloni, H., Rossi, B. M., and Fonseca, F. P.: Prognostic factors in carcinoma of the penis: multivariate analysis of 145 patients treated with amputation and lymphadenectomy. *J Urol*, 156: 1637, 1996.

[40] Ficarra, V., Zattoni, F., Cunico, S. C., Galetti, T. P., Luciani, L., Fandella, A. et al.: Lymphatic and vascular embolizations are independent predictive variables of inguinal lymph node involvement in patients with squamous cell carcinoma of the penis: Gruppo Uro-Oncologico del Nord Est (Northeast Uro-Oncological Group) Penile Cancer data base data. *Cancer*, 103: 2507, 2005.

[41] Leijte, J. A., Kroon, B. K., Valdés Olmos, R. A., Nieweg, O. E., and Horenblas, S.: Reliability and safety of current dynamic sentinel node biopsy for penile carcinoma. *Eur Urol*, 52: 170, 2007.

[42] Catalona, W. J.: Modified inguinal lymphadenectomy for carcinoma of the penis with preservation of saphenous veins: technique and preliminary results. *J Urol*, 140: 306, 1988.

[43] Cabanas, R. M.: An approach for the treatment of penile carcinoma. *Cancer*, 39: 456, 1977.

[44] Morton, D. L., Wen, D. R., Wong, J. H., Economou, J. S., Cagle, L. A., Storm, F. K. et al.: Technical details of intraoperative lymphatic mapping for early stage melanoma. *Arch Surg*, 127: 392, 1992.

[45] Horenblas, S., Jansen, L., Meinhardt, W., Hoefnagel, C. A., de Jong, D., and Nieweg, O. E.: Detection of occult metastasis in squamous cell carcinoma of the penis using a dynamic sentinel node procedure. *J Urol*, 163: 100, 2000.

[46] Kroon, B. K., Horenblas, S., Estourgie, S. H., Lont, A. P., Valdes Olmos, R. A., and Nieweg, O. E.: How to avoid false-negative dynamic sentinel node procedures in penile carcinoma. *J Urol*, 171: 2191, 2004.

[47] Hadway, P., Smith, Y., Corbishley, C., Heenan, S., and Watkin, N. A.: Evaluation of dynamic lymphoscintigraphy and sentinel lymph-node biopsy for detecting occult metastases in patients with penile squamous cell carcinoma. *BJU Int*, 100: 561, 2007.

[48] Kroon, B. K., Lont, A. P., Valdés Olmos, R. A., Nieweg, O. E., and Horenblas, S.: Morbidity of dynamic sentinel node biopsy in penile carcinoma. *J Urol*, 173: 813, 2005.

[49] Leijte, J. A., Hughes, B., Graafland, N. M., Kroon, B. K., Olmos, R. A., Nieweg, O. E. et al.: Two-center evaluation of dynamic sentinel node biopsy for squamous cell carcinoma of the penis. *J Clin Oncol*, 27: 3325, 2009.

[50] Leijte, J. A., Kerst, J. M., Bais, E., Antonini, N., and Horenblas, S.: Neoadjuvant chemotherapy in advanced penile carcinoma. *Eur Urol*, 52: 488, 2007.

[51] Horenblas, S., van Tinteren, H., Delemarre, J. F., Moonen, L. M., Lustig, V., and van Waardenburg, E. W.: Squamous cell carcinoma of the penis. III. Treatment of regional lymph nodes. *J Urol*, 149: 492, 1993.

[52] Zhu, Y., Zhang, S. L., Ye, D. W., Yao, X. D., Dai, B., Zhang, H. L. et al.: Prospectively packaged ilioinguinal lymphadenectomy for penile cancer: the disseminative pattern of lymph node metastasis. *J Urol,* 181: 2103, 2009.

[53] Bartelink, H., Breur, K., Hart, G., Annyas, B., van Slooten, E., and Snow, G.: The value of postoperative radiotherapy as an adjuvant to radical neck dissection. *Cancer,* 52: 1008, 1983.

[54] Graafland, N. M., van Boven, H. H., Van Werkhoven, E., Moonen, L. M., and Horenblas, S. Prognostic significance of extranodal extension in pathological node-positive patients with penile carcinoma. *The Journal of urology* . 2010

[55] Lopes, A., Bezerra, A. L., Serrano, S. V., and Hidalgo, G. S.: Iliac nodal metastases from carcinoma of the penis treated surgically. *BJU Int*, 86: 690, 2000.

In: Essentials and Updates in Urologic Oncology
Editor: Philippe E. Spiess

ISBN: 978-1-62081-494-9
© 2013 Nova Science Publishers, Inc.

Chapter XXXI

Management of Advanced Penile Cancer

Timothy E. Kubal[1], Philippe E. Spiess[1] and Andries M. Bergman[2]

[1]Department of Genitourinary Oncology, H. Lee Moffitt Cancer Center,
Tampa, Florida, US
[2]Department of Medical Oncology, Netherlands Cancer Institute,
Amsterdam, Netherlands

Abstract

Over the past two decades, there has been a timely progression in our therapeutic approach to the management of advanced penile squamous cell cancer within the United States. This chapter will document the evolution from single- to multi-agent chemotherapeutic approaches for locally advanced and metastatic penile cancer. In addition, we will highlight advances in diagnostic modalities for the detection of metastatic disease and increasingly employed multimodal approaches of chemotherapy and surgery (+/- radiotherapy) for patients with locally advanced and metastatic penile cancer.

Introduction

Penile squamous cell carcinoma is rare in the United States with an estimated 1250 new cases in 2010 and 310 predicted deaths (1). While multiple sociodemographic factors lead to a larger number of cases (26,000) diagnosed globally (2), an increasing proportion of newly diagnosed penile cancer cases present with early stage disease and are amenable to penile preserving approaches with curative intent such as local excision, laser ablation, or partial penectomy. In a smaller proportion of cases, patients present with locally advanced bulky nodal or distant metastatic disease. However due to the paucity of cases treated at any individual center, trials in this patient subset are scarce. Despite this lack of randomized trials, the treatment of patients with advanced penile cancer has evolved from single agent chemotherapy regimens, with modest clinical efficacy and significant treatment related toxicity to current multi-agent regimens, with reduced attributable toxicity when used in both the neo-adjuvant and/or adjuvant settings (palliative). In consequence, these changes have led to a significant improvement in the clinical outcomes as well as reduced treatment related morbidity. In the present chapter, we will discuss the historical and sequential evolution in our therapeutic approach to the management of advanced penile cancer.

Overview of Systemic Therapy for Advanced Penile Cancer

Single Agent Therapy

Initial chemotherapeutic regimens for advanced penile cancer focused on the utilization of single agents, with modest activity at the detrimental cost of significant toxicity (Table 1). Sklaroff et al. reported a series of eight patients treated with methotrexate at multiple dose levels, five of whom received high dose methotrexate. Three of the eight patients experienced a partial or complete response but these were noted to be short lived, with multiple recurrences. These three responders subsequently died at 7, 8, and 12 months following the initiation of systemic therapy (3). Ahmed et al. reported a series of fourteen patients treated with infusional bleomycin over a ten year period beginning in 1975, with a 21% response rate and only a single patient developing a complete response and prolonged survival. This moderate activity in patients with advanced disease was accompanied by significant toxicity, with two patients experiencing pulmonary toxicity and eight patients significant mucositis (4). As an extension of this trial, Ahmed et al. reported on patients sequentially treated with bleomycin, cisplatin, and methotrexate where patients received a single agent until demonstrated progression or intolerable side effects at which point they were changed to a different agent. In some cases, a third agent was continued until documented progression or dose limiting toxicities. Although these drugs were not applied in the same order for each patient, it was notable that patients who progressed on one agent could be transitioned to another class of drugs and still achieved a significant response to therapy (5). While this study demonstrated responses as long as 42 months, significant toxicity was apparent, with three reported treatment related deaths (one death secondary to bleomycin induced lung disease and two secondary to sepsis), and one patient developing pulmonary insufficiency requiring cessation of bleomycin.

Table 1. Select Reports of Single-agent Chemotherapy Regimens for Penile Cancer

Author	Agent	Patients	Responders	Median Duration of Response
Sklaroff et al (3)	Methotrexate	8	3/8	3 months (2-11 months)
Ahmed et al (4)	Bleomycin	14	3/14	3 months
Ahmed et al (5)	Methotrexate	13	8/13	3 months (2-31 months)
	Cisplatin	12	3/12	8 months (2-8 months)
	Bleomycin	14	3/14	3 months (2-4 months)

While early single agent therapy had both limited responses and somewhat limited therapeutic duration, single agent methotrexate has proven promising in a subgroup of patients with advanced penile verrucous carcinoma. Given the sexual and psychological implications pertaining to total penectomy, Sheen et al. treated six patients with single agent methotrexate via intra-vascular infusion (6). Methotrexate was delivered into the lower abdominal aorta at 50 mg over a 24 hour period by continuous infusion through a femoral artery catheter. Response was assessed clinically with cessation of the infusion after an average of 11 days of therapy. Development of a skin rash over the area of infusion was noted in all patients. Four of six patients experienced a complete response, with the remaining two patients experiencing a partial response to therapy. Both partial responders eventually underwent penectomy with one patient dying of metastatic disease which on biopsy was found to be moderately differentiated squamous cell carcinoma of the penis rather than verrucous carcinoma. The remaining five patients were alive at last follow-up, between 3 and 17 years following treatment with single agent methotrexate. Given the aforementioned issues associated with penectomy, the efficacy of single agent therapy in this patient subset is of therapeutic consideration among patients with advanced penile verrucous carcinoma.

Multi-Agent Therapy

Following the demonstration of the efficacy of several agents in advanced penile cancer (5), multiple groups embarked on trials of systemic agents delivered concurrently (Table 2) most frequently consisting of cisplatin, methotrexate, and bleomycin (CMB). Dexeus et al. treated 14 patients with inoperable, metastatic squamous cell carcinoma of the male genital tract, 12 of whom had a penile cancer primary, with 4 week cycles of CMB demonstrating a response rate of 72%. Two of fourteen patients experienced a complete response, with one patient alive without evidence of disease more than two years following the initiation of chemotherapy. A partial response was noted in the remaining eight responders however, these responses were short lived, with rapid progression of disease after failure of chemotherapy. The mean overall survival in these patients was only 10 months. Furthermore, treatment related morbidity was significant with evidence of bleomycin toxicity in five patients (7). Corral et al. also evaluated the efficacy of CMB in thirty patients with advanced SCC of the genitourinary tract, twenty one of whom had penile cancer, with a 57% overall response rate and a comparable median survival of only 11.5 months following the initiation of chemotherapy (8). Among the patients with penile cancer, there were eight partial responses and four complete responses. Notably, six patients who were rendered disease-free at some point during therapy had a prolonged overall survival of 27.8 months compared to only 6.7 months in the patients who did not achieve a disease free status at any point during therapy. Side-effects were generally manageable in this cohort, however the toxicity of this regimen was highlighted in a subsequent study of 45 patients treated with CMB by Haas et al.(9). In this study, 13 patients achieved a partial or complete response to CMB however, there were five treatment related deaths secondary to infectious complications in one patient and pulmonary related mortalities in the four others. Another death due to pulmonary toxicity occurred in a group of 13 patients treated with CMB by Hakenberg et al.(10). Thus, despite a significant response rate in patients treated with CMB, many of the responses were of short duration and accompanied by significant toxicity and potential treatment related mortality.

Table 2. Select Reports of Multi-agent Chemotherapy Regimens for Penile Cancer

Author	Regimen	Patients	Responders	Reported Outcomes
Dexeus et al. (7)	CMB	14	10/14 (72%)	Median Response Duration: 5.9 months
Corrall et al. (8)	CMB	21	12/21 (57%)	Median OS: 6.7 months in nonresponders. 27.8 months in responders
Haas et al. (9)	CMB	45	13/45 (29%)	Median OS: 7 months
Shammas et al. (11)	Cisplatin + 5-FU	8	2/8 (25%)	Surival Range: Nonresponders: 2-28 months. Responders >32, >57 months
Hussein et al. (12)	Cisplatin + 5-FU	6	6/6 (100%)	OS: 6 to >32 months.
Pagliaro et al. (13)	TIP	30	15/30 (50%)	Median OS:17.1 months in patients who had died at the time of publication. Range of >14 to >59 months in surviving patients at time of publication.

CMB: Cisplatin, Methotrexate, Bleomycin
TIP: Paclitaxel, Ifosfamide, Cisplatin
OS: Overall Survival

An alternative multiagent regimen of cisplatin on day 1 and 5-fluorouracil infused continuously for a maximum of five days was employed by several groups (11, 12). A combination of their respective results revealed responses in 7 of 14 patients, with a combination approach that included radiation and surgery. Interestingly, four of seven responders experienced a survival of greater than 2 years.

Given the severe toxicities associated with CMB and most notably the pulmonary complications related to bleomycin, the most recent trial in patients with advanced penile cancer employed paclitaxel, ifosfamide, and cisplatin (13). Thirty patients were treated with four courses of therapy every 3-4 weeks. Fifteen of thirty patients had an objective response, with twenty-two patients proceeding to surgical resection. Nine patients treated with chemotherapy followed by surgery were alive without recurrence at time of publication, with an average median follow-up of 34 months. The regimen was well tolerated, with no treatment related deaths. Given the toxicities associated with previous multi-agent regimens, this represents a significant advance in the therapeutic armamentarium for advanced penile cancer. However, while chemotherapy alone has produced some durable responses, a multimodal approach consisting of systemic therapy and consolidative surgical resection offers the greatest promise.

Concept of Multimodal Therapy

Historically, most patients have progressed with single modal therapy consisting of surgery or systemic chemotherapy. Given the small number of patients treated at any single center and lack of large clinical trials in advanced penile cancer, extrapolation from the scientific literature pertaining to the treatment related outcomes of squamous cell carcinoma at other sites suggested the potential merit of a multimodal approach for patients with locally advanced and metastatic penile cancer. This offered the potential to reduce both morbidity and mortality. A number of trials were thus undertaken to investigate the concept of neo-adjuvant and adjuvant chemotherapy followed by surgical resection.

Neo-Adjuvant Chemotherapy

In the subsequent decade, multiple agents were found to have some activity in advanced penile cancer however few of these agents had enough therapeutic efficacy to cure patients with advanced disease. Surgical interventions could be employed with curative intent however extensive radical lymph node dissection and hemi-pelvectomy were accompanied by unacceptable morbidity and mortality (14). Furthermore, historical surgical series of patients with bulky nodal disease managed in this fashion have been disappointing. Patients with unilateral metastases to superficial inguinal lymph nodes have a 5 year survival rate of over 80% with surgical management alone however, as disease progresses to: (1) bilateral superficial inguinal, (2) deep inguinal, or (3) pelvic lymph nodes, the five year survival is significantly worse as demonstrated in a large series in which the five year survival for patients with unilateral inguinal nodal involvement was 86% versus 60% for those with bilateral inguinal lymph node disease and 0% for patients with pelvic lymph node metastases (15). Despite these unfavorable reported outcomes, there remains a role for inguinal lymph node dissection in patients with advanced disease. Figure 1 represents a schematic diagram of how neoadjuvant chemotherapy can be integrated in the management of advanced penile cancer. In the previously mentioned study by Pagliaro et al., thirty patients with clinical N2 and N3 disease were treated neoadjuvantly with paclitaxel, ifosfamide, and cisplatin (TIP), with 50% of patients having a significant clinical response and twenty two patients undergoing subsequent surgical resection. The median overall survival of patients with pelvic nodal metastasis was 19 months (13). While these numbers cannot be directly compared to those reported by Ravi (15), it is likely that survival was significantly prolonged by the combination of neoadjuvant chemotherapy followed by surgical resection within this patient population, most notably in three patients found to have a complete pathologic (i.e. no viable cancer) at the time of surgery.

Other than the regimen employed at the M. D. Anderson Cancer Center by Pagliaro et al., several other chemotherapeutic regimens have been proposed in the neoadjuvant setting (Table 3). Pizzocaro and Piva treated five patients with fixed, non-mobile inguinal lymph nodes with neoadjuvant vincristine, bleomycin, and methotrexate (VBM) weekly for a total of 12 weeks (16). Three patients had a partial response and following radical inguinal lymph node dissection were alive at 20, 27, and 72 months follow-up. The two patients who had a minimal response to neoadjuvant chemotherapy progressed and died of disease within several months of undergoing radical inguinal lymph node dissection. Bermejo et al. reviewed the natural history of ten patients who underwent neoadjuvant chemotherapy with CMB, TIP, or paclitaxel/carboplatin (PC) followed by subsequent inguinal lymph node dissection. Three of the patients who received TIP had no nodal metastases at the time of surgery, with four of ten patients alive at 5 years, with a median survival in the remaining patients of fourteen months (17). Leijte et al. performed a similar review of twenty patients treated with five different neoadjuvant chemotherapeutic regimens over a 34 year period, with the therapeutic goal being clinical downstaging (i.e. regression). Twelve of twenty patients were responsive to neoadjuvant chemotherapy, with two complete responses and nine patients undergoing subsequent surgical consolidation. In the patients responsive to neoadjuvant chemotherapy, the 5 year survival was 56% while all non-responders died within 9 months of chemotherapy. Three patients treated with CMB died secondary to treatment related toxicity, echoing the prior reports on its potential morbidity (18).

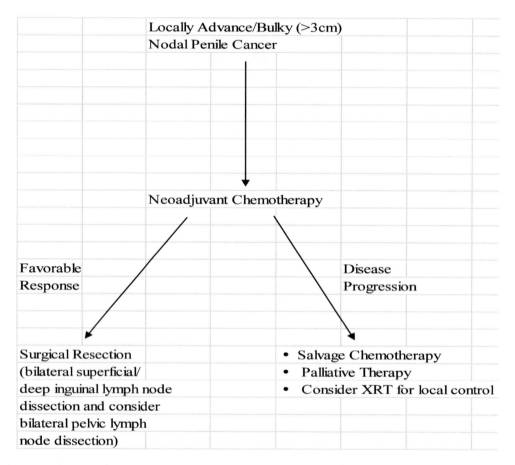

Figure 1. Schematic diagram illustrating the integration of neoadjuvant chemotherapy followed by surgical resection.

Theodore et al. used an alternative neoadjuvant regimen of cisplatin and irinotecan in patients with metastatic penile cancer (19). While this regimen did not improve survival in patients with metastatic disease, three of seven patients experienced a pathologic complete response, with no evidence of metastatic disease at time of inguinal lymph node dissection. Culkin and Beer combined the neoadjuvant studies utilizing cisplatin based regimens and found an overall response rate of 69% (24 of 35 patients). Fifteen of these patients were able to undergo subsequent surgical resection, with eight patients alive without evidence of disease at 1 to 10 years of follow-up (20). Pizzocarro (21) employed a regimen similar to that employed by Vermorken (22) to treat and improve the outcomes of patients with squamous cell cancer of the head and neck, with the regimen consisting of cisplatin, fluorouracil, and docetaxel. Six consecutive patients with unresectable or recurrent nodal metastases were treated with paclitaxel on day 1 followed by cisplatin on day 1 and 2 and continuous infusion of 5-Fluorouracil daily on days 2-5. Five of six patients exhibited a response to therapy and three patients were alive and free of disease greater than 2 years following neoadjuvant chemotherapy and consolidative surgical resection.

Table 3. Select Reports of Neoadjuvant Chemotherapy Approaches to Penile Cancer

Author	Regimen	Patients	Responders	Reported Outcomes
Pizzocaro and Piva (16)	VBM	5	3/5 (60%)	Responders alive at 20-72 months followup at time of publication.
Bermejo et al (17)	CMB, TIP, PC	10	5/10 (50%)	Median OS: 26 months
Leijte et al (18)	Bleomycin, VBM, CMB, 5-FU/Cisplatin, Cisplatin/Irinotecan	20	12/20 (60%)	5 year OS: 32%
Theodore et al (19)	Cisplatin/Irinotecan	7	3/7 (43%)	Outcomes not reported
Pizzocaro et al (21)	TPF	6	5/6 (83%)	Survival from chemotherapy: (4-46 months). 3 patients alive at time of publication.
Pagliaro et al (13)	TIP	30	15/30 (50%)	Median OS:17.1 months in patients who had died at the time of publication. Range of >14 to >59 months in surviving patients at time of publication.

VBM: Vincristine, Bleomycin, Methotrexate
CMB: Cisplatin, Methotrexate, Bleomycin
PC: Paclitaxel, Carboplatin
TPF: Paclitaxel, Cisplatin, 5-FU
TIP: Paclitaxel, Ifosfamide, Cisplatin
OS: Overall Survival

Future directions in systemic regimens for locally advance/metastatic penile cancer will likely include the use of epidermal growth factor receptor (EGFR) inhibitors which have demonstrated some efficacy in the management of squamous cell carcinoma of the head and neck. Carthon et al. reviewed 13 patients with advanced penile cancer who received erlotinib alone, cetuximab or cetuximab plus platinum based chemotherapy, with a median overall survival of 9.8 months (range: 0.5-48.3 months) and 4 of 13 patients surviving beyond 13 months (23). The strong expression of EGFR seen in the majority of primary tumors in this study is promising and indicative of the merit of this approach, which is likely to be examined in future Phase II/III prospective clinical trials.

In an effort to improve our ability to detect occult nodal involvement and to determine which patients would benefit from an inguinal lymph node dissection, several trials have investigated the efficacy of non-invasive imaging/surgical techniques in the detection of occult metastatic disease (Table 4). Tabatabaei et al. evaluated the clinical merit of lymphotropic nanoparticle enhanced MRI with Ferumoxtran-10 in the diagnostic evaluation of patients with penile cancer (24).

Seven patients with penile squamous cell carcinoma underwent nanoparticle MRI prior to their scheduled inguinal lymph node dissection. A total of 113 lymph nodes were resected at the time of surgery, with 13 nodes harboring occult metastatic disease on histopathologic analysis. The sensitivity and specificity of MRI for detecting occult nodal metastases was 100% and 97%, respectively. Scher et al. performed a study evaluating the merit of PET/CT as a staging modality among thirteen patients with suspected penile cancer, with eight patients subsequently found to have penile cancer.

Six of these patients were suspected to have penile cancer based on PET/CT imaging alone. While this study provides some optimism in the diagnostic assessment of primary penile lesions, the greater clinical question for PET/CT remains can it help identify occult metastatic disease. In this regard, the study assessed five patients in which a total of sixteen metastatic inguinal lymph nodes resected as confirmed by histopathologic evaluation. Ninety-four percent of the metastatic lymph nodes were identified by PET/CT, with only a single false negative lymph node.

In patients without penile cancer or in those with negative inguinal lymph nodes, there were no false positives identified by PET/CT (25). Similar results were obtained in a study by Graafland et al. in which patients with clinically suspected inguinal nodes underwent PET/CT prior to undergoing inguinal lymph node dissection. Imaging was performed in fourteen patients (i.e. twenty-eight inguinal areas), with ten of eleven positive inguinal regions for metastatic disease and all seventeen negative inguinal regions for metastatic disease correctly predicted by PET/CT (26).

Table 4. Summary of Non-invasive Diagnostic Surgical Techniques for Evaluating Inguinal Lymph Nodes

Diagnostic
• Nanoparticle MRI
• PET-CT
• Imaging guided (US, CT, MRI) percutaneous lymph node biopsy
Surgical
• Dynamic sentinel node biopsy
• Laparoscopic (pure/robotic assisted) inguinal lymph node dissection

CT, computerized tomography; MRI, magnetic resonance imaging; PET, positron emission tomography; US, ultrasound.

Both PET/CT and MRI are evolving technologies which may represent adjunctive tools to the physical examination in the evaluation and management of penile cancer. These emerging diagnostic tools should be integrated in the staging of penile cancer patients including patients with questionable inguinal lymphadenopathy of uncertain clinical significance. In addition, the multimodal approach of neoadjuvant chemotherapy followed by extirpative surgical resection in penile cancer patients with locally advanced or bulky nodal metastases is rapidly being adopted as the preferred therapeutic approach.

Adjuvant Chemotherapy

Few studies have systematically evaluated the effectiveness of adjuvant chemotherapy following surgical resection however patients with multiple inguinal nodal metastases or pelvic lymph node involvement may benefit from additional systemic therapy. (Table 5) details some of the clinical/pathological features for which adjuvant chemotherapy should be considered. Ravi reviewed 201 patients treated for penile carcinoma with primary penile tumor resection and inguinal lymph node dissection (15). Patients with greater than 3 positive inguinal lymph nodes had a 5 year survival of only 50%. No patients with pelvic lymph node involvement survived up to 5 years. The patients with multiple inguinal or pelvic lymph node metastases who did not receive neoadjuvant chemotherapy were at high risk of recurrence or disease progression, suggesting that these patients should be strongly encouraged to receive adjuvant systemic chemotherapy following inguinal lymph node resection (I'm not sure if you can make this statement. There is very little evidenve for this; I would say: can be considered, despite little evidence). Maiche reported on a series of nineteen patients who received adjuvant bleomycin or VBM following surgical resection for penile cancer. Eleven of nineteen patients had distant metastatic disease at the time of diagnosis, including the presence of pulmonary, hepatic, and/or bone metastases, with an overall survival for this cohort ranging between 5 to 61 months (27). Pizzocaro and Piva reported a series of twelve patients receiving adjuvant chemotherapy with VBM following inguinal lymph node dissection in the clinical context of pathology proven lymph node metastases. Only one of these twelve patients experienced a disease recurrence at a median follow-up of 42 months (16).

**Table 5. Clinical/pathological Features for which Adjuvant
Chemotherapy should be Considered**

Bulky nodal disease (pN2/3)
Extranodal extension
Suspected unresected disease (along with consideration of post-operative radiation therapy)
Lymphovascular invasion

Radiotherapy

Limited data is available on the merit of radiotherapy in patients with advanced penile cancer. The largest study on this topic was conducted by Ravi et al. in which 120 patients with lymph node positive penile cancer received local radiotherapy (28). Forty-one patients received palliative radiation therapy to fixed inguinal lymph nodes with a five year disease-free survival of only 2%. Similarly, 12 patients received post-operative inguinal radiation therapy for perinodal infiltration with only a single patient (8%) free of disease at 5 years. Most notable were the results in thirty three patients (38 inguinal areas) with mobile nodes greater than 4 cm in size who were treated with neoadjuvant radiotherapy followed by inguinal lymph node dissection. Only 3 of 38 subsequent inguinal dissections revealed extranodal extension on histopathologic examination, with only a single patient developing a post-operative inguinal recurrence and a five year disease-free survival of 70%. This study concluded that pre-operative radiotherapy may improve local control in patients with nodes greater than 4 cm in diameter and hence should be at least considered in this subset of patients. Concurrent systemic chemotherapy and radiotherapy has not been tested extensively for squamous cell carcinoma of the penis; however, it has been evaluated for squamous cell carcinomas of other sites (e.g. anus, vulvar), with significant efficacy when used concomitantly. The standard of care for squamous cell carcinoma of the anus was established through trials by the UK Coordinating Committee on Cancer Research and the European Organization for Research and Treatment of Cancer (29,30), both of which showed a significant survival benefit of radiotherapy with concurrent 5-fluorouracil and mitomycin versus radiotherapy alone. Combined systemic chemotherapy and radiotherapy has also proven effective for vulvar carcinoma as demonstrated through multiple clinical trials by the Gynecologic Oncology Group (GOG). In GOG protocol 101, forty women with unresectable N2/N3 vulvar cancer were treated with concurrent chemoradiotherapy utilizing 5-fluorouracil and cisplatin. Ninety-five percent of these patients achieved resectability following chemoradiotherapy, with a complete pathological response in 41% of treated patients (31). Thus, while the current role of radiation in advanced penile cancer remains highly debatable in patients with bulky nodal or widespread metastatic penile cancer, it remains feasible that the concurrent use of chemotherapy and radiotherapy in the neoadjuvant or adjuvant setting may offer some promise.

Conclusions

The definitive treatment of advanced squamous cell carcinoma of the penis remains in constant evolution. Over the proceeding four decades, multiple agents have been identified as active in advanced penile cancer. The response rates to these single agents were modest and short lived in most cases leading to the development of multi-agent regimens including CMB, VBM, cisplatin/5-FU and most recently TIP. These multi-agent regimens generally produce a greater therapeutic response, including some durable responses using CMB, however this is at the expense of severe toxicity and the potential of treatment related mortality. The more recently described TIP regimen offers significant response rates, with an acceptable toxicity profile and in this regard should be considered the first line regimen for patients with advanced penile cancer.

Most promising is the development of multimodal treatment approaches that combine chemotherapy and consolidative surgical resection in patients with advanced penile cancer. Radiation therapy may also play a role in the multimodal approach to advanced penile cancer. Similarly, evolving non-invasive diagnostic tools and targeted therapies including EGFR inhibitors aimed at the phenotypic characteristics of these tumors may redefine the medical/surgical care of penile cancer in the many years to come.

References

[1]   Jemal A, Siegel R, Xu J, Ward E. Cancer statistics, 2010. *CA Cancer J Clin*. 2010 Sep-Oct;60(5):277-300.
[2]   Bleeker MC, Heideman DA, Snijders PJ, Horenblas S, Dillner J, Meijer CJ. Penile cancer: epidemiology, pathogenesis and prevention. *World J Urol*. 2009 Apr;27(2):141-50.
[3]   Sklaroff RB, Yagoda A. Methotrexate in the treatment of penile carcinoma. *Cancer*. 1980 Jan 15;45(2):214-6.

[4]   Ahmed T, Sklaroff R, Yagoda A. An appraisal of the efficacy of bleomycin in epidermoid carcinoma of the penis. *Anticancer Res.* 1984 Jul-Oct;4(4-5):289-92.

[5]   Ahmed T, Sklaroff R, Yagoda A. Sequential trials of methotrexate, cisplatin and bleomycin for penile cancer. *J Urol.* 1984 Sep;132(3):465-8.

[6]   Sheen MC, Sheu HM, Jang MY, Chai CY, Wang YW, Wu CF. Advanced penile verrucous carcinoma treated with intra-aortic infusion chemotherapy. *J Urol.* 2010 May;183(5):1830-5.

[7]   Dexeus FH, Logothetis CJ, Sella A, Amato R, Kilbourn R, Fitz K, et al. Combination chemotherapy with methotrexate, bleomycin and cisplatin for advanced squamous cell carcinoma of the male genital tract. *J Urol.* 1991 Nov;146(5):1284-7.

[8]   Corral DA, Sella A, Pettaway CA, Amato RJ, Jones DM, Ellerhorst J. Combination chemotherapy for metastatic or locally advanced genitourinary squamous cell carcinoma: a phase II study of methotrexate, cisplatin and bleomycin. *J Urol.* 1998 Nov;160(5):1770-4.

[9]   Cisplatin, methotrexate and bleomycin for the treatment of carcinoma of the penis: a Southwest Oncology Group study. *J Urol.* 1999 Jun;161(6):1823-5.

[10]   Hakenberg OW, Nippgen JB, Froehner M, Zastrow S, Wirth MP. Cisplatin, methotrexate and bleomycin for treating advanced penile carcinoma. *BJU Int.* 2006 Dec;98(6):1225-7.

[11]   Shammas FV, Ous S, Fossa SD. Cisplatin and 5-fluorouracil in advanced cancer of the penis. *J Urol.* 1992 Mar;147(3):630-2.

[12]   Hussein AM, Benedetto P, Sridhar KS. Chemotherapy with cisplatin and 5-fluorouracil for penile and urethral squamous cell carcinomas. *Cancer.* 1990 Feb 1;65(3):433-8.

[13]   Pagliaro LC, Williams DL, Daliani D, Williams MB, Osai W, Kincaid M, et al. Neoadjuvant paclitaxel, ifosfamide, and cisplatin chemotherapy for metastatic penile cancer: a phase II study. *J Clin Oncol.* 2010 Aug 20;28(24):3851-7.

[14]   Block NL, Rosen P, Whitmore WF, Jr. Hemipelvectomy for advanced penile cancer. *J Urol.* 1973 Dec;110(6):703-7.

[15]   Ravi R. Correlation between the extent of nodal involvement and survival following groin dissection for carcinoma of the penis. *Br J Urol.* 1993 Nov;72(5 Pt 2):817-9.

[16]   Pizzocaro G, Piva L. Adjuvant and neoadjuvant vincristine, bleomycin, and methotrexate for inguinal metastases from squamous cell carcinoma of the penis. *Acta Oncol.* 1988;27(6b):823-4.

[17]   Bermejo C, Busby JE, Spiess PE, Heller L, Pagliaro LC, Pettaway CA. Neoadjuvant chemotherapy followed by aggressive surgical consolidation for metastatic penile squamous cell carcinoma. *J Urol.* 2007 Apr;177(4):1335-8.

[18]   Leijte JA, Kerst JM, Bais E, Antonini N, Horenblas S. Neoadjuvant chemotherapy in advanced penile carcinoma. *Eur Urol.* 2007 Aug;52(2):488-94.

[19]   Theodore C, Skoneczna I, Bodrogi I, Leahy M, Kerst JM, Collette L, et al. A phase II multicentre study of irinotecan (CPT 11) in combination with cisplatin (CDDP) in metastatic or locally advanced penile carcinoma (EORTC PROTOCOL 30992). *Ann Oncol.* 2008 Jul;19(7):1304-7.

[20] Culkin DJ, Beer TM. Advanced penile carcinoma. *J Urol*. 2003 Aug;170(2 Pt 1):359-65.

[21] Pizzocaro G, Nicolai N, Milani A. Taxanes in combination with cisplatin and fluorouracil for advanced penile cancer: preliminary results. *Eur Urol*. 2009 Mar;55(3):546-51.

[22] Vermorken JB, Remenar E, van Herpen C, Gorlia T, Mesia R, Degardin M, et al. Cisplatin, fluorouracil, and docetaxel in unresectable head and neck cancer. *N Engl J Med*. 2007 Oct 25;357(17):1695-704.

[23] Carthon BC PC, Pagliaro LC. Epidermal growth factor receptor (EGFR) targeted therapy in advanced metastatic squamous cell carcinoma (AMSCC) of the penis [abstract #254]. In: *American Society of Clinical Oncology Genitourinary Cancers Symposium, San Francisco (CA)*, March 5-7, 2010.

[24] Tabatabaei S, Harisinghani M, McDougal WS. Regional lymph node staging using lymphotropic nanoparticle enhanced magnetic resonance imaging with ferumoxtran-10 in patients with penile cancer. *J Urol*. 2005 Sep;174(3):923-7; discussion 7.

[25] Scher B, Seitz M, Reiser M, Hungerhuber E, Hahn K, Tiling R, et al. 18F-FDG PET/CT for staging of penile cancer. *J Nucl Med*. 2005 Sep;46(9):1460-5.

[26] Graafland NM, Leijte JA, Valdes Olmos RA, Hoefnagel CA, Teertstra HJ, Horenblas S. Scanning with 18F-FDG-PET/CT for detection of pelvic nodal involvement in inguinal node-positive penile carcinoma. *Eur Urol*. 2009 Aug;56(2):339-45.

[27] Maiche AG. Adjuvant treatment using bleomycin in squamous cell carcinoma of penis: study of 19 cases. *Br J Urol*. 1983 Oct;55(5):542-4.

[28] Ravi R, Chaturvedi HK, Sastry DV. Role of radiation therapy in the treatment of carcinoma of the penis. *Br J Urol*. 1994 Nov;74(5):646-51.

[29] Epidermoid anal cancer: results from the UKCCCR randomised trial of radiotherapy alone versus radiotherapy, 5-fluorouracil, and mitomycin. UKCCCR Anal Cancer Trial Working Party. UK Co-ordinating Committee on Cancer Research. *Lancet*. 1996 Oct 19;348(9034):1049-54.

[30] Bartelink H, Roelofsen F, Eschwege F, Rougier P, Bosset JF, Gonzalez DG, et al. Concomitant radiotherapy and chemotherapy is superior to radiotherapy alone in the treatment of locally advanced anal cancer: results of a phase III randomized trial of the European Organization for Research and Treatment of Cancer Radiotherapy and Gastrointestinal Cooperative Groups. *J Clin Oncol*. 1997 May;15(5):2040-9.

[31] Montana GS, Thomas GM, Moore DH, Saxer A, Mangan CE, Lentz SS, et al. Preoperative chemo-radiation for carcinoma of the vulva with N2/N3 nodes: a gynecologic oncology group study. *Int J Radiat Oncol Biol Phys*. 2000 Nov 1;48(4):1007-13.

Section 8. Adrenal Cancer

W. Bradford Carter
Section Editor

In: Essentials and Updates in Urologic Oncology
Editor: Philippe E. Spiess

ISBN: 978-1-62081-494-9
© 2013 Nova Science Publishers, Inc.

Chapter XXXII

Adrenal Cancer

*W. Bradford Carter,[1] Jeremiah L. Deneve,[1] John D. Tourtelot,[2]
Jamie T. Caracciolo,[3] Sarah E. Hoffe,[4] Michael D. Chuong[4]
and Howard S. Lilienfeld[2]*

Department of Surgical Oncology[1] Endocrinology[2], Radiology[3],
and Radiation Oncology[4], Moffitt Cancer Center; Tampa, Florida, US

Abstract

Adrenal cortical cancer (ACC) is a rare tumor with an incidence of 1-2 per million population. Although most are identified incidentally on cross-sectional imaging, timely identification and early surgical treatment is critical for optimized treatment outcomes. Sixty percent of ACC autonomously produced adrenal cortical hormones, primarily cortisol or androgens and often present with clinical syndromes such as Cushing's syndrome or virilization. Cross-sectional imaging provides the best assessment of malignant potential. Imaging characteristics of benign neoplasms include low-density lesions (Hounsfield units < 10 on noncontrast CT, size < 4 cm, homogeneity, and rapid washout of contrast. Lipid rich adenomas show signal suppression on chemical shift MRI and very low SUV uptake on PET imaging. Since most adrenal masses are found incidentally, metabolic screening for hormone production should be performed in all cases, including patients without clinical evidence of hormone excess. Surgical resection is indicated for adrenal lesions with suspicion of malignancy and/or those exhibiting autonomous hormone production. While minimally invasive techniques may be appropriate for smaller tumors, oncologic principles should be followed.

Introduction

Adrenocortical cancer (ACC) is a rare cancer occurring in 1 or 2 persons per 1 million population [1, 2, 3] but timely identification and early treatment can make a significant difference in the overall survival. Adrenal cortical cancer has a bimodal distribution based on age and typically occurs under 6 and between 30 and 40 years old [1]. Radical surgical excision is indicated for localized (non-metastatic) tumors and is the only opportunity for cure and the only treatment shown to improve disease free survival. [4, 5, 6, 7, 8, 9] A multidisciplinary approach with the adrenal surgeon, medical oncologist, endocrinologist, radiologist and radiation oncologist is important to devise a therapeutic plan with maximal effective potential. Since large, randomized, long-term studies have not been performed on this rare cancer, most of the available data is gathered from experts who have been following small numbers of patients. This chapter will discuss the metabolic and radiologic workup and treatment paradigms for ACC.

Presentation

The adrenal tumor is often found incidentally during an evaluation for another disorder or a biochemical workup for an endocrinopathy i.e. Cushing's syndrome or hirsutism. The incidence of ACC from incidentally found adrenal masses has been reported to range from 4.7 % in a retrospective review of 2005 patients at the Mayo Clinic to 10% [10, 11, 12] . The radiographic findings on CT and MRI evaluations, including size, were most important in making the diagnosis of ACC. [13, 14, 15, 16]

While many patients with ACC are non-functioning, 60 percent of patients present with endocrinopathies associated with over-production of adrenal cortical hormones. [1, 17, 3] Forty-five percent of these patients have cortisol excess with clinical findings of Cushing's syndrome, and 25% present with hyper-secretion of cortisol and androgens. [1,18] Few present with isolated virilization, feminization, or hyperaldosteronism, but virilization in association with an adrenal neoplasm strongly suggests ACC. Children commonly present with virilization and precocious puberty (84%) but rarely present with isolated glucocorticoid excess. Signs of Cushing syndrome due to corticosteroid excess [19, 20] typically include weight gain with central obesity, supraclavicular fullness, dorsocervical fat pad, striae and moon facies, muscle atrophy and proximal muscle weakness. Hyperaldosteronism (Conn's syndrome) is due to mineralocorticoid excess resulting in hypertension and hypokalemia that may develop rapidly. Signs and symptoms of glucocorticoid excess may be limited in patients with androgen production production due to the anabolic effects, and careful evaluation for glucocorticoid excess should be performed in patients with virilization. [13] Nonfunctioning ACC is more common in older patients and these tumors progress more rapidly. Patients with hypercortisolism appear to have shorter survival, likely due to the morbidity of overt Cushing's syndrome. [21]

Evaluation of Adrenal Tumors

Components of a logical workup for adrenal tumors include determination of hormonally active substances being secreted by the tumor, determining the malignant potential of the tumor, and a search for evidence of metastasis. The starting point (initial consultation) for the surgeon is often incomplete and requires further evaluation and preparation to avoid unexpected and avoidable complications. Radiologic and endocrinologic expertise in adrenal imaging and function are essential for appropriate evaluation and treatment of associated endocrinopathy. Benign adenomas of the adrenal are common, and need not be removed unless autonomously producing adrenal hormones. Understanding the radiologic characteristics indicative of benign, lipid-rich adenomas will prevent unnecessary surgery and negate the ill-conceived suggestion of a fine needle aspiration biopsy. ACC cannot be identified by cytology, and the risk of local seeding of ACC with capsular disruption contra-indicate image guided biopsy for any adrenal lesion with a risk of ACC. [22, 23, 24, 25] Adrenal tumors with more than a minimal malignant potential by imaging characteristics should be surgically removed for diagnosis and treatment, following oncologic principles of surgery, including en bloc resection and surgical resection for margin. [26, 27, 28]

ACC is commonly identified as an adrenal neoplasm discovered incidentally on abdominal cross-sectional imaging performed for symptoms or staging. An adrenal incidentaloma is defined as a mass lesion of the adrenal gland that is over one centimeter in size, found fortuitously on a radiologic study. (sc1) CT and MRI scans make up the majority of the radiologic studies that often initially identify these adrenal masses, [29, 11, 30] which are ordered for numerous reasons ranging from abdominal pain to staging for various malignancies.

Table 1. [11]

Incidental Adrenal Masses
Adenoma (non-secreting)
Pheochromocytoma
Aldosteronoma
Adrenocortical carcinoma
Adrenal Cyst
Hematoma
Ganglioneuroma
Metastasis
Myelolipoma
Sex hormone secreting tumors (very rare)
Nodular adrenal hyperplasia

Most adrenal incidentalomas are benign and relatively small. In a series of 12,000 autopsies it was noted that the majority of adrenal masses recorded were between 2 and 6 cm. in diameter [11, 31] . The Cleveland Clinic published a retrospective case series of non-contrast CT scan findings documenting the size, radiological characteristics and surgical histopathologic findings of adrenal neoplasms. The mean size of an adenoma was 2.8 cm, statistically smaller than adrenocortical carcinomas with a mean of 10.1 cm [32] (table 2). The incidence of incidentally identified adrenal lesions on CT increases with age. In the general population, the incidence of discovery of an adrenal mass is 4%, but in patients between the ages of 20 and 29, the incidence is 0.2%, increasing to 7% in the over-70 age group. [4] (sc1,) The incidental discovery of an adrenal neoplasm should prompt additional investigation to determine its malignant potential and to determine if the tumor produces autonomous hormonal hypersection.

Adrenal Imaging

Cross-sectional imaging characteristics provide the best evaluation of malignant potential. The presence of metastasis confirms malignancy, but other characteristics raise the index of suspicion for ACC.

Imaging of the adrenal glands is largely performed by cross sectional imaging modalities including computed tomography (CT) and magnetic resonance imaging (MRI). Ultrasonography (US) has a limited role in evaluation of adrenal masses, though occasionally a suprarenal mass may be detected at abdominal or renal US performed for other clinical indications. Nuclear medicine studies, such I-131 MIBG scans, are often utilized once an adrenal lesion is detected and/or there is clinical suspicion for pheochromocytoma. Newer radiopharmaceuticals are also available in select cases for the evaluation of adrenal adenoma. F-18 FDG positron emission tomography (PET) may help differentiate between benign and malignancy lesions based on uptake levels.

When an adrenal mass is detected, characterization can be performed by several different imaging techniques. The study selected is usually determined by institutional preference /experience and other clinical factors such as patient history and presentation (i.e. known malignancy with suspicion of metastatic disease or uncontrollable hypertension). However, adrenal masses are often detected incidentally at contrast-enhanced abdominal CT performed for other reasons such as abdominal pain or trauma. In this case, many masses are deemed indeterminate and, subsequently, a dedicated examination is requested for further characterization.

Unenhanced abdominal CT is often utilized to characterize an adrenal mass and has been shown to reliably differentiate between lipid rich adrenal adenomas and non-adenomas with extremely high specificity [14]. Lipid rich adrenal adenomas demonstrate unenhanced attenuation values less than 10 Hounsfield units (HU) due to the presence of intracellular lipids, as opposed to adrenocortical carcinomas which demonstrate unenhanced attenuation values in the range of 40 HU [33]. Unenhanced and contrast-enhanced CT with absolute percentage washout calculation can also be performed to characterize an adrenal mass. This technique requires acquisition of unenhanced (U), early (E; 60 seconds), and delayed (D; 15 minutes) phase contrast-enhanced imaging. On digital image display workstations with electronic caliper functionalities, regions of interest are placed within an adrenal mass to quantify attenuation values and determine the absolute percentage washout calculation defined as [(E-D)/(E-U)] x 100. If unenhanced imaging is not available, relative percentage washout calculation defined as (E-D)/E x 100 can be performed. Adrenal adenomas have been shown to demonstrate more rapid washout of intravenous contrast material than do non-adenomas including adrenocortical carcinoma. With high sensitivity and specificity, absolute washout values (AWV) greater than 60% or relative washout values (RWV) greater than 40% indicate adenoma [15]. Conversely, malignant tumors typically demonstrate relative washout values less than 40% as these tumors tend to retain contrast material longer. In fact, a small retrospective study of proven adrenocortical carcinomas reported that all demonstrated relative washout values less than 40% [33].

Chemical shift MRI, also known as in and opposed phase T1-weighted gradient echo (GRE) imaging, may be employed in the characterization of an adrenal mass. Due to the presence of intracellular lipids within lipid rich adrenal adenomas, chemical shift MRI can distinguish between these lesions and non-adenomas. Unlike spin-echo or fast/turbo spin-echo (SE or FSE/TSE) techniques, GRE imaging lacks a 180 degree refocusing pulse in large part allowing for findings at chemical shift MRI. Intracellular lipid and water protons, responsible for creation of MR signal and subsequently images, precess at different frequencies such that at a predetermined echo time (TE) based on magnetic field strength, they will be directed in exactly opposite directions (opposed or "out of phase"). Therefore, any voxel containing both lipid and water will demonstrate signal suppression, or cancellation, on chemical shift MRI. This phenomenon also occurs at any fat-water interface, such as that between the kidney and perinephric fat, and is referred to as India ink artifact.

The degree of signal suppression can be quantified and used to help distinguish between adenomas and non-adenomas. Signal intensity index is the most commonly utilized quantitative measure of signal suppression. Regions of interest are placed within an adrenal mass to quantify signal intensity of the mass during the in phase and out of phase acquisitions. Signal intensity index is then calculated as (SI in phase − SI out of phase)/ (SI in phase) x 100. Adenomas with a higher amount of intracellular lipid demonstrate greater signal cancellation on the out of phase acquisition with lower opposed phase SI and therefore higher signal intensity index. Alternatively, lack of signal cancellation resulting in a low signal intensity index at chemical shift MRI indicates that an adrenal mass is not a lipid rich adrenal adenoma and could be malignant. In a study of 102 adrenal tumors, researchers reported accuracy of 100% in distinguishing between adenoma and malignant tumors with a threshold index of 16.5% [34]. In addition to chemical shift MRI and traditional T1 and T2-weighted spin-echo imaging, diffusion-weighted imaging (DWI) has more recently been applied to abdominal imaging as neoplasms typically demonstrating increased signal intensity to due restricted diffusion of water molecules within the tumor. However, more studies are necessary to determine if this technique can accurately distinguish between benign and malignant tumors.

Morphologic features of an adrenal mass are often the first and most predictive determinant of a benign etiology versus malignancy. Primary adrenocortical carcinomas are typically large, heterogeneous masses which often are locally invasive and may metastasize. Size and internal heterogeneity have been reported to be the most reliable indicators of adrenocortical carcinoma [35]. Most adrenocortical carcinomas exceed 5 cm in size and may exert local mass effect upon the ipsilateral kidney, liver, pancreas, or stomach. Internal heterogeneity due to necrosis or hemorrhage and irregular, ill-defined margins are typical features of adrenocortical carcinoma. Conversely, adrenal adenomas usually measure less than 3-4 cm and demonstrate internal homogeneity with well defined margins and are often rounded or ovoid in shape. Calcifications may be seen in roughly one-third of adrenocortical carcinomas. Adrenocortical carcinomas may invade the IVC, more commonly with right-sided tumors, but this is not a pathognomonic feature of ACC as other tumors such as renal cell carcinoma, hepatocellular carcinoma, and metastases may also demonstrate this finding. Common sites of metastatic disease include the liver, lung, lymph nodes, and bone.

As discussed above, certain imaging findings at CT or MRI may be helpful in suggesting a preoperative diagnosis when interpreted in the appropriate clinical scenario. Internal areas of necrosis will be hypodense approximating fluid attenuation and non-enhancing at CT, while demonstrating increased signal intensity at T2-weighted MRI. Foci of hemorrhage appear hyperdense (approximately 50-60 HU) at unenhanced CT with increased signal intensity at T1-weighted MRI. Adrenocortical carcinomas demonstrate heterogeneous enhancement which is often peripheral with areas of internal nodularity. Adrenocortical carcinomas do not demonstrate signal suppression at chemical shift MRI, as opposed to lipid rich adrenal adenomas which will suppress on the out-of-phase acquisition. Absolute or relative percentage washout (RPW < 40%) are less than that of adrenal adenomas. In cases of IVC invasion, bland or tumor thrombus presenting as a filling defect that typically expands the IVC may be differentiated by the lack of or presence of enhancement, respectively. Local tumor recurrence can be seen following adrenalectomy presenting as an irregular, heterogeneous enlarging nodule or mass similar in appearance to the primary tumor often occurring at surgical clips placed at initial resection.

F-18 FDG PET has more recently become a helpful adjunct in lesion characterization and preoperative staging of patients with a suspicious adrenal mass or known primary malignancy. Qualitative and quantitative measures of metabolic activity reflected by the degree of FDG uptake within a lesion can often predict benignity versus malignancy. Qualitative or visual evaluation of a lesion may compare uptake within an adrenal mass to uptake within the normal liver. Quantitative measures include adrenal-liver SUV ratio or absolute SUV of an adrenal mass to predict malignancy. When PET is utilized alone or in conjunction with unenhanced CT, accuracy in differentiating between benign and malignancy disease has been reported to be 95-99% [36].

Adrenocortical carcinoma and metastatic disease demonstrate several similar imaging characteristics including propensity for larger size, internal heterogeneity due to necrosis and hemorrhage, unenhanced CT attenuation values greater than 10-20 HU with lower absolute or relative washout values than adenomas, and lack of signal suppression at chemical shift MRI. Certainly, metastatic disease must be considered first in patients with known extra-adrenal primary malignancy. Metastatic disease to the adrenal glands is often bilateral, as opposed to primary adrenocortical carcinoma. While ACC can metastasize, the presence of metastases elsewhere should increase suspicion that an adrenal mass represents an additional site of metastatic disease. Occasionally, collision tumors can occur whereby an extra-adrenal malignancy metastasizes to an adrenal gland containing a benign lesion such as adenoma. In this case, one may see features of benign adrenocortical neoplasm and features of malignancy such as large size and heterogeneity.

Several other common adrenal masses have specific imaging characteristics which allow for confident diagnosis. Adrenal hyperplasia usually presents with bilateral adreniform thickening of the adrenal glands that is often stable over time and can be hyperfunctional. The presence of macroscopic or bulk fat with negative HU on CT or signal suppression on fat saturation MR imaging techniques ("fat sat") indicates myelolipoma, an adrenal tumor containing myeloid (bone marrow) and fatty elements. Pheochromocytomas classically demonstrate markedly increased signal intensity on T2-weighted MRI and accumulate MIBG on nuclear medicine scans. Adrenal hemorrhage will demonstrate increased attenuation on CT, increased signal intensity on T1-weighted MRI, and should resolve or decrease in size over time. Adrenal hemorrhage often occurs in the setting of trauma, anticoagulation, or sepsis, but an underlying lesion should be excluded. Adrenal cysts demonstrate similar imaging characteristics to simple cysts elsewhere in the body including fluid attenuation/signal intensity and lack of enhancement. Aside from adrenal cysts, most benign and malignant lesions will enhance following administration of iodinated or gadolinium based contrast agents and, therefore, enhancement alone is not a predictive feature of malignancy. Finally, lipid poor adrenal adenomas, which may represent up to 30% of adrenal adenomas, will not demonstrate signal suppression at chemical shift imaging due to minimal intracellular fat, but usually will show other imaging characteristics suggestive of benignity such as small size, homogeneity, and washout values similar to lipid rich adenomas.

As the most common adrenal mass, adrenal adenoma should lead the differential diagnosis of an incidental adrenal mass. However, several imaging characteristics should raise concern for malignancy including large size, heterogeneity, and irregular margins. Lesion properties at unenhanced CT, multiphasic contrast-enhanced CT, or chemical shift MRI also direct the differential diagnosis and subsequent treatment strategy. PET can also provide helpful information in differentiating between benign and malignant disease as well as tumor staging.

Table 2.

Adrenal Lesion	Diagnostic imaging characteristics	Comment
Primary adrenocortical carcinoma	• Large > 5cm, irregular, heterogeneous tumor with internal necrosis and hemorrhage • Unenh CT > 40 HU • AWV < 60%, RWV < 40% • Lack of drop out on chemical shift MRI • Heterogeneous enhancement pattern	• Often locally invasive tumor which may metastasize • May present with IVC thrombosis, more commonly on the right
Metastatic disease	• Large, irregular, heterogeneous mass • Often bilateral and commonly seen with other sites of disease	• Most commonly from lung, breast, GI, renal, pancreas
Adrenal adenoma	• Small < 3-4cm, ovoid, homogeneous tumor • Unenh CT < 10HU • AWV > 60%, RWV > 40% • Signal drop out at chemical shift MRI	• Most common adrenal mass which is often detected incidentally • Can be hyperfunctional • 30% may be lipid poor • Collision tumors occur rarely
Adrenal hyperplasia	• Bilateral adreniform thickening of the adrenals • May show signal drop out at chemical shift MRI due to adenomatous nodules	• Demonstrate stability over time at follow up imaging • May be hyperfunctional
Hemorrhage	• Hyperdense on CT • Hyperintense on T1-w MRI • Resolves over time	• Often seen in trauma, anticoagulation, and sepsis • Exclude underlying mass
Cyst/pseudocyst	• Fluid attenuation or signal intensity • Lack of enhancement	• Often sequela of hemorrhage or infection
Myelolipoma	• Macroscopic fat on CT or fat saturated MRI	• Larger lesions at risk for spontaneous hem
Pheochromocytoma	• Hyperintense on T2-w MRI • Positive MIBG scan	• Typical clinical presentation or elevated catecholamine • Extra-adrenal pheo = paraganglioma

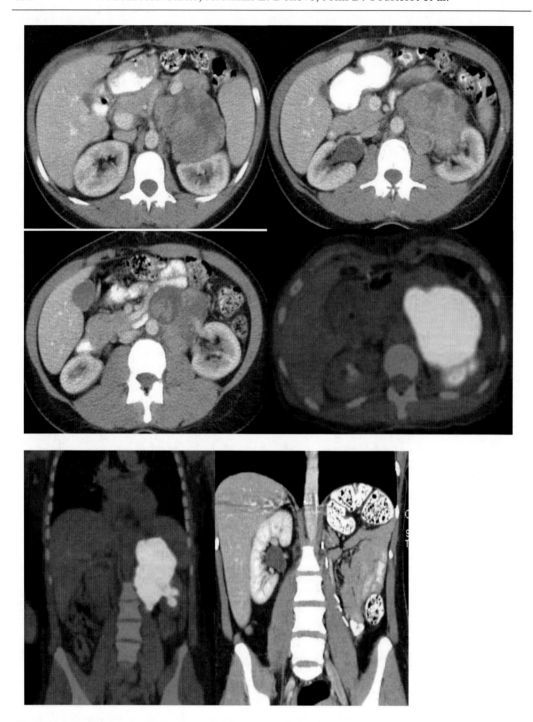

Figure 1. Axial contrast-enhanced CT (a-c) demonstrate large left adrenocortical carcinoma displacing the pancreas anteriorly and compressing the ipsilateral kidney (a), invading the left renal hilum (b) with renal artery (b) and renal vein (c) encasement. (d) Axial and (e) coronal F-18 FDG-PET demonstrate marked avidity and uptake throughout the mass with urinary obstruction. (f) Coronal contrast-enhanced CT demonstrates surgical clips following adrenalectomy and nephrectomy.

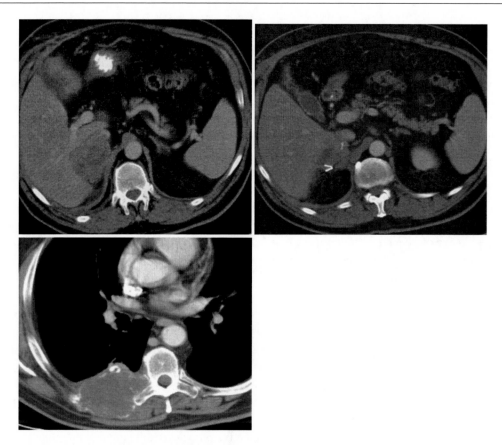

Figure 2. (a) Contrast enhanced CT demonstrates a large, heterogeneous, irregular suprarenal mass in patient status post adrenalectomy for adrenocortical carcinoma consistent with local tumor recurrence. Note the normal left adrenal gland. (b) Caudal to the mass, surgical clips from adrenalectomy are seen. (c) Superiorly in the lower chest, a large, destructive rib metastasis is seen.

Biochemical Evaluation of Adrenal Tumors

Both malignant and benign tumors of the adrenal gland may produce excess hormone. Biochemically active tumors of the adrenal gland include pheochromocytomas, and aldosterone and cortisol secreting adenomas. Rarely other biochemicals are secreted including androgens or estrogens, as well as intermediate metabolites associated with non-classical nodular adrenal hyperplasia [11] . A biochemical evaluation should be performed for all adrenal neoplasms, and functional tumors should be surgically resected. Further, pre- and post-operative management will be influenced by the presence of excess hormone production, and a complete understanding of the biochemical function is essential in the management of these tumors.

Pheochromocytomas are rare in the general population and account for about 5 percent of adrenal incidentalomas. [11, 29] Undiagnosed and untreated pheochromocytoma are potentially life-threatening, particularly during general anesthesia and surgical resection, and a biochemical evaluation for pheochromocytoma should be performed in all of these tumors, even in absence of associated signs or symptoms classically associated with this tumor.

Classic symptoms include episodic or sustained hypertension, often associated with pallor and a severe headache, flushing, profuse sweating, and palpitations (Table).

Screening studies for pheochromocytoma include a 24-hour urine sample for normetanephrine and metanephrine. Although catecholamines and VMA (vanyllil malendelic acid) are often included with these tests, the specificity and sensitivity of these additional tests are poor, and do not add significant value to the metanephrines in terms of screening. The urine metanephrines have a sensitivity of 91 percent for detection with a specificity of 98 percent [29, 11, 37, 38]. Alternately, plasma metanephrine and normetanephrine levels will yield a sensitivity of 96 to 100% [29, 37, 39] at the cost of a lower specificity ranging from 85 to 89 percent [29, 37, 39]. These tests are subject to false positive results, particularly if patients are taking vasoactive antihypertensive medications such as alpha- or beta-blockers, or acetominophen. Metanephrine or normetanephrine levels exceeding 3 times the normal range is conclusive of pheochromocytoma.

Although 10% of adrenal pheochromocytomas are malignant, the ability to determine malignancy is difficult except in the presence of documented metastasis. Traditional histologic findings of capsular or vascular invasion do not necessarily confirm malignancy, and the cytologic appearances are similar in benign and malignant lesions. A combination of worrisome features such as vascular and capsular invasion, along with a high mitotic index and a high proliferation rate (i.e. >5% Ki-67 staining) suggest malignancy. Clinical evidence of local invasion and extensive neovascular development may suggest malignancy as well as a high metabolic activity on FDG-PET imaging.

Preoperative preparation for surgical resection for pheochromocytoma should include alpha blockade. Non-selective alpha blockade using dibenzylene has traditionally been used, but success with terazosin or cardura (alpha selective blockade) and calcium channel blockers have been reported with success. Dibenzylene is given over a minimum of two to four weeks, with increasing doses until mild postural hypotension is achieved. Beta blockade for 48 hrs prior to surgery to prevent excessive chronotropy is also recommended. The duration of preoperative blockade is important to improve volume repletion, and to facilitate the restoration of higher affinity alpha receptors that will improve post operative return to normal vascular tone and stable blood pressure.

Table 3.

Signs and symptoms of a pheochromocytoma
Episodic or sustained hypertension
Pallor
Retinopathy
Increased temperature
Tremor
Palpitations
Headache
Diaphoresis
Excessive sweat

Over-production of aldosterone is rarely found in ACC, and most cases of primary hyperaldosteronism (Conn's syndrome) are bilateral due to adrenal hyperplasia. Biochemically proven overproduction of aldosterone in an adrenal neoplasm is almost certainly an aldosterone producing adenoma, although cases of ACC have been reported. Most patients with hyperaldosteronism present with hypertension, and many patients present with hypokalemia. [29] (Draft ref.1,30). Only 1% of adrenal neoplasms produce unregulated aldosterone, which often leads to cardiovascular complications [29, 40]. Screening is recommended for all patients with adrenal neoplasm, and can be accomplished with a concurrent serum aldosterone and plasma renin activity levels [29, 41, 42]. If the ratio of aldosterone to renin is over 20 with an aldosterone level over 15 ng/dL, primary aldosteronism should be verified with further testing to establish autonomy and unilateral aldosterone secretion. (table 6) [29] . Autonomy is confirmed with salt loading, such as the saline infusion test, with failure to suppress aldosterone levels. Aldosterone producing adenomas may be resected to correct hypertension or hypokalemia. Prior to surgical resection, lateral production of aldosterone should by confirmed by using selective venous catheterization of the adrenal veins. A ratio of > 3:1 confirms lateral production of aldosterone from the adrenal neoplasm.

Table 4. Signs and Symptoms of Primary Aldosteronism

Headaches
Severe weakness, visual impairment, seizure
Hypokalemia
Hypertensive encephalopathy
With hypokalemia
•   Constipation
•   Polyuria
•   Polydipsia
•   Weakness and fatigue
•   Palpitations
Hypertension (higher systolic readings in comparison to essential hypertension
Ischemic cardiomyopathy (more thickened walls in comparison to essential hypertension)
Exercise induced myocardial ischemia
Cardiac arrhythmias
Decreased intrarenal vascular resistance with glomerular hyperfiltration

References: [29 41 43 44]

Table 5. Biochemical evaluation for Primary Aldosteronism

Screening plasma aldosterone to plasma renin activity ratio (am specimen, patient seated). Ratio greater than 20 is considered positive if the aldosterone level is over 15 ng./dL (416 pmol/L)
Confirmation by salt loading/saline infusion or clonidine suppression
Lateralization by adrenal venous sampling should be performed to confirm aldosterone producing adenoma (versus bilateral nodular adrenal hyperplasia)

Ref. [29 45]

Autonomous secretion of cortisol occurs in about 5.3 percent of patients presenting with an adrenal incidentaloma [29, 11] , but 40-50% of ACC produce excess cortisol. Screening for excess cortisol production includes a 24-hour urine collection for cortisol and creatinine levels. Supra-physiologic release of cortisol from an adrenal tumor (Cushing's syndrome) should suppress the release of ACTH, and a fasting am plasma cortisol level is commonly elevated with a suppressed ACTH. To confirm, a high dose dexamethasone suppression test is performed, most easily accomplished using an 8 mg overnight suppression. (Since the patient has a known adrenal mass, a 1 mg test to rule out a pituitary source is unnecessary). In equivocal cases of excess cortisol, two subsequent midnight salivary cortisol levels may demonstrate excess production.

Patients with signs of virilization or lesions suspicious for ACC on imaging studies should also be screened for adrenal production of androgens (DHEAS, androstenedione, testosterone, and 17-OH progesterone) and serum estradiol in men and post menopausal women. Identification of excess production of two cortical hormones is indicative of ACC.

Table 6. Signs and symptoms of Cushing's syndrome

Rapid weight gain (central obesity)
Hyperhidrosis
Psychiatric disorders (depression, anxiety, euphoria, psychosis)
Insomnia
Amenorrhea or oligomenorrhea
Infertility
Polyuria and polydipsia
Musculoskeletal aches and proximal muscle weakness
Moon facies, supraclavicular and dorsocervical fat pads
Telangiectasia
Thinning of skin with easy bruising
Purple or red striae
Hirsutism
Insulin resistance (impaired fasting glucose, diabetes mellitus, Acanthosis nigricans)
Hypertension
Osteoporosis
Biochemical evaluation for hypercortisolism
Screening by 24 hr urinary cortisol level or fasting am plasma cortisol and ACTH levels. Two successive midnight salivary cortisol levels.
Confirmation of autonomy by high dose, overnight dexamethasone suppression test – 8 mg oral dose at 10 pm preceding fasting am (7-8 AM) cortisol level. A dexamethasone level may also be obtained to confirm adequate absorption of the dexamethasone dose.

Pathology

It is difficult to confirm an ACC on histologic evaluation. Certain features should be present such as clear cells, necrosis, increased mitotic figures, and invasion, but these features may be lacking. Aubert in a modified Weiss system suggests a grading system, which currently is commonly used. (1) (Aubert et al Weiss system revisited: a clinicalpathologic and immunohistochemical study of 49 adrenocortical tumors Am J SSurg Pathology 26:1612-1619). Ki-67 staining, an index of proliferation is used for evaluation of mitosis and a proliferative index of >10% is highly suggestive of malignancy. At present there are no discriminatory markers that will confirm ACC. Since cytology cannot distinguish benign adenomas from malignant tumors, FNA should not be performed unless to rule out the possibility of metastatic disease. Pheochromocytoma must be ruled out with appropriate biological evaluation and imaging to proceed with a biopsy for suspected adrenal metastasis in a patient with a known extra-adrenal primary malignancy. Since seeding of the tumor is quite likely if adrenal cortical carcinoma is present, a needle biopsy should not be performed except in the case of confirmation of adrenal metastasis

Staging of ACC by TNM criteria (WHO sanctioned)

TNM classification of adrenal cortical carcinoma		
Tumor	Nodes	Metastasis
T1 Tumor < 5 cm, no invasion of surrounding tissue	N0 - No lymph nodes involved	M0 No distant metastases
T2 Tumor > 5 cm, no invasion	N1 - Regional lymph nodes involved	M1 Distant metastases
T3 Local tumor growth without infiltration of adjacent organs		
T4 Infiltration of surrounding organs		

Adrenocortical carcinoma (ACC) is a relatively rare occurring disease with an incidence of 1-2 per million individuals diagnosed annually.[46] Given the rarity of presentation, there is no standardized treatment regimen and no prospective randomized clinical trial is currently feasible. Surgical resection forms the cornerstone of therapy and offers the only potential for cure. Complete margin negative resection is necessary for the best possible outcome as patients who undergo complete resection have 49% overall 5 year survival rate compared to 9% 5 year survival rate for incomplete resection. [47]

Open surgical resection is recommended for patients suspected of harboring malignancy based on pre-operative imaging characteristics and biochemical hormonal markers. Open adrenalectomy is the procedure of choice for large tumors (larger than 10 cm), regional lymph node enlargement or invasion of adjacent organs. [48] Open adrenalectomy can be performed via an upper midline incision or subcostal approach allowing maximal tumor exposure as well as major vascular control when necessary. Adequate exposure is of the utmost importance in order to perform a microscopic margin negative resection (R0) as this is one of the strongest predictors of survival. Bilimoria et al, in a review of 3982 patients with ACC from the National Cancer Data Base over a 15 year period, described a 51.2 month median survival for those who underwent R0 resection compared to a 7.0 month median survival for incomplete resection. [49] Technical considerations to consider when performing adrenalectomy for suspected ACC include minimal handling of the tumor while minimizing blunt dissection. It is important to leave the tumor capsule intact to minimize tumor spillage, intra-peritoneal spread and reduce the risk of local recurrence. Frequently, en bloc resection of adjacent organ involvement is required. In situations of contiguous liver or kidney involvement for locally advanced adrenal masses, mobilization of these organs is required with proximal and distal vascular control necessary and may necessitate thoracoabdominal exposure. For left adrenal masses, mobilization of the left colon, spleen and pancreas is required. For locally advanced adrenal masses with encasement of the aorta, celiac axis or proximal superior mesenteric artery on pre-operative imaging, complete resection may not be possible. However, when tumor thrombus is present in the inferior vena cava (IVC) or renal vein, complete resection is possible but tumor extirpation may require venovenous bypass or cardiac bypass. [50]

Laparoscopic adrenalectomy was first performed in 1992 [51] and has rapidly become the procedure of choice for benign functioning and nonfunctioning adrenal tumors. The advantage that laparoscopic adrenalectomy provides over open adrenalectomy are many but most notably lower complication rates, less blood loss, less pain with shorter hospital stay and earlier return to activity. [52, 53] For these reasons and others, the role of laparoscopic adrenalectomy in management of ACC has been investigated. There remains considerable debate as to the utility of laparoscopy in the management of adrenal malignancy. For patients with an unsuspected primary ACC, laparoscopic resection is associated with unacceptably high tumor spillage and peritoneal seeding, as high as 50% by experienced laparoscopists [54] with a high recurrence rate. [55] In addition to local recurrences after laparoscopic adrenalectomy, trocar site metastasis after curative resection has also been reported. [56] For patients with suspected ACC, open adrenalectomy is recommended and the decision to perform laparoscopic adrenalectomy should be approached with caution. For patients with symptomatic solitary adrenal metastasis from a lung, kidney or other solid organ primary, there may be a role for laparoscopic adrenalectomy. Given improvements in imaging, detection of adrenal metastasis are frequently more common. These adrenal metastases are often confined within the capsule and may be amenable to a margin negative resection. [57] Some authors have suggested that resection of these metachronous adrenal metastases may improve survival. [58, 59] Resecting these adrenal metastases laparoscopically offers the potential of symptomatic control without the longer recovery or potential morbidity of open adrenalectomy. Laparoscopic adrenalectomy remains a viable treatment alternative for palliative resection of metastatic disease to the adrenal gland.

Despite an aggressive surgical approach, 70-85% of patients recur locally or develop distant metastasis after complete resection. [60, 61] The role of debulking locally recurrent or metastatic disease after prior adrenalectomy remains a matter of debate. One advantage of tumor debulking is that it may help control symptoms of hormonal excess for functioning adrenal tumors.[62] Others argue, however, that incomplete resection of these recurrences or metastatic disease sites does not improve overall prognosis. [63, 64] Nonetheless, surgical resection of local recurrences or metastatic disease amenable to resection has been associated with improved survival in some retrospective series. [48, 65] Complete margin negative surgical resection of locally recurrent ACC is the preferred method of treatment for bulky recurrences in those patients that can tolerate additional procedures.

For patients who undergo multiple debulking operations for recurrence or are unfit to undergo additional resection of locally recurrent or metastatic disease, adjuvant treatment options such as cryotherapy or radiofrequency ablation (RFA) exist. [66] RFA uses alternating electrical current in the radiofrequency range to generate heat which produces its therapeutic effect. RFA offers a safe, predictable treatment option and is associated with minimal morbidity and short recovery period. Wood and colleagues treated 8 ACC patients with 15 primary or metastatic tumors using RFA. Mean tumor size was 4.3 cm with a median follow-up of 10.3 months. Tumors less than 5 cm were most responsive to RFA with 53% having evidence of stable disease at follow up and 20% (3/15) having near complete resolution of the target lesion on follow up imaging. Alternatively, cyroablation exerts its therapeutic effect through application of subfreezing temperatures using argon gas under high pressure. Cryoablation treatment involves placement of multiple catheters within the target lesion and results in tumor destruction by alternating two 10 minute freeze cycles followed by 8 minute thaw cycles. Although limited clinical experience exists, however, there may be a limited role for cryotherapy in select patients with ACC metastasis not amenable to surgical resection. Other adjuvant treatment alternatives for patients whom have undergone multiple debulking procedures for recurrence include radiotherapy to the surgical bed. ACC is often considered radioresistant; however, adjuvant radiotherapy after surgical resection may help reduce local recurrence and should be considered in those patients at high risk for local recurrence such as those with incomplete resection.

Surgical resection offers the only potential for cure in patients with ACC. Open adrenalectomy is the procedure of choice for patients suspected of having primary or metastatic ACC. Laparoscopic adrenalectomy is generally not recommended for primary ACC but may have a role in resection of isolated solitary adrenal metastasis from another primary. Surgical debulking is recommended in patients who are fit to undergo additional resection for recurrence. RFA is also a potential adjuvant to surgical resection for recurrent or metastatic disease not amenable to surgical resection. Lastly, a multidisciplinary treatment approach is advised to optimize patient outcome

Medical Management of ACC

Mitotane (o,p'-DDD)

Since mitotane was introduced in 1970 it has been frequently used but long term outcome data is scarce because of the rarity of this tumor. It has direct cytotoxic effects on the adrenal cortical cells mainly attacking fascicular and reticular cells while sparing glomular cells, therefore having little affect on aldosterone function but a major destructive effect on glucocorticoid function.

Lubitz showed significant response rate in 1973 with 7/18 patients showing tumor regression but other studies could not confirm this energetic response. Fassnacht reviewed mitotane data and estimated a 25% tumor regression and a vast majority had hormonal control.

It appears that mitotane has a narrow therapeutic window and serum levels attained between 14 mg/l-20mg/l are optimal for control and limitation of side affects.(table)

The dosage should be started slowly to avoid side affects and we usually begin at 500 mg daily and advance 500 mg every 4-5 days until the patient reaches 3gms daily. At this point, a mitotane level is drawn, and the dose is adjusted to maintain levels within this target range. Mitotane is fat soluble, can be released from adipose stores for a prolonged period of time, and serum levels remain positive for months after discontinuation of oral dosing. Mitotane also increases the metabolism of glucocorticoids and higher replacement doses of steroids are required, usually 2-3 fold increases of full replacement doses of glucocorticoids (usually 30-40 mg-equivalents of hydrocortisone daily).

There remains controversy about mitotane treatment. Because of the high early recurrence rate of 85% for ACC, adjuvant therapy has been proposed. This approach in small series showed conflicting data about efficacy. More recently however, Terzolo showed a significant improvement in disease free survival and overall survival in patients receiving mitotane compared to a population that did not. Further studies are needed, but our current approach is to give mitotane as adjuvant therapy in patients with Stage II or greater disease. Since the peak of recurrence is within two years of initial treatment, we target an adjuvant therapy window of 2-3 years of treatment.

In patients with persistent, inoperable or metastatic disease, mitotane is used in combination therapy with other chemotherapy agents, primarily etopsode and anthroacycline based regimens or streptozotocin. Local control may also be attempted with other modalities such as external beam radiotherapy, targeted radiotherapy, radiofrequency ablation, or cryoablative techniques.

Table. Side Effects of Mitotane

◆   Gastrointestinal: nausea, vomiting, diarrhea, anorexia, mucositis
◆   CNS: lethargy, somnolence, vertigo, ataxia confusion, depression, dizziness, decreased
◆   memory, polyneuropathy
◆   Adrenal insufficiency
◆   Primary hypogonadism in men
◆   Gynecomastia
◆   Skin rash
◆   Increase of hepatic enzymes (in particular -GT)
◆   Increase in hormone binding globulins (CBG, SHBG, TBG, vitamin D binding protein)
◆   Disturbance of thyroid parameters (interference with binding of T4 to TBG,)
◆   Hypercholesterolemia, hypertriglyceridemia
◆   Prolonged bleeding time
◆   Leucopenia
◆   Thrombocytopenia, anemia

Glucocorticoids

Greater than 60% of patients with ACC present with excess hormonal production and many patients present with excess glucocorticoid production and florid Cushings syndrome. Preoperatively all patients should have a full hormone workup to identify the abnormal hormonal production which can be used as a marker for tumor recurrence. If patients have Cushing's syndrome, the opposite adrenal gland will be suppressed and therefore post-operative adrenal insufficiency will be present. Steroid coverage should be started at the time of surgery and since most patients will start on Mitotane, steroid replacement should be continued indefinitely. If significant tumor bulk remains, steroids may not be needed. Decadron is commonly used in this scenario to improve the opportunity to monitor endogenous cortisol production from residual or recurrent, functional ACC. If excess cortisol production persists, then steroids will be discontinued but monitored closely for potential adrenal insufficiency.

Excess production of steroids must be controlled, if possible, since the catabolic effects of glucocorticoid excess decreases survival. Steroid enzymatic blocking drugs can be used to limit production of glucocorticoids, but their effectiveness is limited. Ketoconazole(600-1200mgs daily) is the preferred initial medication because of its limited side effect profile, but other agents such as metapyrone or aminoglutimide have been used. Rarely, combinations of these drugs have been tried with limited significant improvement in cortisol control. Careful monitoring of electrolytes, cortisol, and chemistry panels must be performed. The presence of active glucocorticoid excess decreases survival and increases morbidity.

Chemotherapy

Etoposide based chemotherapy regimens have used with some success in ACC. The FIRM-ACT trial (currently open to accrual) compares mitotane and steptozocin in combination therapy to a mitotane/etoposide/doxorubicin/cisplatin regimen. Outside of this trial (yet unpublished) little data is available determine efficacy of chemotherapy regimens. Current practice guidelines suggest Mitotane for adjuvant chemotherapy for stage II or III disease. Unresectable recurrent or persistent disease should be treated in combination with Mitotane, and an etoposide- or streptozotocin-based regimen. Limited efficacy data is emerging with use of multi-kinase inhibitors in patients with ACC, including IGF-1 receptor blockade. Early indications suggest additional disease control may be achievable with new, targeted therapies.

Radiotherapy for Adrenal Cortical Carcinoma

Historically, adrenocortical carcinomas (ACC) have been considered to be radioresistant. The evidence upon which this is based has included small retrospective studies showing that radiotherapy does not result in improved local control [67-69]. These studies were performed, however, with what we now consider older treatment technologies that limited the potential of maximizing dose delivery to the intended tumor bearing target while minimizing normal tissue dose. With modern radiation therapy techniques that more precisely deliver higher doses, interest has emerged to once again consider the potential utility of radiation therapy to improve outcomes in a disease with high rates of recurrence post resection.

Central to the renewed interest to integrate a radiotherapy approach is our ability to delineate targets with CT-based treatment planning. No longer must radiation oncologists use large volume fields based on fluoroscopic images. Advances in technology now allow for the transfer of CT data into planning software to reconstruct the location of the intended targets as well as the normal tissues. As a result, patients are treated with techniques such as intensity-modulated radiation therapy (IMRT) that divides the photon beam into individual beamlets, tightly conforming the high dose region to the intended target volume. Furthermore, image-guided radiation therapy (IGRT) permits daily localization of the target prior to dose delivery with the use of either kilovoltage orthogonal images or cone beam CT generated on the treatment machine itself.

For treatment of abdominal tumors such as ACC, respiratory-associated tumor motion should be considered. The region surrounding the adrenal gland is prone to significant changes with respect to superior to inferior, anterior to posterior, and medial to lateral tumor positions during respiration. During CT simulation, which is performed for treatment planning, a 4D scan can be acquired in the treatment position within the patient's custom immobilization device. When the scan completes its reconstruction, the tumor position between maximum inspiration and expiration are visualized, allowing the position of the tumor to be tracked throughout the breathing cycle. The radiation oncologist can then delineate the full trajectory of the target to ensure it receives adequate dose. With modern radiation techniques, optimizing target volume delineation is more important than ever before since failure to do so may result in a marginal miss [70].

Once the target motion has been quantified, the question then arises as to which treatment delivery technique will be most appropriate for the individual patient. Radiation treatment machines can be programmed to only turn "on" during a certain phase of the breathing cycle, a term called respiratory gating. Because of the selective temporal activation of the photon beam, respiratory gating allows for increased normal tissue sparing [71, 72]. A second option is to use active breathing control during which the patient wears a monitoring device that so that the treatment machine can be activated only when the patient's breathing is in the desired phase [73-75]. A third option is to use abdominal compression, such as with a weight belt, to limit diaphragmatic excursion [76-79].

Data published within the last 5 years supports the role of adjuvant radiotherapy to decrease local recurrence. Fassnacht et al performed a retrospective review of patients in the German ACC Registry [80]. Screening identified 14 patients who were then matched with control patients that were uniform for resection status, adjuvant mitotane treatment, stage, and tumor size. Results showed that only 2 of 14 patients in the radiotherapy group experienced a local recurrence compared to 11 of 14 control patients. Although disease-free and overall survivals were not significantly different, the probability to be free of local recurrence 5 years after surgery differed significantly (79% vs. 12%, p< 0.01).

Based on their experience, these authors subsequently reviewed the published literature and have issued radiotherapy recommendations. Given the rarity of this disease, and that both local and distant recurrence rates can be as high as 85% despite complete surgical resection, they advocate that adjuvant tumor bed irradiation may prevent local tumor recurrence. Since there are no prospective data to guide treatment decisions, they advise tumor bed irradiation in all patients who have undergone resection with microscopically positive margins (R1) as well as all patients in whom the margin status is uncertain within 3 months of surgery. If patients have a complete resection of locoregionally advanced disease and/or positive lymph nodes, adjuvant tumor bed treatment should be considered. In addition, adjuvant radiotherapy should be considered if the tumor is >8cm, has evidence of vascular tumor invasion, or has a KI-67 index of >10%. Intraoperative focal tumor spillage or dissemination of necrotic fluid as well as violation of the tumor capsule would be indications to consider adjuvant therapy. No irradiation is advocated if diffuse tumor spillage occurs throughout the abdominal cavity or if patients have large tumor thrombus in the vena cava.

In the case of gross residual disease, a second surgery is recommended; however, if further resection is not an option, radiotherapy in combination with mitotane should be considered. Cerquetti et al have established the ability of mitotane to sensitize ACC cells to ionizing radiation by involvement of the cyclin B1/CDK complex in G2 arrest and mismatch repair enzymes modulation [81]. Only a few studies, however, have reported outcomes of patients treated concurrently with mitotane and radiotherapy. The German group cautions that concomitant mitotane can aggravate the adverse effects of radiotherapy such that doses of mitotane $\leq$ 3g per day are used. Liver enzymes need to be monitored with consideration of discontinuing the drug if the levels reach $\geq$ 3 fold the baseline aspartate and alanine aminotransferase levels.

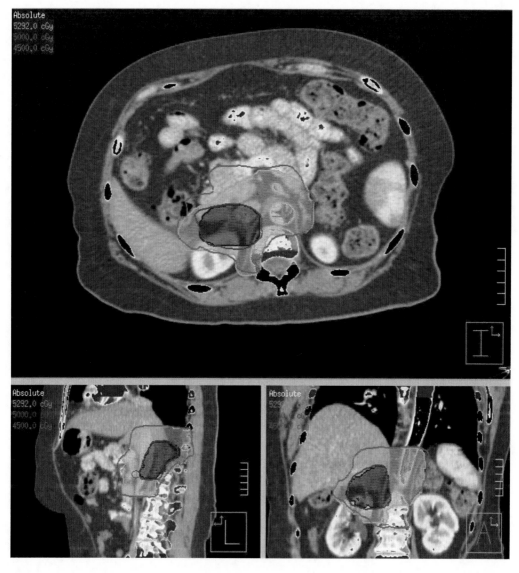

Figure 3. Typical IMRT isodose lines demonstrating high conformality of dose to the target volume with significant sparing of normal surrounding tissues.

In terms of treatment volumes, the German group evaluated sites of locoregional recurrence and recommend covering areas of microscopic tumor spread including the lymphatic drainage of the adrenal gland [82]. Similar to a previous report from Markoe et al, they advocate designing a clinical target volume as follows: 1) dorsal: the diaphragm and parts of the thoracic wall in case of infiltration; 2) medial: the para-aortic/paracaval lymph nodes if involvement was demonstrated or if there is felt to be a high risk of this; 3) lateral: as far as the preoperative tumor extension with adequate margins; 4) cranial: up to the diaphragm crus/apex; and 5) inferior: down to the aortic crest with coverage of at least the kidney hilum [83]. Standard fractionation (1.8-2.0 Gy/fraction) is recommended to a minimum dose of 40 Gy and up to 50-60 Gy. Not only can radiotherapy be effective in decreasing locoregional recurrences, but it can also be offered to patients with unresectable disease or with symptomatic metastases. Patients with painful bone metastases, superior vena cava obstruction, and cerebral metastases likely will benefit from treatment as well.

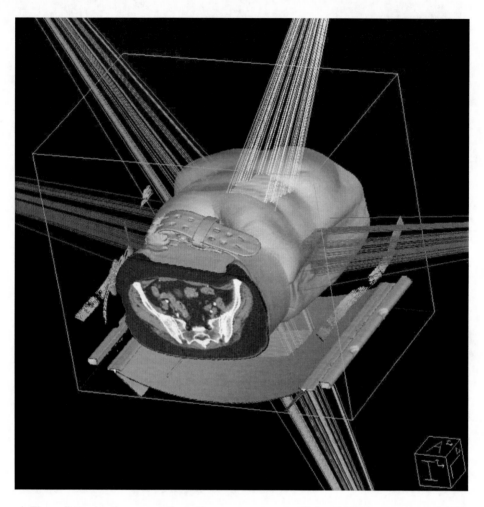

Figure 4. Three-dimensional representation of beam arrangement utilizing IMRT for treatment of ACC.

In the U.S., Sabolch et al recently reviewed the University of Michigan experience and strongly advocate that adjuvant radiotherapy should be considered after surgical resection [84]. The authors reviewed all records of ACC patients treated between 1989-2008, including 58 patients with 64 instances of treatment (37 for primary disease and 27 for recurrent disease). This is the largest published series incorporating radiotherapy, with 10 patients receiving adjuvant and 16 receiving definitive irradiation for unresectable disease. Omission of radiotherapy was associated with 4.7 times increased risk of local failure compared with treatment regimens that involved radiotherapy (95% C.I., 1.2-19.0; p=0.030). The authors also noted that tumors with a maximum size >10 cm were 4.3 times more likely to fail locally than those with smaller tumors (95% C.I., 1.5-13.0; p=0.004). Similar to the German investigators, the Michigan group did not find any difference in overall survival between patients treated with surgery alone compared to those treated with radiotherapy.

For unresectable disease or focal metastases, stereotactic body radiation therapy (SBRT) may offer even more treatment options. Using 1-5 high dose fractions delivered to a small target volume, SBRT has several advantages over standard RT. First, superior local tumor control with minimal toxicity has been demonstrated in various extracranial sites [85-89]. High dose per fraction radiotherapy has an ablative effect thought to be secondary to increased apoptosis of tumor-associated vascular endothelium [90]. Second, treatment over several days is clearly more convenient for the patient. Third, systemic therapy initiation can be expedited in select patients with poor prognosis.

Although multi-institutional prospective randomized data is lacking in the management of ACC, the high rates of locoregional recurrence in the adjuvant setting warrant consideration of radiotherapy. With modern techniques, focused radiotherapy can be delivered with improved accuracy and less morbidity. Future work will need to incorporate these advanced techniques with larger patient numbers to better elucidate the full therapeutic potential of radiotherapy in the treatment of adrenocortical carcinoma.

Surveillance

Routine imaging including CT and FDG-PET is mandatory to discern either local or distant recurrence and should be performed every three months. In addition, for patients who present with excess hormone production, routine evaluation of this hormone should be measured every 3 months. Rising levels may indicate recurrence, and should prompt imaging localization. If isolated, additional surgical extirpation is indicated for recurrence.

References

[1]   Ng L, Libertino JM. Adrenocortical carcinoma: diagnosis, evaluation and treatment. *J Urol* 2003; 169(1):5-11.

[2]   Hsing AW, Nam JM, Co Chien HT, et al. Risk factors for adrenal cancer: an exploratory study. *Int J Cancer* 1996; 65(4):432-6.

[3]   Allolio B, Fassnacht M. Clinical review: Adrenocortical carcinoma: clinical update. *J Clin Endocrinol Metab* 2006; 91(6):2027-37.

[4]   Mantero F, Terzolo M, Arnaldi G, et al. A survey on adrenal incidentaloma in Italy. Study Group on Adrenal Tumors of the Italian Society of Endocrinology. *J Clin Endocrinol Metab* 2000; 85(2):637-44.

[5]   Reznik Y, Lefebvre H, Rohmer V, et al. Aberrant adrenal sensitivity to multiple ligands in unilateral incidentaloma with subclinical autonomous cortisol hypersecretion: a prospective clinical study. *Clin Endocrinol (Oxf)* 2004; 61(3):311-9.

[6]   Lacroix A, Bourdeau I, Lampron A, et al. Aberrant G-protein coupled receptor expression in relation to adrenocortical overfunction. *Clin Endocrinol (Oxf)* 2010; 73(1):1-15.

[7]   Lampron A, Bourdeau I, Oble S, et al. Regulation of aldosterone secretion by several aberrant receptors including for glucose-dependent insulinotropic peptide in a patient with an aldosteronoma. *J Clin Endocrinol Metab* 2009; 94(3):750-6.

[8]   Zwermann O, Suttmann Y, Bidlingmaier M, et al. Screening for membrane hormone receptor expression in primary aldosteronism. *Eur J Endocrinol* 2009; 160(3):443-51.

[9]   Ye P, Mariniello B, Mantero F, et al. G-protein-coupled receptors in aldosterone-producing adenomas: a potential cause of hyperaldosteronism. *J Endocrinol* 2007; 195(1):39-48.

[10]   Terzolo M, Ali A, Osella G, et al. Prevalence of adrenal carcinoma among incidentally discovered adrenal masses. A retrospective study from 1989 to 1994. Gruppo Piemontese Incidentalomi Surrenalici. *Arch Surg* 1997; 132(8):914-9.

[11]   Young WF, Jr. Management approaches to adrenal incidentalomas. A view from Rochester, Minnesota. *Endocrinol Metab Clin North Am* 2000; 29(1):159-85, x.

[12]   Thompson GB, Young WF, Jr. Adrenal incidentaloma. *Curr Opin Oncol* 2003; 15(1):84-90.

[13]   Dackiw AP, Lee JE, Gagel RF, et al. Adrenal cortical carcinoma. *World J Surg* 2001; 25(7):914-26.

[14]   Boland GW, Lee MJ, Gazelle GS, et al. Characterization of adrenal masses using unenhanced CT: an analysis of the CT literature. *AJR Am J Roentgenol* 1998; 171(1):201-4.

[15]   Dunnick NR, Korobkin M. Imaging of adrenal incidentalomas: current status. *AJR Am J Roentgenol* 2002; 179(3):559-68.

[16]   Demeure MJ, Somberg LB. Functioning and nonfunctioning adrenocortical carcinoma: clinical presentation and therapeutic strategies. *Surg Oncol Clin N Am* 1998; 7(4):791-805.

[17]   Vassilopoulou-Sellin R, Schultz PN. Adrenocortical carcinoma. Clinical outcome at the end of the 20th century. *Cancer* 2001; 92(5):1113-21.

[18]   Wajchenberg BL, Albergaria Pereira MA, Medonca BB, et al. Adrenocortical carcinoma: clinical and laboratory observations. *Cancer* 2000; 88(4):711-36.

[19]   Michalkiewicz E, Sandrini R, Figueiredo B, et al. Clinical and outcome characteristics of children with adrenocortical tumors: a report from the International Pediatric Adrenocortical Tumor Registry. *J Clin Oncol* 2004; 22(5):838-45.

[20]   Koch CA, Pacak K, Chrousos GP. The molecular pathogenesis of hereditary and sporadic adrenocortical and adrenomedullary tumors. *J Clin Endocrinol Metab* 2002; 87(12):5367-84.

[21]   Abiven G, Coste J, Groussin L, et al. Clinical and biological features in the prognosis of adrenocortical cancer: poor outcome of cortisol-secreting tumors in a series of 202 consecutive patients. *J Clin Endocrinol Metab* 2006; 91(7):2650-5.

[22]   Weiss LM, Medeiros LJ, Vickery AL, Jr. Pathologic features of prognostic significance in adrenocortical carcinoma. *Am J Surg Pathol* 1989; 13(3):202-6.

[23]   Medeiros LJ, Weiss LM. New developments in the pathologic diagnosis of adrenal cortical neoplasms. A review. *Am J Clin Pathol* 1992; 97(1):73-83.

[24]   Aubert S, Wacrenier A, Leroy X, et al. Weiss system revisited: a clinicopathologic and immunohistochemical study of 49 adrenocortical tumors. *Am J Surg Pathol* 2002; 26(12):1612-9.

[25]   McCorkell SJ, Niles NL. Fine-needle aspiration of catecholamine-producing adrenal masses: a possibly fatal mistake. *AJR Am J Roentgenol* 1985; 145(1):113-4.

[26] van Heerden JA, Roland CF, Carney JA, et al. Long-term evaluation following resection of apparently benign pheochromocytoma(s)/paraganglioma(s). *World J Surg* 1990; 14(3):325-9.

[27] Plouin PF, Chatellier G, Fofol I, et al. Tumor recurrence and hypertension persistence after successful pheochromocytoma operation. *Hypertension* 1997; 29(5):1133-9.

[28] Li ML, Fitzgerald PA, Price DC, et al. Iatrogenic pheochromocytomatosis: a previously unreported result of laparoscopic adrenalectomy. *Surgery* 2001; 130(6):1072-7.

[29] Young WF, Jr. Clinical practice. The incidentally discovered adrenal mass. *N Engl J Med* 2007; 356(6):601-10.

[30] Kloos RT, Korobkin M, Thompson NW, et al. Incidentally discovered adrenal masses. *Cancer Treat Res* 1997; 89:263-92.

[31] Copeland PM. The incidentally discovered adrenal mass. *Ann Surg* 1984; 199(1):116-22.

[32] Hamrahian AH, Ioachimescu AG, Remer EM, et al. Clinical utility of noncontrast computed tomography attenuation value (hounsfield units) to differentiate adrenal adenomas/hyperplasias from nonadenomas: Cleveland Clinic experience. *J Clin Endocrinol Metab* 2005; 90(2):871-7.

[33] Slattery JM, Blake MA, Kalra MK, et al. Adrenocortical carcinoma: contrast washout characteristics on CT. *AJR Am J Roentgenol* 2006; 187(1):W21-4.

[34] Fujiyoshi F, Nakajo M, Fukukura Y, et al. Characterization of adrenal tumors by chemical shift fast low-angle shot MR imaging: comparison of four methods of quantitative evaluation. *AJR Am J Roentgenol* 2003; 180(6):1649-57.

[35] Johnson PT, Horton KM, Fishman EK. Adrenal mass imaging with multidetector CT: pathologic conditions, pearls, and pitfalls. *Radiographics* 2009; 29(5):1333-51.

[36] Boland GW, Blake MA, Holalkere NS, et al. PET/CT for the characterization of adrenal masses in patients with cancer: qualitative versus quantitative accuracy in 150 consecutive patients. *AJR Am J Roentgenol* 2009; 192(4):956-62.

[37] Sawka AM, Jaeschke R, Singh RJ, et al. A comparison of biochemical tests for pheochromocytoma: measurement of fractionated plasma metanephrines compared with the combination of 24-hour urinary metanephrines and catecholamines. *J Clin Endocrinol Metab* 2003; 88(2):553-8.

[38] Perry CG, Sawka AM, Singh R, et al. The diagnostic efficacy of urinary fractionated metanephrines measured by tandem mass spectrometry in detection of pheochromocytoma. *Clin Endocrinol (Oxf)* 2007; 66(5):703-8.

[39] Lenders JW, Pacak K, Walther MM, et al. Biochemical diagnosis of pheochromo-cytoma: which test is best? *JAMA* 2002; 287(11):1427-34.

[40] Kudva YC, Sawka AM, Young WF, Jr. Clinical review 164: The laboratory diagnosis of adrenal pheochromocytoma: the Mayo Clinic experience. *J Clin Endocrinol Metab* 2003; 88(10):4533-9.

[41] Mulatero P, Stowasser M, Loh KC, et al. Increased diagnosis of primary aldosteronism, including surgically correctable forms, in centers from five continents. *J Clin Endocrinol Metab* 2004; 89(3):1045-50.

[42] Montori VM, Young WF, Jr. Use of plasma aldosterone concentration-to-plasma renin activity ratio as a screening test for primary aldosteronism. A systematic review of the literature. *Endocrinol Metab Clin North Am* 2002; 31(3):619-32, xi.

[43] Sechi LA, Di Fabio A, Bazzocchi M, et al. Intrarenal hemodynamics in primary aldosteronism before and after treatment. *J Clin Endocrinol Metab* 2009; 94(4):1191-7.

[44] Napoli C, Di Gregorio F, Leccese M, et al. Evidence of exercise-induced myocardial ischemia in patients with primary aldosteronism: the Cross-sectional Primary Aldosteronism and Heart Italian Multicenter Study. *J Investig Med* 1999; 47(5):212-21.

[45] Young WF, Jr. Minireview: primary aldosteronism--changing concepts in diagnosis and treatment. *Endocrinology* 2003; 144(6):2208-13.

[46] Allolio B, Hahner S, Weismann D, et al. Management of adrenocortical carcinoma. *Clin Endocrinol (Oxf)* 2004; 60(3):273-87.

[47] Haak HR, Hermans J, van de Velde CJ, et al. Optimal treatment of adrenocortical carcinoma with mitotane: results in a consecutive series of 96 patients. *Br J Cancer* 1994; 69(5):947-51.

[48] Schteingart DE, Doherty GM, Gauger PG, et al. Management of patients with adrenal cancer: recommendations of an international consensus conference. *Endocr Relat Cancer* 2005; 12(3):667-80.

[49] Bilimoria KY, Shen WT, Elaraj D, et al. Adrenocortical carcinoma in the United States: treatment utilization and prognostic factors. *Cancer* 2008; 113(11):3130-6.

[50] Mingoli A, Nardacchione F, Sgarzini G, et al. Inferior vena cava involvement by a left side adrenocortical carcinoma: operative and prognostic considerations. *Anticancer Res* 1996; 16(5B):3197-200.

[51] Gagner M, Lacroix A, Bolte E. Laparoscopic adrenalectomy in Cushing's syndrome and pheochromocytoma. *N Engl J Med* 1992; 327(14):1033.

[52] Cobb WS, Kercher KW, Sing RF, et al. Laparoscopic adrenalectomy for malignancy. *Am J Surg* 2005; 189(4):405-11.

[53] Gagner M, Pomp A, Heniford BT, et al. Laparoscopic adrenalectomy: lessons learned from 100 consecutive procedures. *Ann Surg* 1997; 226(3):238-46; discussion 246-7.

[54] Miller BS, Ammori JB, Gauger PG, et al. Laparoscopic resection is inappropriate in patients with known or suspected adrenocortical carcinoma. *World J Surg*; 34(6):1380-5.

[55] Kebebew E, Siperstein AE, Clark OH, et al. Results of laparoscopic adrenalectomy for suspected and unsuspected malignant adrenal neoplasms. *Arch Surg* 2002; 137(8):948-51; discussion 952-3.

[56] Shen WT, Kebebew E, Clark OH, et al. Reasons for conversion from laparoscopic to open or hand-assisted adrenalectomy: review of 261 laparoscopic adrenalectomies from 1993 to 2003. *World J Surg* 2004; 28(11):1176-9.

[57] Sarela AI, Murphy I, Coit DG, et al. Metastasis to the adrenal gland: the emerging role of laparoscopic surgery. *Ann Surg Oncol* 2003; 10(10):1191-6.

[58] Kim SH, Brennan MF, Russo P, et al. The role of surgery in the treatment of clinically isolated adrenal metastasis. *Cancer* 1998; 82(2):389-94.

[59] Giraudo G, Del Genio G, Porpiglia F, et al. [Laparoscopic adrenalectomy in multiple endocrine tumors, in secreting and non-secreting lesions]. *Minerva Chir* 2004; 59(1):1-5.

[60] Assie G, Antoni G, Tissier F, et al. Prognostic parameters of metastatic adrenocortical carcinoma. *J Clin Endocrinol Metab* 2007; 92(1):148-54.

[61] Henley DJ, van Heerden JA, Grant CS, et al. Adrenal cortical carcinoma--a continuing challenge. *Surgery* 1983; 94(6):926-31.

[62] Jensen JC, Pass HI, Sindelar WF, et al. Recurrent or metastatic disease in select patients with adrenocortical carcinoma. Aggressive resection vs chemotherapy. *Arch Surg* 1991; 126(4):457-61.

[63] Crucitti F, Bellantone R, Ferrante A, et al. The Italian Registry for Adrenal Cortical Carcinoma: analysis of a multiinstitutional series of 129 patients. The ACC Italian Registry Study Group. *Surgery* 1996; 119(2):161-70.

[64] Icard P, Louvel A, Chapuis Y. Survival rates and prognostic factors in adrenocortical carcinoma. *World J Surg* 1992; 16(4):753-8.

[65] Bellantone R, Ferrante A, Boscherini M, et al. Role of reoperation in recurrence of adrenal cortical carcinoma: results from 188 cases collected in the Italian National Registry for Adrenal Cortical Carcinoma. *Surgery* 1997; 122(6):1212-8.

[66] Wood BJ, Abraham J, Hvizda JL, et al. Radiofrequency ablation of adrenal tumors and adrenocortical carcinoma metastases. *Cancer* 2003; 97(3):554-60.

[67] Schulick RD, Brennan MF. Long-term survival after complete resection and repeat resection in patients with adrenocortical carcinoma. *Ann Surg Oncol* 1999; 6(8):719-26.

[68] Kasperlik-Zaluska AA, Migdalska BM, Zgliczynski S, et al. Adrenocortical carcinoma. A clinical study and treatment results of 52 patients. *Cancer* 1995; 75(10):2587-91.

[69] Bodie B, Novick AC, Pontes JE, et al. The Cleveland Clinic experience with adrenal cortical carcinoma. *J Urol* 1989; 141(2):257-60.

[70] Mendenhall WM, Amdur RJ, Palta JR. Intensity-modulated radiotherapy in the standard management of head and neck cancer: promises and pitfalls. *J Clin Oncol* 2006; 24(17):2618-23.

[71] Giraud P, Garcia R. [Respiratory gating for radiotherapy: main technical aspects and clinical benefits]. *Bull Cancer* 2010; 97(7):847-56.

[72] Keall PJ, Kini VR, Vedam SS, et al. Potential radiotherapy improvements with respiratory gating. *Australas Phys Eng Sci Med* 2002; 25(1):1-6.

[73] Dawson LA, Eccles C, Bissonnette JP, et al. Accuracy of daily image guidance for hypofractionated liver radiotherapy with active breathing control. *Int J Radiat Oncol Biol Phys* 2005; 62(4):1247-52.

[74] Dawson LA, Brock KK, Kazanjian S, et al. The reproducibility of organ position using active breathing control (ABC) during liver radiotherapy. *Int J Radiat Oncol Biol Phys* 2001; 51(5):1410-21.

[75] Wong JW, Sharpe MB, Jaffray DA, et al. The use of active breathing control (ABC) to reduce margin for breathing motion. *Int J Radiat Oncol Biol Phys* 1999; 44(4):911-9.

[76] Eccles CL, Dawson LA, Moseley JL, et al. Interfraction Liver Shape Variability and Impact on GTV Position During Liver Stereotactic Radiotherapy Using Abdominal Compression. *Int J Radiat Oncol Biol Phys* 2010.

[77] Eccles CL, Patel R, Simeonov AK, et al. Comparison of liver tumor motion with and without abdominal compression using cine-magnetic resonance imaging. *Int J Radiat Oncol Biol Phys* 2011; 79(2):602-8.

[78] Heinzerling JH, Anderson JF, Papiez L, et al. Four-dimensional computed tomography scan analysis of tumor and organ motion at varying levels of abdominal compression during stereotactic treatment of lung and liver. *Int J Radiat Oncol Biol Phys* 2008; 70(5):1571-8.

[79] Wunderink W, Mendez Romero A, de Kruijf W, et al. Reduction of respiratory liver tumor motion by abdominal compression in stereotactic body frame, analyzed by tracking fiducial markers implanted in liver. *Int J Radiat Oncol Biol Phys* 2008; 71(3):907-15.

[80] Fassnacht M, Hahner S, Polat B, et al. Efficacy of adjuvant radiotherapy of the tumor bed on local recurrence of adrenocortical carcinoma. *J Clin Endocrinol Metab* 2006; 91(11):4501-4.

[81] Cerquetti L, Bucci B, Marchese R, et al. Mitotane increases the radiotherapy inhibitory effect and induces G2-arrest in combined treatment on both H295R and SW13 adrenocortical cell lines. *Endocr Relat Cancer* 2008; 15(2):623-34.

[82] Polat B, Fassnacht M, Pfreundner L, et al. Radiotherapy in adrenocortical carcinoma. *Cancer* 2009; 115(13):2816-23.

[83] Markoe AM, Serber W, Micaily B, et al. Radiation therapy for adjunctive treatment of adrenal cortical carcinoma. *Am J Clin Oncol* 1991; 14(2):170-4.

[84] Sabolch A, Feng M, Griffith K, et al. Adjuvant and Definitive Radiotherapy for Adrenocortical Carcinoma. *Int J Radiat Oncol Biol Phys* 2010.

[85] Onishi H, Araki T, Shirato H, et al. Stereotactic hypofractionated high-dose irradiation for stage I nonsmall cell lung carcinoma: clinical outcomes in 245 subjects in a Japanese multiinstitutional study. *Cancer* 2004; 101(7):1623-31.

[86] Chang DT, Schellenberg D, Shen J, et al. Stereotactic radiotherapy for unresectable adenocarcinoma of the pancreas. *Cancer* 2009; 115(3):665-72.

[87] Koong AC, Christofferson E, Le QT, et al. Phase II study to assess the efficacy of conventionally fractionated radiotherapy followed by a stereotactic radiosurgery boost in patients with locally advanced pancreatic cancer. *Int J Radiat Oncol Biol Phys* 2005; 63(2):320-3.

[88] Koong AC, Le QT, Ho A, et al. Phase I study of stereotactic radiosurgery in patients with locally advanced pancreatic cancer. *Int J Radiat Oncol Biol Phys* 2004; 58(4):1017-21.

[89] Schellenberg D, Goodman KA, Lee F, et al. Gemcitabine chemotherapy and single-fraction stereotactic body radiotherapy for locally advanced pancreatic cancer. *Int J Radiat Oncol Biol Phys* 2008; 72(3):678-86.

[90] Brown JM, Koong AC. High-dose single-fraction radiotherapy: exploiting a new biology? *Int J Radiat Oncol Biol Phys* 2008; 71(2):324-5.

Section 9. Robotic Surgery in Urologic Oncology

Julio Pow-Sang
Section Editor

In: Essentials and Updates in Urologic Oncology
Editor: Philippe E. Spiess

ISBN: 978-1-62081-494-9
© 2013 Nova Science Publishers, Inc.

Chapter XXXIII

Evolving Role of Robotic Surgery in Prostate Cancer

Rafael Ferreira Coelho* and Vipul R. Patel±

Global Robotics Institute, Florida Hospital Celebration Health,
Celebration, Florida, US

Abstract

With the widespread diffusion of prostate-specific antigen (PSA) testing, prostate cancer is nowadays frequently diagnosed in younger and healthier men, with organ confined disease. For patients with organ confined disease numerous treatment alternatives are now available. These patients desire treatments that not only provide excellent oncological and functional outcomes but that can also offer short hospitalization times, low morbidity and minimal convalescence while maintaining their quality of life. The introduction of the da Vinci robotic Surgical System (Intuitive Surgical, Inc., Sunnyvale, CA) has been a key step towards minimally invasive approach to RP due to its technological peculiarities, including 10x magnified three-dimensional visualization, motion scaling with tremor filtration, improved surgical ergonomics and miniature wristed, articulating instruments with 7-degrees of freedom. The surgical technique is described in detail. We report on intra-operative and post-operative outcomes, complications as well as oncologic and functional outcomes from our series of robotic prostatectomy. We review and discuss contemporary published series of robotic prostatectomy.

* Rafael Ferreira Coelho M.D., Global Robotics Institute, Florida Hospital Celebration Health, Celebration, Fl, Department of Urology, University of Sao Paulo, Faculty of Medicine., Email: coelhouro@yahoo.com.br
± Vipul R. Patel, M.D., Medical Director Global Robotics Institute and Urologic Oncology Program: Florida Hospital Celebration Health, Associate Professor of Urology at University of Central Florida, Address: Global Robotics Institute, 410 Celebration Place Suite 302, Celebration, FL 34747, USA, Phone- 407-303-4673, Fax- 407-303-4674, Email- Vipul.patel.md@flhosp.org

1. Introduction - Evolution of Minimally Invasive Laparoscopic Prostatectomy

Data from the Surveillance, Epidemiology and End Results (SEER) registry indicate that the incidence of prostate cancer in men under 50 has increased over the past 10 years, with an annual percent increase of 9.5%. Prostate cancer accounts today for nearly 33% of all newly diagnosed cancers in men (1). For patients with organ confined disease numerous treatment alternatives are now available. However, since Walsh et al (2) first introduced the anatomic nerve sparing technique for radical prostatectomy (RP), it has become the gold standard and most widespread treatment for clinically localized prostate cancer, providing excellent long cancer control. (3)

With the widespread diffusion of prostate-specific antigen (PSA) testing, prostate cancer is nowadays frequently diagnosed in younger and healthier men, with organ confined disease. These patients desire treatments that not only provide excellent oncological and functional outcomes but that can also offer short hospitalization times, low morbidity and minimal convalescence while maintaining their quality of life. This concept has paved the way for exploring into minimally invasive approaches for the surgical management of prostate cancer. A minimally invasive surgical approach for RP was first described by Schuessler and colleagues, in 1997 (4). These authors performed the first successful laparoscopic radical prostatectomy (LRP). With their initially experience these authors noted the challenging nature of the operation and showed no clear benefits compared to open RP (RRP). The operation was advanced in the late 1990s, as European surgeons tackled the difficult learning curve and reported feasibility with results comparable to the open surgical approach (5,6). Despite this, the technical demands of the surgery and the protracted learning curve has prevented the widespread adoption of LRP by most urologic surgeons, especially in US.

The introduction of the da Vinci robotic Surgical System (Intuitive Surgical, Inc., Sunnyvale, CA) has been a key step towards minimally invasive approach to RP due to its technological peculiarities, such as 3D vision, 7 degrees of freedom and magnification. Robotic-assisted laparoscopic radical prostatectomy (RALP) offers the additional advantages of 10x magnified three-dimensional visualization, motion scaling with tremor filtration, improved surgical ergonomics and miniature wristed, articulating instruments with 7-degrees of freedom. The first robotic prostatectomy was performed in 2000 by Binder and Kramer in Germany (7). Menon, Guillonneau and Vallancien refined the technique at Henry Ford Hospital later in that same year and its growth has been exponential since then (8). Currently, almost one decade after the introduction of RALP, several technical modifications have been added to the original surgical technique and the procedure is currently standardized.

2. Surgical Technique – Step-by-Step (Table 1) (9)

RALP can be performed via a transperitoneal or pre-peritoneal technique. The transperitoneal approach is the most common utilized and is also the preferred by the authors. The peritoneal cavity can be accessed by using either a Veress needle or Hasson techniques and the abdomen is then insufflated to a maximum pressure of 15 mmHg. Six trocars are placed under direct vision, as shown in Figure 1. The patient is then placed in a 25 degree steep Trendelenberg position and the robot docked.

Table 1. RALP- Surgical Steps

Surgical Step	Lens	Right Robotic Instrument	Left Robotic Instrument	Fourth Robotic Arm	Assistant Port
Step 1: Incision of the peritoneum and entry into the retropubic space of retzius	0° binocular lens	Monopolar scissor (25 W)	PK (plasma kinetic) forceps (26 W)	Prograsp	Microfrance grasper and suction
Step 2: Incision of the endopelvic fascia (EPF) and identification of the dorsal venous complex (DVC)	0° binocular lens	Monopolar scissor (25 W)	PK (plasma kinetic) forceps (26 W)	Prograsp	Grasper and suction
Step 3: Ligation of the DVC and Periurethral	0° binocular lens	Robotic needle driver	Robotic needle driver	Prograsp	Laparoscopic scissor and suction
Step 4: Anterior bladder neck dissection	30° binocular lens directed downward	Monopolar scissor (25 W)	PK (plasma kinetic) forceps (26 W)	Prograsp	Microfrance grasper and suction
Step 5: Posterior bladder neck dissection	30° binocular lens directed downwards	Monopolar scissor (25 W)	PK (plasma kinetic) forceps (26 W)	Prograsp	Microfrance grasper and suction
Step 6: Athermal Seminal vesicle dissection	30° binocular lens directed downwards	Monopolar scissor (25 W)	PK (plasma kinetic) forceps (26 W)	Prograsp	Microfrance grasper and suction
Step 7: Denonvillier's fascia and posterior dissection	30° binocular lens directed downwards	Monopolar scissor (25 W	PK (plasma kinetic) forceps (26 W)	Prograsp	Microfrance grasper and suction
Step 8: Nerve-sparing: "Athermal early retrograde release of the neurovascular bundle"	30° binocular lens directed downwards	Monopolar scissor (25 W)	PK (plasma kinetic) forceps (26W)	Prograsp	Microfrance grasper and suction
Step 9: Apical dissection	30° binocular lens directed downwards	Monopolar scissor (25 W)	PK (plasma kinetic) forceps (26W)	Prograsp	Microfrance grasper and suction
Step 10: Modified posterior reconstruction of the rhabdosphincter and Urethrovesical anastomosis	30° binocular lens directed downwards	Robotic needle driver	Robotic needle driver	Prograsp	Suction and scissor

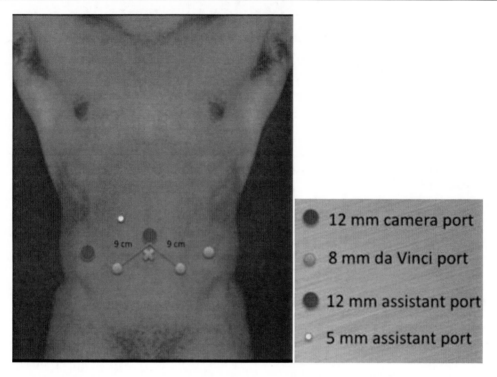

Figure 1. Port Placement.

The robotic and laparoscopic instruments and sutures used during RALP are presented in table 2.

Table 2. Surgical Instruments

Laparoscopic Instruments and Trocars
– Laparoscopic Scissors
– Laparoscopic needle driver
– Laparoscopic Weck Clip appliers
– Microfrance grasper
– Suction
– Endocath Bag
– Laparoscopic Trocars (5mm, 12mm)
Robotic Instruments
– Monopolar scissors
– PK (Plasma Kinetic) Forceps
– Robotic needle drivers
– Prograsp
Sutures
– 0 Caprosyn suture on CT 1 needle (12 inches) – DVC and periurethral suspension stitch
– 3-0 monocryl suture on RB 1 needle (6 inches) – Bladder neck reconstruction
– Two 5 inches 3-0 monocryl sutures of different colors on RB 1 needles tied together- Posterior reconstruction
– Two 8 inches 3-0 monocryl sutures on RB 1 needles of different colors tied together- Vesicourethral anastomosis

Step 1: *Incision of the peritoneum and entry into the retropubic space of retzius*

A transverse peritoneal incision is made through the median umbilical ligament and is extended on both sides in an inverted U fashion to the level of the vas deferens on either side. The assistant and the fourth arm provide the counter-traction. The peritoneum is dissected to the following boundaries: the pubic bone superiorly, the median umbilical ligaments laterally and the vas deferens inferolaterally. The key step is to find the pubic tubercle and follow it laterally to the vasa. It is important to dissect the peritoneum all the way up to the base of the vasa for optimum release of the bladder to allow tension free vesicourethral anastomosis.

Step 2: *Incision of the endopelvic fascia (EPF) and identification of the dorsal venous complex (DVC)*

The important landmarks are the bladder neck, the base of the prostate, the levator muscles and the apex of the prostate. The EPF is best opened at the base of the prostate using cold scissors. This is the area with the largest amount of space between the prostate and the levators and the point at which the prostate has most mobility. Once adequate exposure has been obtained, the EPF is then opened immediately lateral to the reflection of the puboprostatic ligaments bilaterally. Proceeding from the base to the apex, the levator fibers are pushed off of the prostate until the DVC and urethra are visualized. (Fig 2)

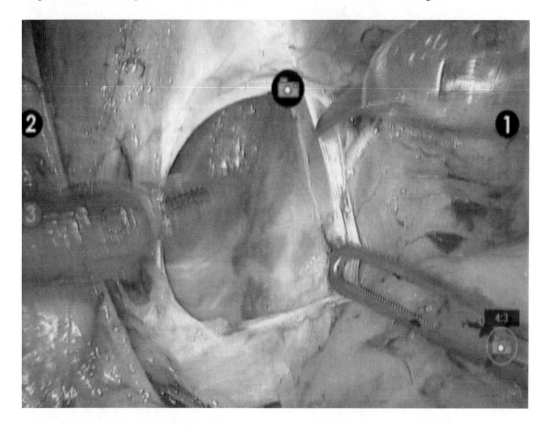

Figure 2. Incision of the endopelvic fascia.

Step 3: *Ligation of the DVC and Periurethral Suspension Stitch (10)*

Robotic needle drivers are placed via the robotic ports. Many different sutures and types of needles are used for this purpose; however, we have tended to use a 0 Caprosyn suture on a large CT1 needle. We hold the needle about 2/3 back at a slight downward angle and place the needle in the visible notch between the urethra and DVC. The needle is pushed straight across at 90° and then the wrist is turned to curve around the apex of the prostate. The suture strength needs to be sufficient to allow the needle holders to pull up tight and perform a slip knot. We prefer to use the slip knot as it prevents the suture from loosening as it is tied.

A periurethral retropubic suspension stitch is then placed. This stitch is positioned holding the needle two-thirds of the way back in a 90° angle and passed from right side to left between the urethra and DVC, and then through the periostium on the pubic bone. The stitch is passed again trough the DVC and through the pubic bone, in a figure eight, and then tied with mild amount of tension. (Figure 3)

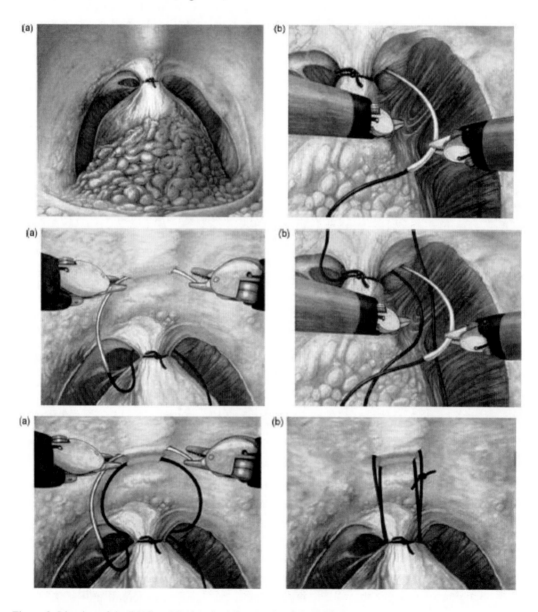

Figure 3. Ligation of the DVC and Periurethral Suspension Stitch (10).

Step 4: *Anterior bladder neck dissection*

The laparoscope is then changed to a 30° down-facing lens for the bladder neck dissection.. The bladder neck is identified by cessation of the fat extending from the bladder at the level of the prostatovesical junction (Figure 4). Another technique is to pull on the urethral catheter and visualize the balloon snagging against the prostate. However, this can be unreliable and misleading after transurethral resection of the prostate or with a median lobe or large prostate. The bladder is dissected off the prostate in the midline using a sweeping motion of the monopolar scissor while visualizing the bladder fibers. The key is to stay in the midline to avoid lateral venous sinuses till the anterior bladder neck is opened and then dissect on either side of the bladder neck. Once the anterior urethra is divided, the Foley catheter is retracted out of the bladder using the fourth arm, and upward traction is applied to expose the posterior bladder neck.

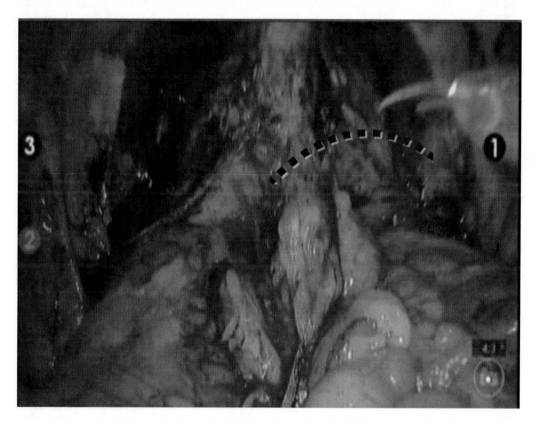

Figure 4. Anterior bladder neck dissection – The urinary catheter is pull and the prostatovesical junction is identified.

Step 5: *Posterior bladder neck dissection*

After incision of the anterior bladder neck, any remaining peripheral bladder attachments should be divided to flatten out the area of the posterior bladder neck and allow precise visualization and dissection of the posterior plane. The full thickness of the posterior bladder neck should be incised at the precise junction between the prostate and the bladder. (**Fig 5**) The lip of the posterior bladder neck is then grasped with the Prograsp (fourth arm) and used for gentle traction to visualize the natural plane between the prostate and bladder. The dissection is directed posteriorly and slightly cranially (towards the bladder) to expose the seminal vesicles. It is important to avoid dissecting caudally (towards the prostate) as there is a possibility of entering the prostate and missing the seminal vesicles completely. The most lateral bladder attachments to the prostate are controlled with hemolock clips and divided. By clipping these attachments, bleeding from large venous sinuses is prevented while maximal exposure is gained prior to beginning the seminal vesicle dissection.

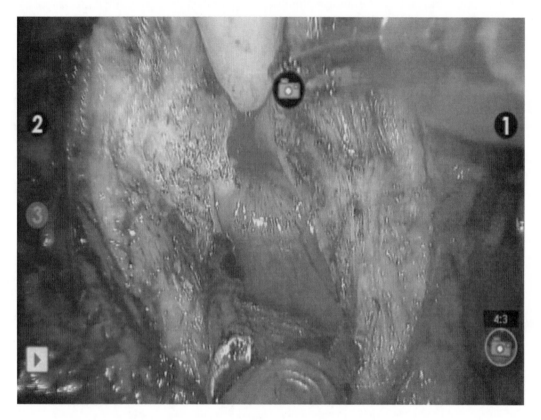

Figure 5. Posterior bladder neck dissection –The precise junction between the prostate and the bladder is identified.

Step 6: *Athermal Seminal vesicle dissection* (11)

The anterior layer of Denonvilliers' fascia is opened with sharp dissection to expose the anterior surfaces of the vas deferens and seminal vesicles. One of the vas deferens is elevated with the fourth arm to improve exposure. Dissection proceeds in the midline between the vas deferens until an avascular plane on the medial surface of one of the seminal vesicles is identified. (Figure 6) Once the tip of the seminal vesicle is identified, it is elevated by the fourth arm rolling it out medially from behind the vas deferens and away from the cavernous nerve. The vas deferens is then clipped and divided just below the level of the tip of the seminal vesicle. The vascular supply to the vesicle is then evident entering the lateral aspect of its tip.

This is controlled with a second hemolock clip placed immediately adjacent to the seminal vesicle tip. Once divided the seminal vesicle can be elevated with the fourth arm and finally released with sharp dissection. If further vessels are identified entering the lateral aspect of the vesicle another hemolock clip can be placed. These steps are repeated on the contralateral side to mobilize the other seminal vesicle.

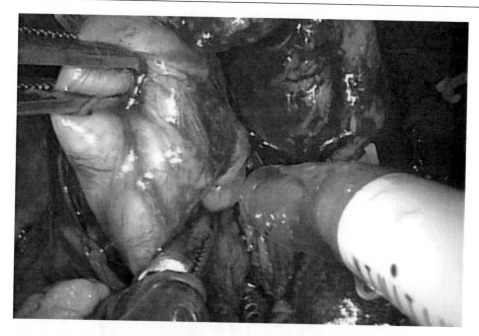

Figure 6. Seminal Vesicle Dissection - The left vas deferens is retracted with the fourth arm. The medial avascular plane of the left seminal vesicle has been identified.

Step 7: *Denonvillier's fascia and posterior dissection*

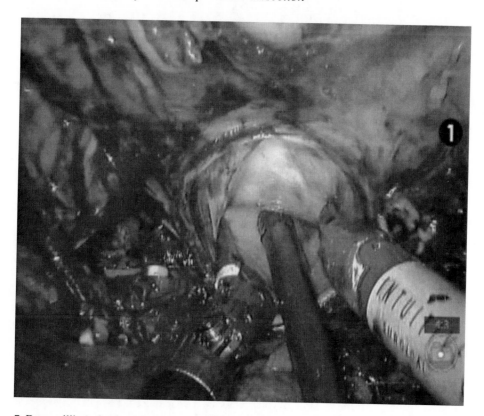

Figure 7. Denonvillier's fascia and posterior dissection.

It is important to dissect the seminal vesicles all the way to the base to allow for appropriate elevation of the prostate and identification of the posterior Denonvillier's fascia. The incision of Denonvillier's fascia is made at the base of the seminal vesicles. The correct plane can be identified by the presence of a clear pearly white plane that is relatively avascular between the posterior prostatic capsule and the rectum. When entered correctly, the plane is avascular and spreads easily with the scissors with minimal bleeding. The posterior space is dissected widely to fully release the prostate and facilitate its rotation during the nerve sparing. (Fig 7)

Step 8: *Nerve-sparing: "Athermal early retrograde release of the neurovascular bundle"* (12)

A complete posterior dissection is critical to successful nerve sparing. It is essential to maximally release the prostate from the rectum all the way to the apex and laterally to the bundles. Prior adequate ligation of the dorsal venous complex is also critical as it decompresses large periprostatic veins that can potentially be a frustrating source of bleeding during the step of nerve preservation.

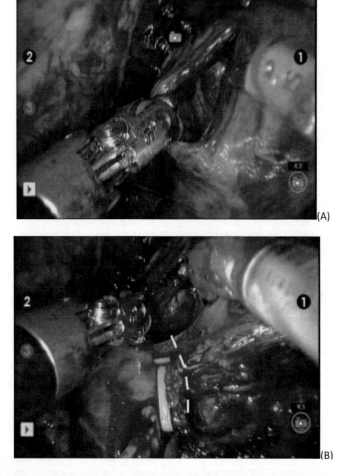

Figure 8. Nerve-sparing: "Athermal early retrograde release of the neurovascular bundle". A) The avascular plane between the neurovascular bundle and prostatic fascia is developed. B) The pedicle is controlled with a hemolock clip placed above the level of the already released bundle.

Our nerve-sparing procedure is performed in a retrograde manner, mirroring the open approach. The neurovascular bundles are released prior to ligation of the prostatic pedicle.

For release of the left neurovascular bundle the assistant grasps the left lateral aspect of the base of the gland and rotates the prostate to the right side. The fourth arm grasps the left side of the bladder and retracts cranially to provide a degree of countertraction. When dissecting the right neurovascular bundle the fourth arm, instead of the assistant, is used to rotate and elevate the prostate. With the prostate rotated medially, the left lateral pelvic fascia is identified in the side and early release of neurovascular bundle is then performed. The lateral pelvic fascia is elevated with the plasma kinetic forceps and incised along the lateral aspect of the prostate. At the level of the apex and mid portion of the prostate the avascular plane between the neurovascular bundle and prostatic fascia is developed (Figure 8a). The plane is continued posteriorly, in a retrograde fashion, between the neurovascular bundle and the prostatic fascia (interfascial nerve-sparing dissection). During the dissection, the neurovascular bundle is stabilized with plasma kinetic forceps and the prostate is gently stroked medially away from the bundle. No thermal energy is used during dissection of the bundle or ligation of the pedicle. The pedicle is controlled with a hemolock clip placed above the level of the already released bundle (figure 8b). The neurovascular bundle is then released distally to the level of the pelvic floor to avoid damaging it during the apical dissection or vesicourethral anastomosis.

Step 9: *Apical dissection*

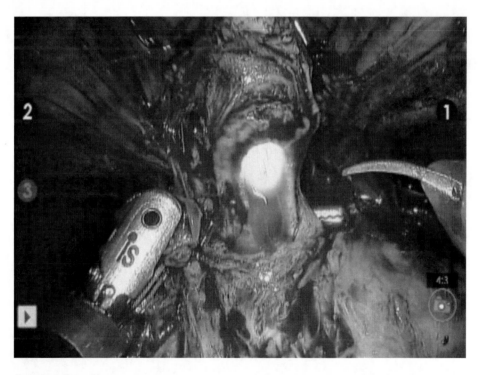

Figure 9. Apical dissection.

The landmarks are the ligated DVC, urethra, apex of the prostate and NVB. It is essential to securely ligate the DVC to prevent bleeding, which may interfere with the apical dissection and division of the urethra under direct vision. Cold scissors are used to divide the DVC and a long urethral stump is developed. Complete dissection of the apex and urethra is facilitated by the robotic magnification. The urethra is then incised at the apex of the prostate under direct vision to completely liberate the prostate. (Figure 9)

Step 10: *Bladder neck reconstruction, modified posterior reconstruction of the rhabdosphincter and urethrovesical anastomosis* (13,14)

A) Bladder Neck Reconstruction

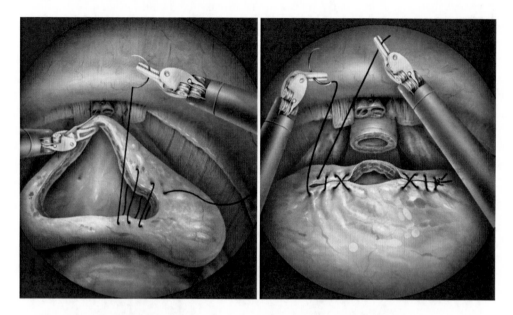

B) Modified posterior reconstruction of the rabdosphincter- Final aspect

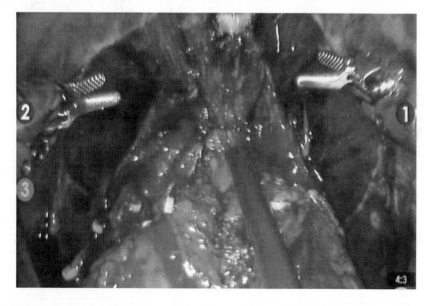

Figure 10. Bladder neck reconstruction, modified posterior reconstruction of the rhabdosphincter and vesicourethral anastomosis. (13,14).

Before starting the bladder neck reconstruction it is essential to check the position of ureteral orifices and their distance from the edge of the bladder neck. Bilateral plication over the lateral aspect of the bladder is then performed using sutures of 3-0 monocryl, with 6 inches length, in a RB-1 needle. The suture begins laterally and runs medially until the bladder neck size matches that of membranous urethra. The same suture subsequently runs laterally, back to the beginning of the suture in the lateral edge of the bladder neck; the suture is then tied. (Figure 10a)

Posterior reconstruction of the rhabdosphincter is performed prior to beginning the vesicourethral anastomosis. The principles are consistent with the two layer reconstruction described previously by Rocco et al with some technical modifications. The reconstruction is performed utilizing two 5 inches 3-0 monocryl sutures (on RB 1 needles) of different colors tied together. The free edge of the remaining Denovilliers' fascia is identified anteriorly to the rectum, just caudal to the bladder neck. This edge is approximated to the posterior aspect of the rhabdosphincter and the posterior median raphe using one arm of the continuous monocryl suture. The second layer of the reconstruction is then performed with the other arm of the monocryl suture approximating the posterior bladder neck to the initial reconstructed layer of rhabdosphincter and to the posterior urethral edge. This suture is then tied with the first arm of the suture, utilized in the first layer of the reconstruction. (Figure 10B)

A continuous modified Van Velthoven vesico-urethral anastomosis is then performed. Two 8 inches 3-0 monocryl sutures of different colors (on RB 1 needles) are tied together with 10 knots to provide a bolster for the anastomosis. The posterior part of the vesicourethral anastomosis is performed with one arm of the suture, in a clockwise direction, from the 5 to 9 o'clock position. This is followed by completion of the anterior anastomosis with the second arm of the suture in a counterclockwise fashion. An 18 Fr Foley catheter is then placed and saline is irrigated to confirm watertight anastomosis. A JP drain is placed around the anastomosis and all the trocars are removed under direct vision.

3. Outcomes

Perioperative Outcomes

The mean operative duration, BMI, estimated blood loss, blood transfusion rates, hospital stay and overall complication rates for current RALP series are presented in Table 3 (15-28).

Operative Time

It is difficult to compare operative time among various series because of variations in reporting this variable to include set-up and/ or pelvic lymph node dissection. However, there is a clear downward trend in the operative time as the surgeon's experience increase. We reviewed our perioperative outcomes for 2500 consecutive RALPs performed by a single surgeon (VRP) (28). The mean operative time decreased from 120 min in the first 300 cases to 78 min in the last 500 patients of the series. For the entire cohort, the mean operative time (from skin incision to fascial closure) was 95 minutes. Similarly, Badani et al. (17) recently reported their experience with 2766 RALPs. For the entire cohort, the mean surgical time (calculated from the time of Veress needle placement to skin closure) and the mean console time were 154 and 116 min, respectively. They compared the results of their first 200 patients (Group 1) with their last 200 patients (Group 2). For Group 1 the mean surgical and console times were 160 and 121 min, respectively; for Group 2 they were 131 and 97 min, respectively. The robotic set-up and docking time also decreased from 45 min in Group 1 to 8 min in Group 2.

Table 3. RALP: Perioperative Outcomes

Authors	Patients (N)	Median/ Mean Age	Mean BMI	Pre-op PSA	Operative Time. min	Mean EBL	% Transfused	Open Conversion	Hospital Length of Stay (days)	Complication Rate
Hu [15]	322	62.1	27.5	-	186	250	1.60%	0%	-	14.60%
Joseph [16]	325	60	-	6.6	130	196	1.30%	0.00%	-	8.60%
Badani [17]	2766	60.2	27.6	6.4	154	142	1.50%	0.10%	1.14	12.20%
Mottrie [18]	184	62	-	8.7	171	200	0.5%	0.54%	-	11.9%
Rozet [19]	133	62	24.8	7.6	166	609	3%	0%	5.4	19.4%
Nelson [20]	629	59.3	-	6.4	-	-	-	-	1.17	17%
Borin [21]	400	61.2	26.8	6.6	-	103.5	-	-	1	-
Zorn [22]	744	59.6	28.1	6.6	234	222	1.20%	1.20%	1.2	-
Schroeck [23]	362	59.2	27.8	5.4	-	150	-	1.60%	-	-
Chan [24]	660	60	-	6.8	207	140	0.80%	0.90%	1.3	-
Krambeck [25]	294	61	-	4.9	236	-	5.1%	-	-	8%
Murphy [26]	400	60.2	27.2	7	186	-	2.50%	0.30%	3.1	15.70%
Rocco [27]	120	63	-	6.9	215	200	-	-	3	-
Patel[28]	2500	61	28	4.9	95	113	0.48%	0% (0.08% LRP)	1.25	5.08%

Estimated Blood Loss and Transfusion Rates

Decreased intraoperative blood loss has been reported to be a hallmark advantage of LRP and RALP. As most intraoperative blood loss originates from the venous sinuses, the tamponade effect created by pneumoperitoneum helps to diminish blood loss.

In a matched-pair analysis comparing 120 RALPs to 240 RRP, Rocco et al. (27) showed that the mean blood loss during RALP was significantly lower than in RRP (200 vs 800 mL; P<0.001). Two recent meta-analysis of studies directly comparing RRP, LRP and RALP confirmed that RALP is associated with less operative blood loss and a lower risk of transfusion than open RP (29-30).

The blood transfusion rates and the mean estimated blood loss in our series of 2500 consecutive RALPs were 0.48% and 113cc, respectively.

Complications

Perioperative complications following RALP have been reported in some recent series. Few studies, however, have used standardized systems to classify surgical complications, which has hampered accurate comparisons between different series or surgical approaches. Based on these limitations, Clavien and colleagues proposed a grading system for surgical complications in 1992 and modified it in 2004 (31). The Clavien grading system is a simple, objective, and reproducible approach for comprehensive surgical outcomes assessment and has been applied more frequently in recent publications reporting complications after RRP, LRP and RALP.

Few series comparing complications after open RP, LRP, and RALP are available and the results are conflicting. Hu et al. (15) compared intraoperative and early postoperative complications in 358 consecutive LRPs and 322 RALPs and showed lower overall complication rates after RALP (27.7% vs 14.6%). By contrast, Rozet et al. (19), in a matched pair analysis of 133 extraperitoneal RALPs and 133 extraperitoneal pure LRPs, reported a higher overall complication rate after RALP (19.4% vs 9.1%, p = 0.01). In turn, Ficarra et al. (29), in cumulative analysis of comparative studies, showed similar complication rates after RALP and LRP (risk ratio [RR]: 1.83; 95% confidence interval [CI], 0.78–4.31; p = 0.16). With regard to the comparison between RRP and RALP, similar complication rates were reported in most of the available publications. Krambeck et al. (25) recently reported comparable perioperative overall complication rates between RALP and RRP (8.0% vs 4.8%, p = 0.064). Similarly, Nelson et al. (20) showed equivalent rates of unscheduled visits (RRP 10% vs RALP 10%, p = 0.95) and readmissions (RRP 5% vs RALP 7%, p = 0.12) due to complications for these two surgical approaches. Finally, the cumulative analysis of comparative studies performed by Ficarra et al. [ref] showed only a nonstatistically significant trend in favor of RALP (RR: 1.33; 95% CI, 0.64–2.74; p = 0.44).

Oncologic Outcomes (Table 4) (16-19, 21-27,32-35)

PSM after RP has been uniformly associated with an increased hazard of biochemical and local disease recurrence as well as the need for secondary treatment. PSM also can cause significant psychological distress to patients because men with PSMs remain more fearful in the long term following surgery compared with those with negative margins (36). Therefore, the status of surgical margins is one of the most important outcomes to be evaluated in any innovative surgical treatment proposed for prostate cancer.

With the advantage of 10 magnified, binocular, three-dimensional visualization, RALP has the potential to reduce the incidence of PSMs, enabling a more precise apical dissection and correct delineation of the neurovascular bundle. Some recent studies showed lower overall and stage-specific PSM rates following RALP when compared to RRP (29,37,38). Smith et al. (37) analyzed the results of 1747 patients undergoing RP (RALP in 1238, RRP in 509) and selected the last 200 consecutive patients in each group. The overall incidence of PSM in the RALP and RRP groups was 15% and 35%, respectively (P < 0.001). The incidence of PSM according to pathological stage was also higher in the RRP than the RALP groups (pT2 tumours, 9.4% for RALP vs 24.1% for RRP, P < 0.001; pT3 tumours, 50% for RALP vs. 60% for RRP). Similarly, in a cumulative analysis of six comparative studies reporting data on margins, Ficarra et al. (29) showed a statistically significant difference in favour of RALP over RRP (relative risk 1.58, 95% CI 1.29–1.94; P <0.001). Considering the PSM rates in patients with pathologically localized cancer, it was re-confirmed that RALP was followed by a lower risk of PSMs (relative risk 2.23, 95% CI 1.36–3.67; P = 0.002). However, by contrast with these results, Schroek et al. (23), comparing 362 consecutive RALPs to 435 RRPs, found no significant difference in PSM rates between RALP and RRP. The risk of bichemical recurrence was also not significantly different after adjusting for clinical (hazard ratio 0.82, 95% CI 0.48–1.38; P = 0.448) and pathological differences (0.94, 0.55–1.61; P=0.824). Similarly, Krambeck et al. (25) showed, in their matched-pair analysis, no difference in the PSM rates between RALP and RRP. The 3-year biochemical progression-free survival was also not significantly different between the groups (RALP 92.4% vs RRP 92.2%; P = 0.69). Finally, a systematic review of thirteen comparative studies (30) showed no significant differences in overall risk or incidence of PSM between RRP and LRP/RALP.

Table 4. RALP: Positive Surgical Margin Rates

Authors	Patients (N)	Pathologic Staging			Positive Surgical Margins		
		pT2	pT3	pT4	pT2	pT3	Overall
Joseph [16]	325	81.00%	19.00%	-	-	-	13.00%
Atug [32]	140	87.9%	9.3%	2.8%	18%	53.8%	18.5%
Badani [17]	2766	77.70%	22.00%	0.30%	13.00%	35.00%	12.30%
Rozet [19]	133	88.5%	11.5%	0	13%	20.9%	19.5%
Mottrie [18]	184	62.5%	37.5%	0	2.5%	37.1%	15.7%
Zorn [22]	744	-	-	-	12.90%	44.80%	18.80%
Borin[21]	400	73.5%	26.5%		6.1%	31.9%	12.5%
Tewari [33]	700	83.5%	13.6%	2.9%	5.4%	-	-
Schroeck [23]	362	79.30%	20.70%	0	-	-	29.30%
Chan [24]	660	80.60%	19.40%	0	11.30%	45.00%	17.90%
Liss [34]	216	68.5%	31.5%	0	5.4%	33%	14.8%
Patel [35]	1500	78.30%	19.50%	1.50%	4.00%	34.00%	9.30%
Murphy [26]	400	70%	29.80%	0.20%	9.60%	42.30%	19.20%
Krambeck[25]	294	90.1%	9.9%		-	-	15.6%
Rocco[27]	120	73%	24%	3%	17%	34%	22%

Besides the surgical approach, different pre, intra and postoperative factors have also been correlated with the incidence of PSM after RALP. Previous studies showed that surgeon's experience and learning curve, for exemple, can affect the oncological outcomes after RALP. Atug et al. (32) evaluated 140 consecutive patients who had RALP by the same surgical team. The patients were divided into three groups based on the time of surgery: group I included the first 33, group II the second 33 and group III the last 34 cases. The PSM rates were 45.4%, 21.2% and 11.7% for groups I, II and III, respectively. The difference among the groups was statistically significant (P =0.005), showing lower PSM rates with increasing of surgeon experience. Similarly, Patel et al. (39), evaluating 500 consecutive RALPs done by one surgeon, reported a PSM rate of 13% in the first 100 patients and 8% in the last 100 of the series. Likewise, Liss et al (34) analyzed the effect of the learning curve in 216 consecutive patients who underwent RALP by one fellowship-trained urological oncologist. There was a small independent 'learning curve' effect representing a lower rate for PSM associated with each increase in 25 patients (odds ratio 0.8, 0.6–1.0) favoured by the significantly decreasing trend in PSM for pT3 cancers over time (P =0.031).

With regard to predictive factors for PSM after RALP, factors correlated with aggressiveness of the cancer, such as clinical stage, pathological stage and tumor volume, appears to predict the PSM rates independently of the nerve-sparing technique adopted by a experienced surgeon. We recently analyzed 876 consecutive patients who underwent RALP performed by a single surgeon with previous experience greater than 1500 cases (40). Stepwise logistic regression was used to identify potential predictive factors for PSM. In the multivariate analysis including pre-operative (age, Body Mass Index (BMI), PSA level, clinical stage, number of positive cores, percentage of positive cores, biopsy Gleason grade, AUA-Symptom Score), clinical stage was the only independent predictive factor for PSM, with a higher PSM rate for T3 vs T1c (OR. 10.7, 2.6–43.8) and for T2 vs T1c (OR 2.9, 1.9–4.6). Considering pre, intra and post-operative variables combined, percentage of tumor, presence of extraprostatic extension, pathological stage and pathological gleason score were associated with increased risk of PSM in the univariable analysis (P<0,001 for all variables). However, in the multivariate analysis, pathological stage (p<0.0001) and percentage of tumor in the surgical specimen (p=0.0022) were the only independent predictive factors for PSM. The PSM rates for pT2 tumors plus bilateral, unilateral or non-nerve sparing procedures were 8.15%, 6.14 and 8.51%, respectively; for pT3 tumors the PSM rates were 27.7%, 26.66% and 30.76%, respectively. Neither of these differences was statistically significant. We believe that surgeon's experience and adequate planning of the nerve-sparing procedure adopted in each patient can explain the lack of difference in the PSM rates comparing bilateral, unilateral or non-nerve sparing procedures in our series. We plan our nerve-sparing procedure individually for each case based on preoperative clinical and biopsy parameters; an incremental or partial nerve-sparing is adopted for patients with high potential for extra-prostatic extension. These results suggest that cancer biology and tumor burden appear to be more important in determining the PSM rates after RALP than the type of nerve-sparing procedure performed by an experienced surgeon adopting a planned nerve-sparing protocol.

Continence Outcomes (Table 5) (16,18,21,22,25-27,33,39,41,42)

Continence rates 1 year after RALP reaches more than 90% in most large single center prospective studies, results at least comparable to RRP series (Table 5). However, the early recovery of urinary continence after RP remains a challenge to be overcome. Reports on early continence from different series differ widely, likely secondary to the lack of a standardized surgical technique and definitions on assessment of continence.

Table 5. RALP: Continence Outcomes

Authors	Patients (N)	Follow-up (months)	Immediate	1 month	3 month	6 month	12 month
Joseph [16]	325	6	24%	56%	93%	96%	-
Menon [41]	1142	12	-	-	-	-	92.00%
Mottrie [18]	184	6	-	43%	-	95%	-
Borin[21]	400	6	-	70.5%	89%	97%	-
Zorn [22]	300	24	-	23.00%	47.00%	68.00%	90.00%
Patel [39]	500	12	27%	-	89%	95%	97%
Tewari[33]	214 (NR)	13	13.1%	35.2%	50.2%	61.9%	82.1%
	304 (AR)	13	27%	59%	76.6%	85.6%	91.2%
	182 (TR)	6	38.4%	82.5%	91.3%	97.1%	-
Murphy [26]	395	>18	-	-	-	-	91.40%
Krambeck[25]	294	12	-	-	-	-	91.8%
Rocco[27]	120	12	-	-	70%	93%	97%
Van der Poel[42]	151	12	-	-	-	54% (any loss of urine)	70% (any loss of urine)

As a result, several technical modifications have been described in an attempt to improve early return of continence after RP.

We have recently described two technical refinements during RALP aiming to improve early continence rates: placement of a periurethral suspension stitch (10) and modified posterior reconstruction of the rabdosphincter (14).

Periurethral Suspension Stitch

Walsh previously described a technical refinement during RRP to divide the DVC with minimal blood loss while avoiding excision or damage to striated sphincter. The maneuver consists of passing a suture through the DVC and through the perichondrium of the pubic symphysis, in a reverse direction, suspending the DVC. According to Walsh, this maneuver can help control the venous bleeding and can provide a recapitulation of the puboprostatic ligaments, supporting the striated sphincter. We have recently described the placement of a periurethral suspension stitch during RALP (figure 3; *Surgical Technique- step 3*) and showed a significant shorter interval to recovery of continence with this technical refinement (10).

We analyzed 331 consecutive patients who underwent RALP, 94 without the placement of a suspension stitch and 237 with the application of a suspension stitch. Continence rates were assessed with a self-administrated validated questionnaire (Expanded Prostate Cancer Index Composite [EPIC]) at 1, 3, 6, and 12 mo after the procedure. Continence was defined as the use of "no pads" and "no leakage of urine," based on patient responses to the EPIC questions. We reported a statistically significant shorter interval to recovery of continence (mean: 7.338 wk; 95% CI: 6.387–8.288 vs. (9.585 wk; 95% CI: 7.558–11.612; log rank test, p = 0.02) and higher continence rates at 3 months after RALP with the placement of the suspension stitch compared to RALP without the suspension stitch (92.8% vs. 83%; p=0.013) (10)

Posterior Reconstruction of Rhabdosphincter

Posterior reconstruction of the rhabdosphincter has been previously described by Rocco and colleagues (43) during RRP and laparoscopic RP and shorter intervals to return of continence were reported using this technical modification. The technique consists in a two layered reconstruction with apposition of the free edge of Denovilliers' fascia and the posterior bladder with the posterior aspect of the rhabdosphincter and posterior median raphe. The purpose of the reconstruction is to preserve the urethral sphincteric complex in the anatomical and functional position in the pelvic floor. This technique has been recently applied during RALP with numerous technical modifications and contradictory results.

We have recently described a modified technique of posterior reconstruction during RALP (14). We analyzed prospectively 803 patients who underwent RALP; 330 without performing posterior reconstruction (group 1) and 473 with posterior reconstruction (group 2). Periurethral suspension stitch, as previously described, was performed in both groups. Continence was defined as the use of "no pads" and "no leakage of urine," based on patient responses to the EPIC questions. In group 1, the continence rates at 4, 12 and 24 weeks postoperatively were 42.7%, 91.8% and 96.3%, respectively; in group 2, the continence rates were 51.6%, 91.7% and 97%, respectively. We found statistically significant higher continence rates at 4 weeks after RALP with posterior reconstruction (51.6 vs. 42.7%;

p=0.016) and lower anastomotic leak rates (0.4% vs. 2.1%; p=0.036) compared to the control group.

Similarly, Tewari et al (33) described an anterior and posterior reconstruction technique (total reconstruction) during RALP and compared their outcomes to RALP performed with no reconstruction (control group) or only with posterior reconstruction. The total reconstruction technique described includes preservation of puboprostatic ligaments and arcus tendineus. the 'Rocco principle' and re-attachment of the arcus tendineus and puboprostatic plate to the bladder neck. The total reconstruction group had continence rates of 38%, 83%, 91%, and 97% at 1, 6, 12, and 24 weeks, respectively. At all the follow-up intervals the continence rate was significantly lower in the control group than in the anterior and total reconstruction groups (P<0.01). The authors concluded that the total reconstruction procedure is a safe and effective way to achieve an early return to continence after RALP.

By contrast with these results, Menon and colleagues (44) showed no improvement in continence rates with reconstruction of the periprostatic tissues. The authors randomized 116 consecutive patients undergoing RALP to urethrovesical anastomosis with or without periprostatic reconstruction. They found no statistical difference in the urinary continence rates at 1, 2, 7 and 30 days after the procedure. However, they did notice a decreased in the incidence of urinary leak, which is a known risk factor for developing bladder neck contracture and urinary incontinence.

We believe that variations in the techniques described for posterior reconstruction during RALP can explain, at least in part, the disparity of results reported in the literature. Each technique involves some individual modifications which precludes definitive conclusions regarding the impact on early recovery of continence. The surgical technique described by Menon et al, for example, was considered by Rocco et al different from their original technique. After reconstructing the Denonvilliers fascia and the posterior wall of the striated sphincter Rocco et al we also suture the reconstructed sphincter to the posterior wall of the bladder, fixing the sphincter 1 to 2 cm dorsocranially to the margin of the new bladder neck. This step, not included in Menon et al study (44), is considered by the authors of the utmost importance because it increases the functional length of the urethral sphincteric complex and brings the urethral sphincteric complex back within the abdomen.

With regard to the comparison of continence rates after RALP, LRP or RRP, very few studies are currently available in the literature and meaningful conclusions about whether any particular approach delivers superior continence outcomes are impractical. Additionally, compilation of data for urinary continence from different RP series is difficult due to variations in definitions, data collection methods and length of follow-up. Nevertheless, better continence rates were suggested after RALP in some studies. Tewari et al. (45) showed, in an unrandomized comparative study, that RALP provides earlier continence recovery than RRP. These authors reported a prospective comparison between 100 RRPs and 200 RALPs, and showed a quicker return of continence after RALP (median 160 vs 44 days; P < 0.05). Similarly, RALP provided a significantly better continence outcome than RRP in a matched-pair analysis by Rocco et al. (27) Posterior reconstruction of the rhabdosphincter was used in both groups and continence was defined as no pad usage or at least one safety pad. The return of continence was significantly (P = 0.007) shorter in men undergoing RALP, with most of them becoming continent within the first 3 months after surgery. The continence rates at 3, 6 and 12 months after RALP and after RRP were 70%, 93% and 97%, and 63%, 83% and 88%, respectively (P = 0.15, 0.011 and 0.014, respectively). By contrast with these results,

Krambeck et al. (25), in a matched-pair comparison of RRP and RALP, showed comparable continence rates at the 1-year follow-up (RALP 91.8%, RRP 93.7%, P = 0.344). Likewise, Parsons and Bennet (30), analysing urinary continence rates within a 1-year follow-up in four comparative studies, showed no significant difference between LRP or RALP and RRP (relative risk 1.07, 95% CI 0.75–1.5, P = 0.70; relative difference 0.03, 95% CI − 0.06 to 0.12, P = 0.49).

Potency Outcomes (Table 6) (16,18, 22, 25-27, 46-48)

Potency is one of the most difficult outcomes to evaluate following RP. Factors other than surgeon or surgical approach have a significant effect on recovery of potency, including patient's age, type and quality of the nerve sparing and use of medications. Also, the assessment of postoperative potency is not standardized, including non validated questionnaires and open interviews. Therefore, direct comparisons between different series are fairly inaccurate, precluding any definitive conclusions.

Table 6. RALP: Potency Outcomes

Authors	Patients (N)	Median/ Mean Age	Type of Nerve Sparing			Follow-up (months	Potency		Overall Potency Rates after Nerve-sparing procedure (considering bilateral AND unilateral NS)			
			Unilateral	Bilateral	NNS		Unilateral NS	Bilateral NS	3 month	6 month	12 month	>18 month
Joseph [16]	325	60	23,6%	70%	6,4%	12	58%	80,60%	-	77,1%	-	-
Menon [41]	1142	60,2	25,00% (unilateral veil)	33,00% (bilateral veil)		>18	-	100%	-	-	70% (bilateral veil NS)	100% (bilateral veil NS)
Mottrie [18]	184	62	13%	64,5%	18,1%	6	47%	70%	-	66,6%	-	-
Zorn [22]	300	59,4	26,40%	59,60%	14%	24	62,00%	83,00%	47%	58%	74%	76,5%
Patel [39]	500	63,2	-	-	-	12	-	-	-	-	78%	-
Tewari [46]	215	60	11%	85%	4%	12	-	87%	-	-	-	-
Krambeck[25]	294	61	91%		9%	12	-	-	-	-	70%	-
Rocco[27]	120	63	-	-	-	12	-	-	31%	43%	61%	-
Murphy[26]	395	60,2	28,2% of potent men	65,3% of potent men	-	12	-	-	-	-	62%	-
Finley[47]	42 (using cautery)	56,5	26%	74%	-	>18	50%	67,8%	8,3%	14,7% (9 months)	43,2%	63,1%
	62 (cautery free)	57	26%	74%	-	>18	80%	93%	32,1%	57,1% (9 months)	76,6%	89,6%
Van der Poel [48]	107	59,6	45,8%	54,2%	-	6	40,8%	63,8%	-	53%	-	-

Different studies have addressed the importance of surgical technique during dissection of the NVBs for preservation of potency after RALP. Ahlering et al (49) demonstrated in a prospective nonrandomized study that the adoption of a cautery-free technique for dissection of NVB allowed significantly higher potency rates postoperatively. The rate of potency rates at 3 months after RALP was 47% (24/51) in the cautery-free group versus just 8.3% (3/36) in the bipolar cautery treated group (P <0.001). Additionally, only 9 of 25 patients (36%) in the cautery-free group reported zero fullness compared with 15 of 22 patients (68%) in the bipolar cautery treated group (P = 0.03).

Based on this study, several athermal antegrade approaches to nerve sparing during RALP have been described. These techniques use either clips or laparoscopic vascular clamps with suturing to control the vascular pedicles before releasing the NVB from the prostate, beginning at the base and moving toward the apex of the gland. While these techniques avoid damaging the bundle with thermal energy they potentially could induce mechanical trauma to the neural tissue. The close proximity of the neurovascular bundle to the base of the prostate places it at risk of inadvertent trauma during these antegrade approaches. Based on this principle, we developed an athermal retrograde release of the NVB during RALP, combining benefits of the traditional open anatomical approach with those of the laparoscopic antegrade approach (12). figure 8; Surgical *Technique- step 8)*. The technique involves releasing the NVB in a retrograde direction, from the apex toward the base of the prostate, during an antegrade RALP. The aim is to clear delineate the path of the bundle avoiding inadvertently injury when controlling the prostatic pedicle. We have recently analyzed mid-term outcomes using our technique of retrograde release of the NVB during RALP and showed higher overall potency rates as well as earlier return of sexual function compared to antegrade nerve-sparing. 346 consecutive patients with preoperative SHIM score >21 who underwent RALP with bilateral nerve sparing were evaluated. Retrograde and antegrade nerve sparing was performed in 200 pts (57.8%) and 146 pts (42.2%), respectively. Nerve-sparing was performed completely athermally in both groups, using Hemolock clips for pedicle ligation. No difference in postero-lateral positive surgical margins (PSM) was found between groups (3.4% vs. 3%; p=0.78). Recovery of erectile function was significantly better in the retrograde nerve-sparing group at 4 weeks (32.1% vs. 37.4%), 6 weeks (50.9% vs. 58.7%), 3 months (75.8% vs. 82.6%), 6 months (82.2% vs. 92.5%) and 12 months (89.7% vs. 96.3%) postoperatively (p<0.05 on all time points).

Whether there is difference in the potency rates after RRP, LRP or RALP is still not clear. It has been proposed that RALP might prevent damage to the NVB, as the three-dimensional magnified vision offered by the Da Vinci Surgical System allows more precise dissection and prevents inadvertent incision, traction or incorporation of the NVB into a suture or clip. Rocco et al. (27) reported higher potency rates after RALP than RRP at 3, 6 and 12 months (RALP 31%, 43% and 61%, respectively; RRP 18%, 31% and 41%, respectively; P = 0.006, 0.045 and 0.003, respectively). Similarly, Tewari et al. (45) reported earlier potency recovery after RALP than RRP. Patients who had a RALP showed an earlier return of erections (50% at a mean follow-up of 180 days, vs 50% at a mean of 440 days after RRP) as well as a quicker return to intercourse (50% at 340 days, vs 50% at 700 days for RRP) than RRP. By contrast with these results, the matched pair analysis by Krambeck et al. (25) showed comparable potency rates between RALP and RRP at 1 year of follow-up (RALP 70.0%, RRP 62.8%, P = 0.081).

Conclusions

Almost one decade after the first RALP was performed, multiple large series are currently mature enough to show safety, efficiency and reproducibility of RALP; RALP is associated with decreased operative blood loss and decreased risk of transfusion in comparative studies with RRP. Excellent functional and oncological outcomes were also reported in large series, with results at least comparable to those presented in high-volume RRP series. Recent studies appear to show advantage of RALP in terms of LOS, PSM rates and early potency and continence rates. However, the current lack of prospective randomized studies precludes definitive conclusions. Additionally, as with any foray into new technology and surgical procedures, the development of technical modifications and surgical refinements are inevitable with increasing experience, explaining the role of surgical volume in ultimately improving the RARP outcomes. During our learning experience we developed several technical modifications which currently allow us to perform the procedure with shorter operative time, improved oncological and functional outcomes and low overall complication rates.

References

[1]   Hayat HJ, Howlander N, Reichman ME, Edwards BK. Cancer statistics, trends and multiple primary cancer analyses from the Surveillance, Epidemiology and End Results (SEER) Program. *Oncologist* 2007; 12: 20–37

[2]   Walsh PC, Donker PJ: Impotence following radical prostatectomy: Insight into etiology and prevention. *J Urol* 1982; 128:492-497.

[3]   Bill-Axelson A, Holmberg L, Ruutu M et al. Radical prostatectomy versus watchful waiting in early prostate cancer. *N Engl J Med.* 2005 12;352(19):1977-84

[4]   Schuessler WW, Schulam PG, Clayman RV, Kavoussi LR: Laparoscopic radical prostatectomy: Initial short-term experience. *Urology* 1997; 50:854-857.

[5]   8.Guillonneau B, Vallancien G: Laparoscopic radical prostatectomy: the Montsouris experience. *J Urol* 2000; 163:418-422

[6]   Rassweiler J, Sentker L, Seemann O, et al: Laparoscopic radical prostatectomy with the Heilbronn technique: An analysis of the first 180 cases. *J Urol* 2001; 166:2101-2108

[7]   Binder J and W Kramer. Robotically-assisted laparoscopic radical prostatectomy. *BJU Int* 2001, 87(4): 408-10.

[8]   Pasticier G, Rietbergen JBW, Guillonneau B, Fromont G, Menon M, Vallancien G. Robotically assisted laparoscopic radical prostatectomy: Feasibility study in men. *Eur Urol.* 2001 40:70–74

[9]   Orvieto MA, Patel VR. Evolution of robot-assisted radical prostatectomy. *Scand J Surg* 2009;98:76–8.

[10] Patel VR, Coelho RF, Palmer KJ, Rocco B. Periurethral suspension stitch during robotic-assisted laparoscopic radical prostatectomy. Description of the technique and continence outcomes. *Eur Urol* 2009; 56: 472–8

[11] Kalan S, Coughlin G, Palmer KJ, Patel VR. Robot-assisted laparoscopic radical prostatectomy: an athermal anterior approach to the seminal vesicle dissection. *J Robotic Surg* 2008, 2:223–226

[12] Coughlin G, Pankaj D, Palmer KJ, Samavedi S, Patel V. Athermal early retrograde release of the neurovascular bundle during nerve-sparing robotic-assisted laparoscopic radical prostatectomy. *J Robot Surg* 2009; 1: 13–7

[13] Lin VC, Coughlin G, Savamedi S, Palmer KJ, Coelho RF, Patel VR. Modified transverse plication for bladder neck reconstruction during robotic-assisted laparoscopic prostatectomy. *BJU Int.* 2009 Sep;104(6):878-8

[14] Coughlin G, Dangle PP, Patil NN et al. Surgery Illustrated – focus on details. Modified posterior reconstruction of the rhabdosphincter: application to robotic-assisted laparoscopic prostatectomy. *BJU Int* 2008; 102: 1482–5

[15] Hu JC, Nelson RA, Wilson TG et al. Perioperative complications of laparoscopic and robotic assisted laparoscopic radical prostatectomy *J Urol* 2006; 175: 541–6

[16] Joseph JV, Rosenbaum R, Madeb R, Erturk E, Patel HR. Robotic extraperitoneal radical prostatectomy: an alternative approach. *J Urol* 2006; 175: 945–50;

[17] Badani KK, Kaul S, Menon M. Evolution of robotic radical prostatectomy: assessment after 2766 procedures. *Cancer* 2007; 110: 1951–8

[18] Mottrie A, Van Migem P, De Naeyer G, Schatteman P, Carpentier P, Fonteyne E. Robot-assisted laparoscopic radical prostatectomy: oncologic and functional results of 184 cases. *Eur Urol* 2007; 52: 746–50

[19] Rozet F, Jaffe J, Braud G et al. A direct comparison of robotic assisted versus pure laparoscopic radical prostatectomy: a single institution experience. *J Urol* 2007; 178: 478–82

[20] Nelson B, Kaufman M, Broughton G et al. Comparison of length of hospital stay between radical retropubic prostatectomy and robotic assisted laparoscopic prostatectomy. *J Urol* 2007; 177: 929–31

[21] Borin JF, Skarecky DW, Narula N, Ahlering TE. Impact of urethral stump length on continence and positive surgical margins in robot-assisted laparoscopic prostatectomy. *Urology* 2007; 70: 173–8

[22] Zorn KC, Gofrit ON, Orvieto MA et al. Da Vinci robot error and failure rates: single institution experience on a single three arm robot unit of more than 700 consecutive robot-assisted laparoscopicradical prostatectomies. *J Endourol* 2007; 21: 1341–4

[23] Schroeck FR, Sun L, Freedland SJ et al. Comparison of prostate-specific antigen recurrence-free survival in a contemporary cohort of patients undergoing either radical retropubic or robot-assisted laparoscopic radical prostatectomy. *BJU Int* 2008; 102: 28–32

[24] Chan RC, Barocas DA, Chang SS et al. Effect of a large prostate gland on open and robotically assisted laparoscopic radical prostatectomy. *BJU Int* 2008; 101: 1140–4

[25] Krambeck AE, DiMarco DS, Rangel LJ et al. Radical prostatectomy for prostatic adenocarcinoma: a matched comparison of open retropubic and robot-assisted techniques. *BJU Int* 2008; 103: 448–53

[26] Murphy DG, Kerger M, Crowe H, Peters JS, Costello AJ. Operative details and oncological and functional outcome of robotic-assisted laparoscopic radical prostatectomy: 400 cases with a minimum of 12 months follow-up. *Eur Urol* 2009; 55: 1358–67

[27] Rocco B, Matei DV, Melegari S et al. Robotic vs open prostatectomy in a laparoscopically naive centre: a matched-pair analysis. *BJU Int* 2009; 103: 448–53

[28] Coelho RF, Palmer KJ, Rocco B, et al. Early Complication Rates in a Single-Surgeon Series of 2500 Robotic-Assisted Radical Prostatectomies: Report Applying a Standardized Grading System. *Eur Urol*. 2010 Feb 13. [Epub ahead of print]

[29] Ficarra V, Novara G, Artibani W et al. Retropubic, laparoscopic, and robot-assisted radical prostatectomy. A systematic review and cumulative analysis of comparative studies. *Eur Urol* 2009; 55: 1037–63

[30] Parsons JK, Bennett JL. Outcomes of retropubic, laparoscopic, and robotic-assisted prostatectomy. *Urology* 2008; 72: 412–6

[31] Dindo D, Demartines N, Clavien PA. Classification of surgical complications: a new proposal with evaluation in a cohort of 6336 patients and results of a survey. *Ann Surg* 2004; 240: 205–13

[32] Atug F, Castle EP, Srivastav SK, Burgess SV, Thomas R, Davis R. Positive surgical margins in robotic-assisted radical prostatectomy: impact of learning curve on oncologic outcomes. *Eur Urol* 2006; 49: 866–71

[33] Tewari A, Jhaveri J, Rao S et al. Total reconstruction of the vesico-urethral junction. *BJU Int* 2008; 101: 871–7

[34] Liss M, Osann K, Ornstein D. Positive surgical margins during robotic radical prostatectomy: a contemporary analysis of risk factors. *BJU Int* 2008; 102: 603–7

[35] Patel VR, Palmer KJ, Coughlin G, Samavedi S. Robot-assisted laparoscopic radical prostatectomy: perioperative outcomes of 1500 cases. *J Endourol* 2008; 22: 2299–305

[36] Pfitzenmaier J, Pahernik S, Tremmel T, Haferkamp A, Buse S, Hohenfellner M. Positive surgical margins after radical prostatectomy: do they have an impact on biochemical or clinical progression? *BJU Int* 2008; 102: 1413–8

[37] Smith JA Jr, Chan RC, Chang SS et al. A comparison of the incidence and location of positive surgical margins in robotic assisted laparoscopic radical prostatectomy and open retropubic radical prostatectomy. *J Urol* 2007; 178: 2385–9

[38] White MA, De Haan AP, Stephens DD, Maatman TK, Maatman TJ. Comparative analysis of surgical margins between radical retropubic prostatectomy and RALP: are patients sacrificed during initiation of robotics program? *Urology* 2009;73:567–71.

[39] Patel VR, Thaly R, Shah K. Robotic radical prostatectomy: outcomes of 500 cases. *BJU Int* 2007; 99: 1109–12

[40] Coelho RF, Chauhan S, Orvieto MA, Palmer KJ, Rocco B, Patel VR. Predictive Factors for Positive Surgical Margins and Their Locations After Robot-Assisted Laparoscopic Radical Prostatectomy.. *Eur Urol*. 2010 Feb 15. [Epub ahead of print]

[41] Menon M, Shrivastava A, Kaul S et al. Vattikuti Institute prostatectomy: contemporary technique and analysis of results. *Eur Urol* 2007; 51: 648–57

[42] van der Poel HG, de Blok W, Joshi N, van Muilekom E. Preservation of lateral prostatic fascia is associated with urine continence after robotic-assisted prostatectomy. *Eur Urol* 2009; 55: 892–901

[43] Rocco F, Carmignani L, Acquati P et al. Restoration of posterior aspect of rhabdosphincter shortens continence time after radical retropubic prostatectomy. *J Urol* 2006; 175: 2201–6

[44] Menon M, Muhletaler F, Campos M, Peabody JO. Assessment of early continence after reconstruction of the periprostatic tissues in patients undergoing computer assisted (robotic) prostatectomy: results of a 2 group parallel randomized controlled trial. *J Urol* 2008; 180: 1018–23

[45] Tewari A, Srivasatava A, Menon M, Members of the VIP Team. A prospective comparison of radical retropubic and robot-assisted prostatectomy: experience in one institution. *BJU Int* 2003; 92: 205–10

[46] Tewari A, Rao S, Martinez-Salamanca JL et al. Cancer control and the preservation of neurovascular tissue: how to meet competing goals during robotic radical prostatectomy. *BJU Int* 2008; 101: 1013–8

[47] Finley DS, Rodriguez E, Skarecky DW, Ahlering TE. Quantitative and qualitative analysis of the recovery of potency after radical prostatectomy: effect of unilateral vs bilateral nerve sparing. *BJU Int* 2009 Nov;104(10):1484-9

[48] van der Poel HG, de Block W. Role of extent of fascial preservation and erectile function after robot-assisted laparoscopic prostatectomy. *Urology* 2009; 73: 816–21

[49] Ahlering TE, Eichel L, Skarecky D. Evaluation of long-term thermal injury using cautery during nerve sparing robotic prostatectomy *Urology*. 2008 Dec;72(6):1371-4

In: Essentials and Updates in Urologic Oncology
Editor: Philippe E. Spiess

ISBN: 978-1-62081-494-9
© 2013 Nova Science Publishers, Inc.

Chapter XXXIV

Robot-Assisted Partial Nephrectomy: Surgical Technique and Contemporary Outcomes

Ryan Turpen and Li-Ming Su

University of Florida Department of Urology, Gainesville, Florida, US

Abstract

Over the past couple of decades, the detection of small, localized renal cell carcinoma has been increasing. As a result, more patients are being referred for surgical management of these incidentally found renal masses. Historically, these patients would have been managed with a radical nephrectomy. However, the paradigm of the management of small renal masses has shifted with an increased emphasis on a nephron-sparing approach. Partial nephrectomy has become an attractive option as it has been shown to provide excellent oncologic control, while at the same time preserving renal function. pure laparoscopic partial nephrectomy remains an extremely technically challenging procedure that is primarily offered at select centers of excellence by experienced laparoscopic surgeons. With the introduction and diffusion of the robotic platform to the field of urology, robot-assisted partial nephrectomy (RAPN) has become an attractive minimally invasive approach for management of renal masses. The technical advantages that robotics provides in comparison to conventional laparoscopy may allow surgeons with limited laparoscopic experience to perform a partial nephrectomy via a minimally invasive approach safely and efficiently.

Introduction

Over the past couple of decades, the detection of small, localized renal cell carcinoma has been increasing [1]. Increased incidence has been greatest in localized tumors when comparing incidence trends by stage [2]. As a result, more patients are being referred for surgical management of these incidentally found renal masses. Historically, these patients would have been managed with a radical nephrectomy. However, the paradigm of the management of small renal masses has shifted with an increased emphasis on a nephron-sparing approach. Partial nephrectomy has become an attractive option as it has been shown to provide excellent oncologic control, while at the same time preserving renal function.

The minimally invasive approach to partial nephrectomy was first described in 1993 when McDougall *et al.* described a laparoscopic technique in a pig model [3]. This approach has since been applied to humans and has shown to provide functional and oncologic outcomes equivalent to the gold standard of open partial [4]. Despite this, sAs a result, its broad application to the urologic community at large remains limited. With the introduction and diffusion of the robotic platform to the field of urology, robot-assisted partial nephrectomy (RAPN) has become an attractive minimally invasive approach for management of renal masses.

The da Vinci® Surgical System (Intuitive Surgical Corp., Sunnyvale, California) has been rapidly adopted into the field of urology, being successfully used for several urologic procedures. The unique three-dimensional visualization, 10x magnification, 6 degrees of freedom at the instrument tip, and elimination of tremor provided by the da Vinci system allow for performance of complex laparoscopic surgical maneuvers with greater ease and precision than conventional laparoscopy.

Indications and Contraindications

The indications for RAPN are similar to that for open and conventional laparoscopic surgery. In general, solitary, clinically localized tumors less than 4 cm are excellent candidates for RAPN, however larger masses (i.e. clinical stage T2) that are peripheral in location may also be approached successfully. Although lesions located peripherally are ideal, some groups have shown that with experience, even central tumors located at the renal hilum can be addressed with RAPN [5]. Multiple tumors may be a relative contraindication to RAPN due to the predictable longer warm ischemia time required to resect multiple tumors and may be more appropriately addressed by open partial nephrectomy or radical nephrectomy. Tumors in a solitary kidney may be approached by RAPN, however this needs to be carefully weighed against alternatives such as open partial nephrectomy that allows cold or no ischemia to reduce the physiologic insult to the solitary renal unit. Absolute contraindications to RAPN include cardiopulmonary compromise precluding general anesthesia or uncorrectable bleeding diathesis.

Preoperative Preparation

Bowel Preparation

One bottle of citrate of magnesium is taken the day before surgery and the patient's diet is limited to clear liquids. A broad-spectrum antibiotic such as cefazolin is administered intravenously 30 minutes before surgery. Aspirin and other anticoagulants are held at least 7-10 days prior to surgery.

Informed Consent

In addition to bleeding, transfusion, and infection, patients undergoing RPN must be aware of the potential for conversion to conventional laparoscopic or open surgery. As with open surgery, patients must be counseled on the risk of incisional hernia, adjacent organ injury (e.g. ureter, colon, small bowel, spleen, liver, pancreas, and lung), as well as conversion to radical nephrectomy. Unique to partial nephrectomy is the risk for development of a post-operative urine leak, especially in endophytic lesions that abut the renal collecting system. Furthermore, the discussion that 6% to as high as 46% of solid, enhancing masses may represent benign tumors when stratified by tumor size, must also be held during pre-operative counseling with the patient [6]. Finally, the risks of general anesthesia must also be presented to the patient, as RAPN cannot be performed under regional anesthesia.

Before entering the operating room, several measures are taken to optimize surgical success.

Operative Preparation

Preparation of required operating room equipment and personnel is necessary to ensure optimal success. Standard laparoscopic equipment, endoscopes and video towers are needed. Vascular bulldog clamps, renorrhaphy sutures, Surgicel® gauze (Ethicon360), laparoscopic ultrasound probe are some of the specialized items unique to RAPN that must be made available in the operating room before the start of the surgery. Thorough preoperative review of cross-sectional imaging to plan patient positioning and handling of the renal mass at time of excision is critical. Key imaging features include renal vasculature (i.e. number of renal arteries and veins), location of renal mass (anterior vs. posterior, superior vs. inferior, endophytic vs. exophytic, hilar vs. peripheral), as well as depth of invasion and approximation to renal collecting system all of which serve as a guide to planning the excision of the mass.

Preparation of the OR personnel including the circulating nurse, scrub technician, and anesthesiologist, is addressed to best ensure success of the surgery. Having a dedicated team versed in laparoscopic and robotic surgery helps to ensure a smooth and efficient surgery. Pre-operative briefings allows for the entire team to identify the patient and planned procedure as well as verbalize any concerns so that these may be addressed and resolved before beginning the surgery.

This includes communication with the anesthesiologist, making them aware of surgical expectations and anticipated challenges such as intravenous access, fluid administration and end-tidal carbon-dioxide monitoring. Lastly, critical to the success of RAPN is the use of a experienced bedside assistant, well versed in laparoscopic renal surgery.

Surgical Technique

Patient Positioning

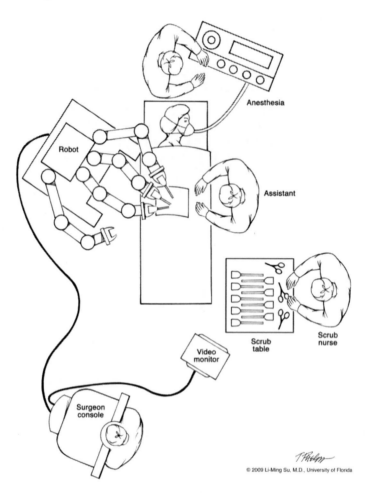

Figure 1. Positioning of da Vinci® Surgical System and OR personnel.

After induction of general endotracheal anesthesia, a foley catheter is placed for bladder decompression prior to positioning. The abdomen is shaved and the midline is marked for extraction site identification. The patient is then placed in either the modified or full flank position based upon location (i.e. anterior vs. posterior) of the renal mass. For posterior tumors, we prefer placing the patient in the full flank position and approaching the kidney via a transperitoneal route. This positioning allows for the kidney to be rotated medially, allowing for adequate visualization of the renal tumor and resection bed during renorraphy. The patient is placed so that the anterior superior iliac spine is located at the level of the breaking point of the table to allow for flexion of the bed to increase space for trocar placement. Sufficient padding at all pressures points is ensured at the time of positioning to reduce neuromuscular injuries. If placed in the full 90° flank position, an axillary role is required.. The patient is then secured to the table with the use of foam padding across the shoulders and hips and heavy cloth tape. A shoulder role is secured between the ipsilateral shoulder and neck. Once fully secured, the patient is test-rolled maximally to the left and right to ensure the patient is well secured to the operating table.

The da Vinci® Surgical System is positioned by approaching the patient at a 45° relative to the OR bed at the level of the ipsilateral costal margin. The positioning of the robotic platform as well as the additional OR personnel is depicted in Figure 1.

Access and Trocar Placement

It is our practice to perform RAPN in a transperitoneal fashion although posterior masses can be approached retroperitoneally as well [7]. We find that with adequate dissection and patient positioning, even posteriorly located masses can be removed via a transperitoneal approach. Pneumoperitoneum is established with the Veress needle at the umbilicus and insufflation pressure is initially set at 15 mm Hg.

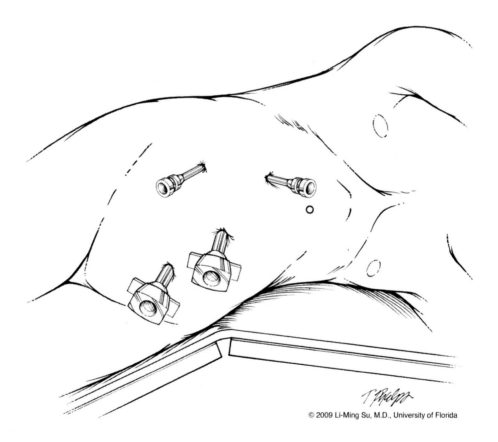

© 2009 Li-Ming Su, M.D., University of Florida

Figure 2. Trocar positioning. For the three-arm approach, a 12-mm camera trocar is placed at the umbilicus with two 8-mm robotic trocars placed in a diamond-shaped configuration pointing towards the kidney. The 12-mm assistant trocar is placed inferior to the robotic camera trocar along the midline. For right-sided tumors, a liver retractor can be placed below the xyphoid process (not depicted).

One of the most critical steps in ensuring a successful RAPN is strategic trocar positioning. Use of the available cross-sectional imaging to serve as a guide for trocar placement is essential. The ideal approach to the renal mass is at a 45° angle in relation to the camera and robotic arms. Whereas this may be easy to conceptualize for anteriorly located masses, when planning trocar placement for more posteriorly located masses, it is important to understand that with mobilization of the kidney, the location of the mass will change dramatically. If one does not plan accordingly, the result can be an extremely acute angle of approach, making mass excision and renorraphy extremely challenging for even the most experienced surgeon.

We prefer a three-arm approach although a four-arm approach has been described and can be utilized [8]. For the three-arm approach, a 12-mm camera trocar is placed at the umbilicus with two 8-mm robotic trocars placed in a diamond-shaped configuration pointing towards the kidney (Figure 2). A single 12-mm assistant trocar is placed below the umbilicus. For right-sided tumors, a 5-mm trocar is placed below the xyphoid process to allow for liver retraction with a locking grasper.

Bowel Mobilization

The colon is mobilized medially be sharply incising the white line of Toldt. A Maryland bipolar forcep is used with the left robotic arm and the curved monopolar scissors are used with the right robotic arm. The incision is generally carried from the pelvic inlet to the upper pole of the kidney, releasing the spleen or liver depending on whether a left or right renal mass is being approached. Special attention must be paid to avoid a thermal injury to the bowel throughout mobilization. The assistant aids in mobilization by applying countertraction medially with use a bowel grasper or the suction-irrigator. Once the superficial layer of peritoneum has been incised, a combination of sharp and blunt dissection is used to continue medial mobilization of the posterior mesocolon off of anterior Gerota's fascia. Care must be taken to avoid creating a rent in the posterior mesentery during blunt dissection. Should an inadvertent rent be created during dissection, closure and repair with Hem-o-lok clips should be performed to reduce the chance of an internal hernia.

Renal Hilar Dissection

Once the bowel has been reflected adequately, the gonadal vein and ureter are visible. The retroperitoneum allows for these structures to be lifted anteriorly to expose the psoas muscle (Figure 3). Dissection is then carried cranially, tracing the gonadal vein along it course to the vena cava on the right and the renal vein on the left. Most commonly, the renal vein is identified first as it lies anterior to the artery. Visualization of arterial pulsations can help to guide in dissection of the renal artery. Use of pre-operative cross-sectional imaging can also be extremely useful to estimate the location of the renal artery relative to the vein. In addition, quantifying the number of renal arteries is important, as there occasionally may be a lower pole artery that is encountered during dissection along the gonadal vein. This is also important for clamping purposes as control of all renal arteries is necessary to ensure adequate ischemia to the excision bed. During dissection and skeletonization of the renal vessels, use of a monopolar hook electrocautery can be of particular benefit as it is a small profile thermal device, reducing the risk of inadvertent arching or cautery to adjacent critical structures.

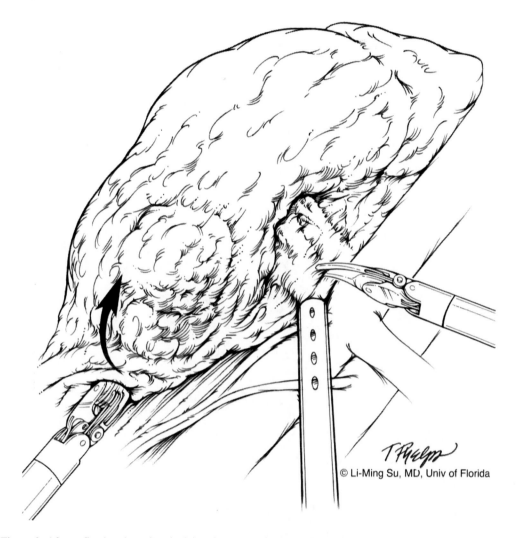

© Li-Ming Su, MD, Univ of Florida

Figure 3. After reflecting the colon, incising the retroperitoneum allows for the ureter to be lifted in a cephalad direction, exposing the psoas muscle. Dissection is then followed along the ureter towards the renal hilum where the hilar vessels are dissected to allow for subsequent clamping.

Tumor Identification

The adipose tissue overlying the kidney and mass is incised and then reflected off the kidney to expose the renal mass. Attention is made to leave the fat immediately overlying the mass intact to submit en bloc with the excised specimen. For exophytic lesions, it is often easy to identify the mass. However, for mesophytic or endophytic lesions, use of a flexible laparoscopic ultrasound probe through the 12-mm assistant trocar can be used to locate the lesion. In addition, even for exophytic lesions, the ultrasound probe is used to delineate the margins of resection. Again, this is all guided by careful intraoperative review of cross-sectional imaging. With the use of the TilePro™ feature of the da Vinci system, both the ultrasound images and even CT images can be imported and seen from within the surgeon console. Once identified, scoring the renal capsule circumferentially around the mass with the monopolar scissors marks the margins of resection (Figure 4). Prior to hilar clamping and mass excision, the sutures that will be used for the renorraphy are introduced and stored in the abdomen to allow for more efficient renal reconstruction and therefore decreased warm ischemia time.

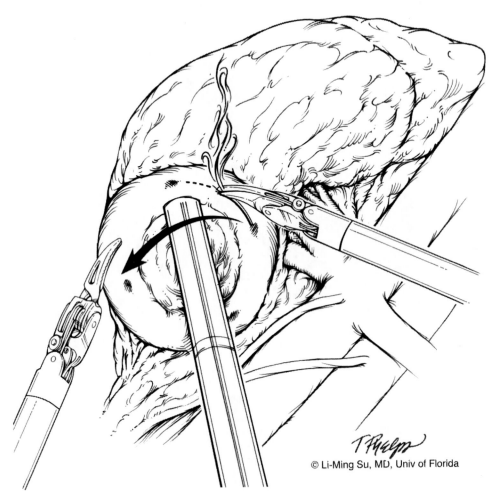

© Li-Ming Su, MD, Univ of Florida

Figure 4. Tumor Identification. Once identified, scoring the renal capsule circumferentially around the mass with the monopolar scissors marks the margins of resection. Use of the laparoscopic ultrasound probe can aid in identification of the edge of the tumor for scoring purposes, especially for more endophytic masses.

Hilar Clamping

Prior to obtaining vascular control of the hilum, 12.5 grams of mannitol followed by 10 mg of lasix is administered intravenously as a free radical scavenger and diuretic to reduce ischemia-related renal injury. We prefer to control each vessel individually with the use of laparoscopic bulldog clamps. Alternatively, a laparoscopic Satinsky can be used to clamp the hilum en bloc. The bedside assistant applies the first bulldog clamp to the renal artery. The operating room circulator is instructed to begin monitoring the duration of warm ischemia after the first bulldog clamp is applied to the renal artery. We routinely apply a second bulldog clamp to the renal artery, ensuring complete occlusion (Figure 5). Inspection of the kidney is then performed to ensure appropriate blanching occurs, indicating adequate arterial control. In the event that blanching does not occur, consideration should be given to a second artery or that the artery controlled may represent only a branch of the main renal artery. On occasion, we will apply a single bulldog clamp to the renal vein. This decision is made after excision of the mass is started in the setting of excessive venous back bleeding. In such instances, control of the renal vein often improves visualization during excision of the mass.

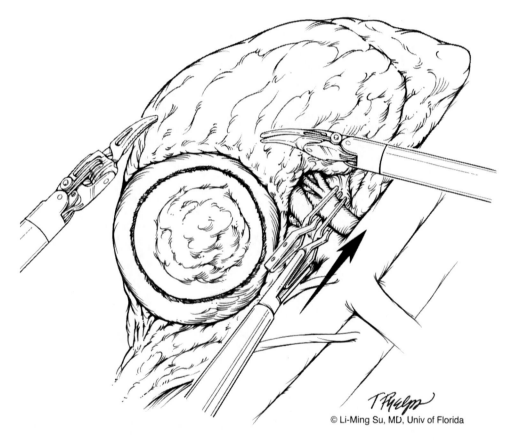

© Li-Ming Su, MD, Univ of Florida

Figure 5. Hilar Clamping. Once the hilar vessels are skeletonized, the bedside assistant applies the first bulldog clamp to the renal artery. We routinely apply a second bulldog clamp to the renal artery, ensuring complete occlusion.

Excision of Mass

Once control of the renal hilum has been established, the mass is sharply excised using the monopolar scissors, along the previously scored margin. Only select use of electrocautery is recommended so as to provide a pristine view of the renal parenchyma during resection of the mass to ensure clean surgical margins of resection. The Maryland bipolar forceps (or alternatively a ProGrasp forceps) is used to manipulate and retract the mass to aid in exposure of the resection plane. In addition the assistant uses the suction-irrigator to provide counter traction aid in visualization of the resection plane during excision of the mass (Figure 6). Any entry into the collecting system is noted for later repair. Once the mass is completely excised, the mass an its overlying fat is placed above the liver on the right, or above the spleen on the left for later retrieval.

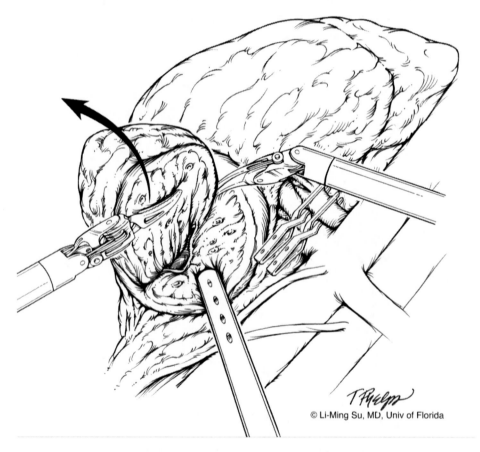

© Li-Ming Su, MD, Univ of Florida

Figure 6. Mass Excision. Once control of the renal hilum has been established, the mass is sharply excised using the monopolar scissors, along the previously scored margin. The Maryland bipolar forceps (or alternatively a ProGrasp forceps) is used to manipulate and retract the mass to aid in exposure of the resection plane. In addition the assistant uses the suction-irrigator to provide counter traction aid in visualization of the resection plane during excision of the mass.

Renorraphy

Once the mass is excised, the cortical edge of the defect is cauterized using the monopolar scissors. The instruments of the second and third robotic arms are exchanged for large robotic needle drivers and a renorraphy is performed. First, a 3-0 polyglactin SH suture cut to 6-7 inches is used as a running continuous suture along the deep margin of the resection site to achieve hemostasis and repair any noted entry into the collecting system (Figure 7).

This suture is secured with use of Lapra-Ty clips (Ethicon Endo-Surgery, Inc., Cincinnati, OH) on either end. Next, renal parenchymal sutures are placed to complete the renorraphy. Using 0 Vicryl sutures on CT1 needles cut 6 inches in length and secured with large Hem-o-lok clips (Teleflex Medical, Kenosha, WI), these sutures are passed across the renal defect approx.-imately 1cm apart (Figure 8). The sutures are tightened to reapproximate the parenchymal edges and then secured in placed with additional Hem-o-lok clips applied by the bedside assistant. Using the robotic needle drivers, the renorraphy can be tightened by sliding the clip against the renal parenchyma to ensure appropriate compression and hemostasis. After the initial hem-o-lok clips are secured and the defect closed, the bulldog clamps are removed and the termination of warm ischemia noted by the circulating nurse (Figure 9). A second Hem-o-lok clip is then applied to the parenchymal sutures for additional security. Spot cautery is used if needed in areas of minor persistent bleeding from the parenchymal edge. Finally, a hemostatic agent such as Floseal® (Baxter, Deerfield, IL) is then applied along with Surgicel® gauze. A Jackson Pratt drain is placed through the lateral robotic trocar site at the end of the operation.

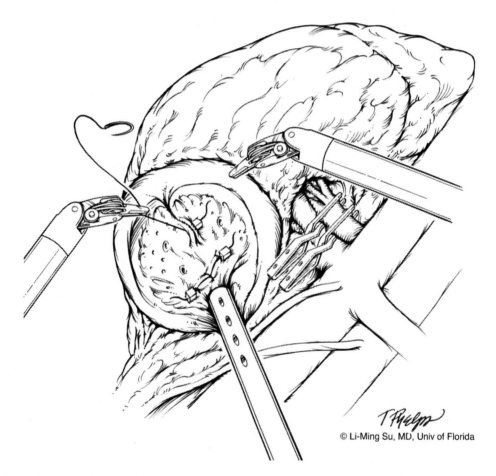

© Li-Ming Su, MD, Univ of Florida

Figure 7. Renorraphy. A running continuous 3-0 polyglactin suture is placed along the deep margin of the resection site to achieve hemostasis and repair any noted entry into the collecting system. The sutures are secured using Lapra-Tys.

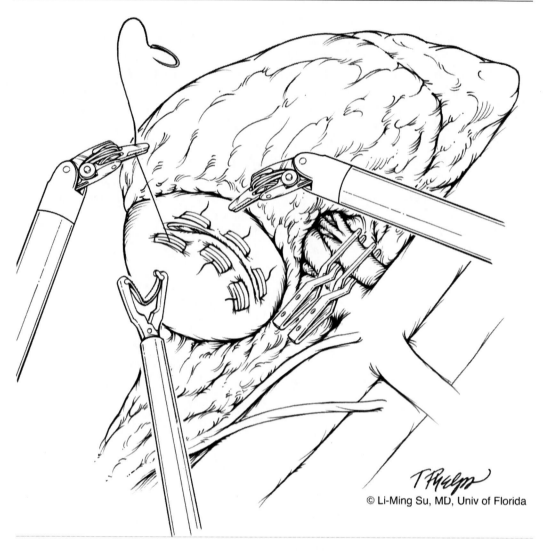

© Li-Ming Su, MD, Univ of Florida

Figure 8. Renorraphy. Renal parenchymal sutures are placed to complete the renorraphy. Using 0 Vicryl sutures on SH needles are passed across the renal defect approximately 1cm apart. The sutures are tightened to reapproximate the parenchymal edges and then secured in placed with Hem-o-lok clips applied by the bedside assistant. Using the robotic needle drivers, the renorraphy can be tightened by sliding the clip against the renal parenchyma to ensure appropriate compression and hemostasis.

Specimen Retrieval and Closure

The specimens that was stored above the liver or spleen is placed in an entrapment sac that is introduced through the assistant port. At time of extraction, this port site can be enlarged and the fascia opened. A fascial closure is performed using 0 Vicryl suture. The remaining trochar sites do not require fascial closure as the risk for developing herniation at these sites is low.

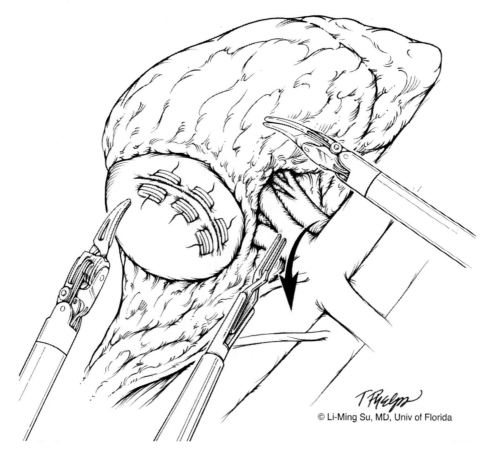

© Li-Ming Su, MD, Univ of Florida

Figure 9. Removal of hilar clamps. After the initial hem-o-lok clips are secured and the defect closed, the bulldog clamps are removed and the termination of warm ischemia noted by the circulating nurse.

Contemporary Outcomes

With the introduction of a novel surgical technique such as RAPN, comparisons to the gold standard must be made to ensure that equivalent or improved outcomes are realized. Open partial nephrectomy (OPN) has long been the gold standard for removal of small renal masses, resulting in excellent long-term cancer control with preserved renal function9. Efforts to decrease the morbidity associated with OPN lead to a move towards a minimally invasive approach to nephron-sparing surgery, resulting in a laparoscopic partial nephrectomy (LPN) approach to small renal masses as first described by McDougall et al [3]. This approach has been shown to result in functional and oncologic outcomes equivalent to those reported with the open approach10. However, the technical demands of LPN, specifically intracorporeal suturing, has made this technique available only at centers of excellence with experienced laparoscopic teams. This has limited the widespread dissemination of LPN as a minimally invasive surgical technique for nephron-sparing surgery. RAPN offers an alternative to LPN, with the potential for simplifying the technique of minimally invasive nephron-sparing surgery. Currently available outcomes of RAPN will be reviewed in the following sections.

Intraoperative Parameters

Operative Time

Reported operating times (OT) for RAPN varied from 140 to 265 minutes in the contemporary series of RAPN (Table 1). In the five series that compared RAPN to LPN [13, 16-18, 20], three showed no difference in OT between RAPN and LPN while one each showed a difference favoring RAPN and LPN. It is worth noting that in most of those series reported that the results reflect the initial experience with RAPN compared to a mature LPN experience. Thus, all except one series were able to show equivalent or improved OTs as compared to LPN despite the relatively inexperience with the robotic approach. In the lone series that reported a shorter OT with the laparoscopic approach, the difference was 30.9 minutes, the clinical significance of which is unclear. In the series reported by Patel *et al.* that compared RAPN in tumors less than and greater than 4 cm, there was no difference in mean OT between the two groups [22].

In addition, Rogers *et al.* reported a mean OT for hilar tumors comparable to all other series, indicating a hilar location does not impact on OT[5]. Finally, in a series evaluating results of RAPN for complex renal tumors, defined as hilar, endophytic, or multiple tumors, Rogers *et al.* reported a mean OT of 192 minutes, again within the range of those reported by all RAPN series [14]. Finally, in the lone series that reported a favorable decrease in OT for RAPN as compared to LPN, Wang *et al.* found a 16 minute decrease in mean OT for the robotic approach versus the laparoscopic approach [20]. Again, the clinical significance of such a difference is unclear. Overall, it appears that the robotic approach to nephron-sparing surgery is equivalent to the published series of LPN .

Warm Ischemia Time

A warm ischemia time (WIT) of less than 30 minutes has long been established as the limit beyond which permanent physiologic insult to the kidney may ensue. Limiting renal ischemia during partial nephrectomy is important so as to minimize kidney damage from free oxygen radical formation and reperfusion injury. The mean WIT in the series reported in Table 1 varied from 17.8 to 32 minutes. It should be noted that in some of the series reviewed, the mean ischemia time included cases in which no ischemia was used for purely exophytic tumors.

For example, in the series reported by Benway *et al.*, although the mean WIT was reported to be 17.8 minutes, when the data is limited to those cases in which clamping was performed, the mean WIT was 22.8 minutes [21]. Once again, the clinical difference of which is unclear, as long-term creatinine clearance data are needed to truly evaluate the impact on functional outcomes. Of those studies comparing RAPN to LPN, two reported a decreased mean WIT for RAPN as compared to LPN while the remaining three showed no statistical difference between modalities [13, 16-18, 20]. Only two of the five studies evaluated a difference in pre-operative and post-operative serum creatinine (SCr) or estimated GFR (eGFR) [13, 16].

Both of these two studies showed no statistical difference in WIT and not surprisingly showed no statistical difference in functional outcome as defined by change in SCr or eGFR at 3 months of follow-up. It would be more appropriate to perform a similar analysis in those studies in which a difference in WIT was seen to determine if that difference translates to long-term functional outcome in terms of SCr and eGFR. Patel *et al.* showed that increased tumor size (>4cm) was associated with a statistically significant increase in the median WIT (25 vs. 20 min, p=0.011), although both groups maintained median WITs of less than 30 minutes [22].

No difference in absolute 24-h postoperative eGFR, change in 24-h postoperative eGFR, mean follow-up eGFR or mean change in follow-up eGFR was seen between the groups, again questioning the significance of the difference in WIT in regards to functional outcomes. In the end, creatinine clearance may be too crude a measure to evaluate impact of renal ischemia to a single renal unit. New serologic and urine markers such as NGAL may provide more insight into acute phase injury caused during partial nephrectomy while under warm ischemia [23].

Estimated Blood Loss

Reported mean estimated blood loss (EBL) ranged from 100 to 329 ml in contemporary series (Table 1). Only one of the five studies comparing RAPN to LPN showed a difference between modalities.

In their series, Benway *et al.* showed a statistically significant difference in EBL of 155 versus 196ml (p = 0.03) in favor of RAPN [17]. However, there was no difference in post-operative changes in hematocrit (-5.5% vs. -6.6%, p = 0.8). There did appear to be a trend of increased rates of transfusion in the RAPN groups as compared to the LPN groups in those studies reporting transfusions. This is perhaps a more clinically relevant end point although whether or not this reached a level of statistical significance is unclear in the studies reviewed.

Postoperative Outcomes

The mean length of stay (LOS) reported in all robotic partial nephrectomy contemporary series ranged from 1.9 to 4.7 days (Table 1). In the authors' experience, most patients are ready for discharge by postoperative day 2. Three of the five studies comparing RAPN and LPN reported a shorter LOS favoring RAPN [16-17, 20]. While two of these three differed by less than a day (2.5 vs. 2.9 [20]) and 2.4 vs. 2.7 [17]), Deane *et al.* reported a difference of 1.1 days[16]. No statistically significance differences have been reported in other postoperative parameters such as mean postoperative hematocrit and serum creatinine between RAPN and LPN.

Table 1.

Parameter	Gettman [11]	Phillips [12]	Aron [13]	Rogers [14]	Bhayani [15]	Deane [16]	Benway [17]	Jeong [18]	Rogers [19]	Wang [20]	Benway [21]	Patel [22]	Rogers [5]
No. RAPN	13	12	12	14	35	11	129	31	148	40	50	71	11
No. LPN	N/A	N/A	12	N/A	N/A	12	118	26	N/A	62	N/A	N/A	N/A
Mean (range) Tumor Size, cm	3.5 (2-6)	1.8 (NR)	2.4 (1.4-3.8)	3.6 (0.8-6.4)	2.8 (1-6)	3.1 (2.5-4)	2.8 (NR)	3.4 (NR)	2.8 (0.8-7.5)	2.5 (1-5)	2.5 (0.3-7.5)	3.55 (0.7-7.9)	3.8 2.3-6.4
Mean (range) OT, min	215 (130-262)	265 (NR)	242 (130-360)	192 (165-214)	142 (69-219)	228.7 (98-375)	189 (NR)	169.9 (NR)	197 (63-392)	140 (87-219)	145.3 (69-219)	256.75 (210-344)	202 (154-253)
Mean (range) EBL, mL	170 (50-300)	240 (NR)	329 (50-1000)	230 (100-450)	133 (25-500)	115 (75-500)	155 (NR)	198.3 (NR)	183 (15-1000)	136 (25-500)	140.3 (25-450)	100 (50-200)	220 (50-750)
Mean (range) WIT, min	22 (15-29)	26 (NR)	23 (13-36)	31 (24-45)	21 (0-40)	32 (30-45)	19.7 (NR)	20.9 (NR)	27.8 (12-60)	20 (13-40)	17.8 (0-40)	22.5 (14-30)	28.9 (20-39)
Positive Margins (%)	1 (7.7)	NR	0 (0)	0 (0)	0 (0)	0 (0)	5 (3.9%)	NR	6 (4.1)	1 (2.5)	1 (2)	3 (4.2)	0 (0)
Mean (range) LOS, days	4.3 (2-7)	2.7 (NR)	4.7 (2-10)	2.6 (2-3)	2.5 (1-7)	2 (NR)	2.4 (NR)	5.2 (NR)	1.9 (1-7)	2.5 (1-4)	NR	2* (2-4)	2.6 (1-4)
Follow-up, mon	2-11	NR	7.4	3	NR	4-37	Up to 12	12*	2-54	NR	NR	0.3-19.3	NR
Recurrence	0	NR	0	0	NR	0	0	1	0	NR	0	0	NR
Complications	Ileus (1)	Conversion to LPN (1), HLPN (1), open (1)	Conversion to LPN (2); PE (1)	None	Conversion to open (1), conversion robotic cryo (1); PE (1); MI (1); transfusion (2)	Post-operative bleed requiring exploration (1)	Urine leak (3); PE (1); MI (1); rectus hematoma (1); transfusion (1); AVM (2); subcapsular hematoma requiring completion nephrectomy	Trans-fusion (1); conversion to robotic radical nephrectomy (1)	Hematoma (1); ileus (3); urine leak (2); rhabdomyolysis (1); conversion to open (2)	Cardio-pulmonary (3); thromboembolic (1); hematoma (1); transfusion (2); cystoscopy and sten (1)	MI (1); DVT (1); transfusion (2)	Enterotomy (1); urine leak (2); transfusion (2); PE (1); bleeding requiring angioembolization (1) and reexploration (1)	Urine leak (2)

OT = operative time; EBL = estimated blood loss; WIT = warm ischemia time; LOS = length of stay; NR = not reported; HLPN = hand-assisted laparoscopic partial nephrectomy; PE = pulmonary embolus; MI = myocardial infarction; AVM = arteriovenous malformation; DVT = deep venous thrombosis

Oncologic Outcomes

To assess the success of a new technique being applied to an oncologic procedure, as is the case with RAPN, its oncologic outcomes must be at least equivalent if not favorable as compared to the standard of care. Outcomes from the minimally invasive approach to nephron-sparing surgery, namely LPN, have been shown to provide equivalent intermediate-term cancer cure and preservation of renal function as compared to OPN [24]. RAPN oncologic outcomes in contemporary series have shown to have an extremely low margin positivity rate, ranging from 0% to 7.7% (Table 1). In the 5 largest series (n ≥ 40) the margin positivity ranged from 2% to 4.2% [17, 19-22]. More importantly, in the short-term oncological outcomes reported in the contemporary series reviewed only one recurrence was reported of the 577 tumors represented (Table 1). Further long-term follow-up is required to ensure that this oncologic control is maintained over time, but preliminary results are promising. In those studies comparing RAPN and LPN, no study reported a statistically significant difference in margin positivity rates between the two modalities.

Complications

The intraoperative and postoperative complication rates for RAPN appear to be low and comparable to those of LPN. The most common complications reported in contemporary series include cardiopulmonary and thromboembolic complications as well as anemia requiring transfusion and urine leak (Table 1). Patel *et al.* showed that even when managing larger renal mass with RAPN there is not an increase in the complication rate, intraoperative or postoperative [22]. However, the only two urine leaks reported in their series were both in the larger renal mass group. Whether a tumor is exophytic, mesophytic, or endophytic would be expected to correlate with urine leak rates although this was not evaluated in the series reviewed. Need for conversion is another intraoperative complication that several of the series discussed. The need to convert from a robotic approach to either a laparoscopic or open approach was attributed to the learning curve in many instances. Indications for conversion included bleeding after removal of vascular clamps, robotic malfunction, inability to visualize a clear margin, positive margin on frozen section, and adherent fat to surface of the tumor.

Cost

Although no formal cost analysis comparing RAPN and LPN has been performed to date, studies evaluating the cost of OPN to LPN have been reported. In three separate studies, LPN was shown to be financially advantageous to OPN [25-27]. The increased intraoperative costs that LPN incurs are more than compensated by the decreased postoperative and in-hospital costs associated with the increased LOS of OPN. In addition, a financial analysis of open versus laparoscopic radical nephrectomy and nephroureterectomy performed by Meraney *et al* showed the minimally invasive approach to be less expensive with increased operator experience and efficiency [28]. Although it can be speculated that RAPN will be significantly more costly than LPN due to the increased financial investment with the robotic platform as well as the recurring costs of system maintenance and instrumentation, it is yet to be determined if this holds true in formal analysis.

Conclusion

The role of robotic surgery in the field of urology continues to expand. Its use in nephron-sparing surgery for localized renal masses has grown considerably since its first description by Stifelman *et al.* in 2005 [29]. Since that time, an increasing number of centers have reported their experiences and outcomes with RAPN. It is evident that RAPN is a safe and feasible minimally invasive approach to management of renal masses in experienced hands. More importantly, the oncologic outcomes appear equivalent to the gold-standard minimally invasive approach of LPN. The technical advantages that robotics provides in comparison to conventional laparoscopy may allow surgeons with limited laparoscopic experience to perform a partial nephrectomy via a minimally invasive approach safely and efficiently. Longer-term follow-up is required to better evaluate the functional and oncologic outcomes over time. In addition, further studies investigating the cost-effectiveness of a robotic approach to partial nephrectomy are warranted.

References

[1]   Chow WH, Devesa SS, Warren JL, et al. Rising incidence of renal cell cancer in the United States. *JAMA*, 1999; 281: 1628-1631.

[2]   Jemal A, Siegel R, Ward E, et al. Cancer Statisitics, 2008. *CA Cancer J Clin*, 2008; 58(2): 71-96.

[3]   McDougall EM, Clayman RV, Chandhoke PS, et al. Laparoscopic partial nephrectomy in the pig model. *J Urol*, 1993; 149(6): 1633-1636.

[4]   Gill IS, Kavoussi LR, Lane BR, et al. Comparison of 1,800 laparoscopic and open partial nephrectomies for single renal tumors. *J Urol*, 2007; 178(1): 41-46.

[5]   Rogers CG, Metwalli A, Blatt AM, et al. Robotic partial nephrectomy for renal hilar tumors: a multi-institutional analysis. *J Urol*, 2008; 180: 2353-2356.

[6]   FrankI, Blute ML, Cheville JC, et al. Solid renal tumors: an analysis of pathological features related to tumor size. *J Urol*, 2003; 170: 2217–2220.

[7]   Wrught JL, Porter JR. Laparoscopic partial nephrectomy: comparison of transperitoneal and retroperitoneal approaches. *J Urol,* 2005; 174(3): 841-845.

[8]   Rogers CG, Laungani R, Bhandari A, et al. Maximizing console surgeon independence during robot-assisted renal surgery by using the Fourth Arm and TilePro. *J Endourol,* 2009; 23(1): 115-12.

[9]   Fergany AF, Hafez KS, Novick AC. Long-term results of nephron sparing surgery for localized renal cell carcinoma: 10-year followup. *J Urol*, 2000; 163(2): 442-445.

[10] Uzzo RG, Novick AC. Nephron sparing surgery for renal tumors: indications, techniques and outcomes. *J Urol,* 2001; 166: 6-18

[11] Shapiro E, Benway BM, Wang AJ, et al. The role of nephron-sparing robotic surgery in the management of renal malignancy. *Curr Opin Urology,* 2009; 19(1): 76-80.

[12] Gettman MT, Blute ML, Chow GK et al. Robotic-assisted laparoscopic partial nephrectomy: technique and initial clinical experience with da Vinci robotic system. *Urology,* 2004; 64: 914–918.

[13] Phillips CK, Taneja SS, Stifelman MD. Robotic-assisted laparoscopic partial nephrectomy: the NYU technique. *J Endourol,* 2005; 19: 441–446.

[14] Aron M, Koenig P, Kaouk JH, et al. Robotic and laparoscopic partial nephrectomy: a matched-pair comparison from a high-volume center. *BJU Int,* 2008; 102: 86–92.

[15] Rogers CG, Singh A, Blatt AM, et al. Robotic partial nephrectomy for complex renal tumors: surgical technique. *Eur Urol,* 2008; 53: 514–523.

[16] Bhayani SB, Das N. Robotic-assisted laparoscopic partial nephrectomy for suspected renal cell carcinoma: retrospective review of surgical outcomes of 35 cases. *BMC Surg,* 2008 ; 8: 16.

[17] Deane LA, Lee HJ, Box GN, et al. Robotic versus standard laparoscopic partial/wedge nephrectomy: a comparison of intraoperative and perioperative results from a single institution. *J Endourol,* 2008; 22: 947–952.

[18] Benway BM, Bhayani SB, Rogers CG, et al. Robot assisted partial nephrectomy versus laparoscopic partial nephrectomy for renal tumors: a multi-institutional analysis of perioperative outcomes. *J Urol,* 2009; 182: 866-873.

[19] Jeong W, Park SY, Lorenzo EI, et al. Laparoscopic partial nephrectomy versus robotic-assisted laparoscopic partial nephrectomy. *J Endourol,* 2009; 23(9) 1457-1460.

[20] Rogers CG, Menon M, Weise ES, et al. Robotic partial nephrectomy: a multi-institutional analysis. *J Robotic Surg,* 2008; 2: 141–143.

[21] Wang AJ, Bhayani SB. Robotic partial nephrectomy versus laparoscopic partial nephrectomy for renal cell carcinoma: single surgeon analysis of >100 consecutive procedures. *Urology,* 2008; 73(2): 306-310.

[22] Benway BM, Wang AJ, Cabello JM, et al. Robotic partial nephrectomy with sliding-clip renorrhaphy: technique and outcomes. *Eur Urol,* 2009; 55: 592-599.

[23] 22. Patel MN, Krane LS, Bhandari A, et al. Robotic partial nephrectomy for renal tumors larger than 4cm. *Eur Urol,* 2010; 57: 310-316.Devarajan, P. Review: Neutrophil gelatinase-associated lipocalin: A troponin-like biomarker for human acute kidney injury. *Nephrology,* 2010; 15: 419-428.

[24] Porpiglia F, Volpe A, Billia M, et al. Laparoscopic versus open partial nephrectomy: analysis of the current literature. *Eur Urol,* 2008; 53(4): 732-742.

[25] Link RE, Bhayani SB, Allaf ME, et al. Exploring the learning curve, pathological outcomes and perioperative morbidity of laparoscopic partial nephrectomy performed for renal mass. *J Urol, 2005*; 173: 1690-1694.

[26] Lotan Y, Cadeddu JA. A cost comparison of nephron-sparing surgical techniques for renal tumor. *BJU Int,* 2005; 95: 1039-1042.

[27] Park S, Pearle MS, Cadeddu JA, et al. Laparoscopic and open partial nephrectomy: cost comparison with analysis of individual parameters. *J Endourol,* 2007; 21: 1449-1454.

[28] Meraney AM, Gill IS. Financial analysis of open versus laparoscopic radical nephrectomy and nephroureterectomy. *J Urol,* 2002; 167:1757-1762.

[29] Stifelman MD, Caruso RP, Nieder AM, et al. Robot-assisted laparoscopic partial nephrectomy. *JSLS,* 2005; 9: 83-86.

In: Essentials and Updates in Urologic Oncology
Editor: Philippe E. Spiess

ISBN: 978-1-62081-494-9
© 2013 Nova Science Publishers, Inc.

Chapter XXXV

Robot-Assisted Radical Cystectomy –Technique and Results

Michael A. Poch, Rebecca L. O'Malley and Khurshid A Guru

Roswell Park Cancer Institute, Buffalo, New York, US

Abstract

The standard management of invasive, non-metastatic bladder cancer is radical cystectomy with pelvic lymph node dissection and reconstruction of the urinary tract. The open surgical approach has demonstrated its efficacy and effectiveness in the management of bladder cancer. Nevertheless, the procedure is still a challenge with a significant risk of increased blood loss and transfusion rate. Also, the convalescence rate is high with a significant rate of post-operative complications. The advent of minimally invasive surgery with laparoscopy and the introduction of robotic technology to assist laparoscopy lead many centers in America and Europe to explore the application of robotics in the management of bladder cancer. Patient selection and preparation of the patient for surgery are critical in the success of the procedure. Equally important is surgical expertise with the requirement of a well trained laparoscopic surgeon supported with an experienced team experienced dedicated to robotic surgery. A systematic approach to the surgery is critical in minimizing intra-operative complications and maximizing an optimal pelvic lymph node dissection. Recent large surgical series are reviewed and summarized.

Introduction

While radical cystectomy and pelvic lymph node dissection remains the gold standard for managing muscle invasive bladder cancer, over the past two decades there has been an increasing interest in approaching the surgery through a minimally invasive technique. The first case reports of laparoscopic radical cystectomy were described in early 1993 [1] and the development of robotic surgery allowed the first robot-assisted radical cystectomy to be performed in 2003 [2]. Robot-assisted radical cystectomy has since evolved over the past decade as an alternative to open radical cystectomy with the potential advantages of decreased blood loss, post operative pain and possible faster recovery of the bowel function.

Table 1.

Author	N	Urinary diversion	Age	Mean OR Time	EBL	Hosp LOS	Complications
Menon et al. 2003 [2]	17	Ileal conduit (3) Neobladder (14)	-	260 308	150	-	Re-exploration for postop bleed (1) Bilharziasis (13)
Beecken et al. 2003 [48]	1	Intracorporeal W neobladder	-	510	200	5	Nil
Yohannes et al. 2003 [49]	2	Ileal conduit	60	690	1118	6	Nil
Hemal et al. 2004 [50]	24	Ileal conduit (4) W pouch (16) T pouch (2) Double chimney (2)	-	290	200	-	Minimal blood loss and morbidity
Sala et al. 2006 [51]	1	Intracorporeal W neobladder	65	720	100	5	Nil
Rhee et al, 2006 [52]	7	Ileal conduit	60	638	479	11	57% Transfusion rate (4) Port site hematoma (1) Ileus (1)
Galich et al. 2006 [53]	13	Ileal conduit (6) Neobladder (5) Indiana pouch (2)	70	697	500	8	Enterovesical fistula + SBO (1) Abscess (1)
Abraham et al. 2007 [20]	14	Ileal conduit (14)	76.5	419	212	5.8	42.8% Transfusion rate 28% Complication rate: Ileus (2) Urine leak (1) MI (1) Incomplete transection of L obturator nerve
Lowentritt et al, 2008 [54]	5	Ileal conduit (4)	69.5	350	300	5	Initial open conversion for hypercapnea (1) not reported
Hemal et al. 2008 [50]	6	Ileal conduit (5) Neobladder (1)	56	330	200	9.2	Partial wound dehiscence secondary to infection (1), Blood loss of 1L requiring 2 units of blood transfusion (1)
Dasgupta et al 2008 [55]	30	Ileal conduit Studer pouch		405	200	11	Ileus, others previously reported in Murphy et al, 2008
Park et al. 200856	1	Ileal Conduit	59	340	600	-	-
Ng et al. 2009 [57]	83	Ileal conduit (47) Indiana pouch (10) Neobladder (26)	70.9	375	460	5.5	Cellulitis, dehiscence, renal failure, ureteral obstruction, urinary fistula/leak, FUO, PNA, UTI, abscess, pyelonephritis, ileus, fungal infn, SBO, C.diff colitis, GI bleed, hematemesis, EC fistula, arrhythmia, MI, transfusion (1), rash, dehydration, DVT, PE
Kasraeian et al. 2010 [58]	9	Neobladder	63	270	400	14	Urinoma (1), pyelonephritis (1), hematoma (1)
Pruthi et al. 2010 [24]	100	Ileal conduit (61) Neobladder (38) No diversion (1)	65.5	276	271	4.9	Major (8), minor (33)

Table 1. (Continued)

Author	N	Urinary diversion	Age	Mean OR Time	EBL	Hosp LOS	Complications
Josephson et al. 2010 [59]	58	Indiana pouch (16) Neobladder (42)	68	480	450	10	Mortality (1) major (4), minor (37)
Manoharan et al. 2010 [60]	14	Neobladder (14)	58	360	310	8.5	Nil
Kauffman et al. 2010 [30]	85	Cutaneous diversion (60) Neobladder (25)	73.5	360	400	-	-
Hayn et al. 2010 [61]	164	Ileal conduit (152) Neobladder (11) Continent cutaneous diversion (1)	68	158	568	-	Major (39), minor (66)

The approach is similar to that of the laparoscopic radical cystectomy with the benefits of improved range of motion of the endowrist and 3-dimensional vision. Table 1 summarizes RARC series reported in English literature.

Technique

The technique for robotic cystectomy was developed based on the principles of open surgery with modifications using the da Vinci Surgical System. Since initial reports of RARC by Menon and colleagues, the technique has evolved and has been reproduced in many centers. Herein the technique adopted in Roswell Park Cancer institute, is described.

Patient Selection

Due to decreased blood loss, opioid requirement and length of stay, as well as comparable intermediate term oncologic outcomes, RARC is a good option for most patients. [3,4] Patients with pulmonary status inadequate to tolerate prolonged Trendelenberg positioning and pneumoperitoneum are poor candidates for RARC. Those with clinical T3 and T4 disease should be carefully selected for RARC following consideration for neoadjuvant chemotherapy.[4] Morbidly obese patients and those who've undergone several prior abdominal surgeries can safely undergo RARC. Due to concerns for oncologic control and technical difficulty, surgeons should not choose these patients for RARC early in the learning curve. [5]

Preoperative Preparation

Extensive discussion and evaluation in order to determine which urinary diversion is preferable should be undertaken. All patients should be marked for a stoma (preferably in consultation with a stoma nurse) regardless of diversion chosen. In female patients, whether preservation of vaginal length and/or one ovary should be undertaken should also be discussed. Preoperative antibiotics are administered in compliance with the AUA best practice statement for twenty-four hours.[6] Deep vein thrombosis prophylaxis is administered via compression stockings for low risk patients and with the addition of 5,000 units of subcutaneous heparin for patients with increased risk factors for venous thromboembolism, according to institutional policy. A nasogastric tube is placed following general anesthesia and a foley is placed on the surgical field. The patient is placed supine on the padded operating room table with the legs in low lithotomy. Well-padded chest straps are used to secure the patient to the table in a crossing fashion. The arms are adducted, padded and secured beneath these straps.

Equipment

The following laparoscopic instruments are usually needed: 2 bowel graspers, 1 endoshears, 1 fan retractor, 1 suction irrigator, 1 needle driver, 1 hem-o-lok clip applier, 1 laparoscopic clip applier, Endo GIA with 2.5mm vascular load staples and one 15mm EndoCatch bag. Each of the following robotic instruments are usually used: 1 long tip grasper, 1 monopolar hook, 1 round tip scissor, 1 bipolar forceps, and 2 needle drivers. The robotic 0 deg and 30 deg lenses are used depending on anatomy. A "vaginal apple" is used to manipulate the vagina/uterus during dissection in female patients.

Port Placement

After Veress needle insufflation of pneumoperitoneum to 15 mm Hg, a supraumbilical 12 mm port is placed 2 cm above the umbilicus for the camera. Two 8 mm robotic ports are placed for the right and left robotic arms, just lateral to each rectus muscle 1-2 cm below the level of the camera port. A 12 mm right assistant's port is placed approximately 5 cm above the right anterior superior iliac spine in the anterior axillary line. A 5 mm port is placed midway between the robotic arm port and camera port approximately 2.5 cm above the camera port. This is used by the right-sided assistant for suction. On the left, an 8 mm port is positioned approximately 5 cm above the left anterior superior iliac spine for the insertion of the 4th robotic arm. After all ports are placed, the da Vinci robotic system is docked between the patient's abducted legs.

Surgical Technique

Initial view of the pelvis reveals relevant anatomic landmarks, including, the sigmoid colon to the left, the bladder in the midline, and the right ureter peristalsing and crossing over the pulsating iliac artery. The lateral paracolic spaces and any sigmoid attachments should be freed. The goal of early dissection is to develop and define avascular spaces, including the periureteric, lateral pelvic and anterio rectal spaces. Important structures are preserved as long as possible to serve as anatomic landmarks ensuring continued orientation in a dissection where tactile feedback is lacking.

Development of Periureteric Space

The posterior peritoneum overlying the ureter is incised. Peristalsis can easily be seen and aid in identification of the ureter as it crosses the bifurcation of the iliac arteries with the 10X magnification and three dimensional, high definition vision of the robotic interface. The periureteric space is developed as the ureter is isolated up to the ureterovesical junction, taking care to preserve the vascular periureteral tissue (Figure 1). Early clipping of the ureter is avoided at this point so that it may continue to serve as an anatomic landmark. The lateral pedicles are more easily identified with the distal ureters intact as is identification of the correct plane thus minimizing positive surgical margins.

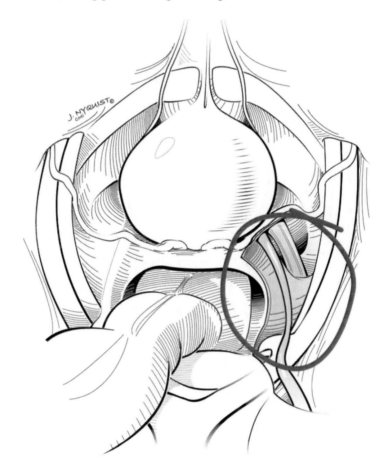

Figure 1. Peri-ureteric Space.

Lateral Pelvic Space

The lateral pelvic space can be developed on the ipsilateral side prior to or after development of the periureteric space on the contralateral side. The anterior rectal space should not be approached however until the lateral pelvic and periureteric spaces have been developed bilaterally. Incision of the posterior peritoneum is carried parallel and lateral to the umbilical ligament onto the anterior abdominal wall above the superior pubic ramus. Dissection continues along the avascular plane that follows the natural curve of the pelvic brim down to the vas deferens (Figure 2). The vas deferens is ligated lateral to the umbilical ligament to gain access to the lateral pelvic space. The bladder remains naturally anteriorly retracted because the urachus and space of Retzius have not yet been dissected. All tissue medial to the pelvic sidewall should be swept toward the bladder and taken with the specimen. Dissection continues toward the endopelvic fascia exposing the obturator vessels and nerve as they course toward the obturator canal as well as the inferior vascular pedicle. The periureteral and lateral pelvic spaces are separated by the ureters and the postero-lateral pedicle arising from the internal iliac vessels. The external iliac vessels and obturator nerve and vessels constitute the lateral borders of both spaces.

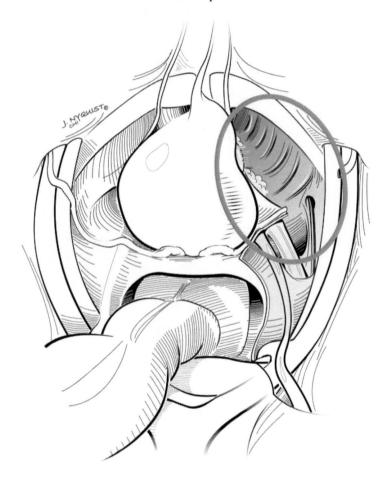

Figure 2. Lateral Pelvic Space.

Anterior Rectal Space

After development of the periureteral and lateral pelvic spaces bilaterally, the anterior rectal space is developed (Figure 3). The two lateral incisions in the posterior peritoneum are joined at the peritoneal reflection of the pouch of Douglas.

This space is then developed distally to the apex of the prostate in the place between the anterior sheath of Denonvillier's fascia and the rectum using blunt and sharp dissection with a cold, round-tip scissor.

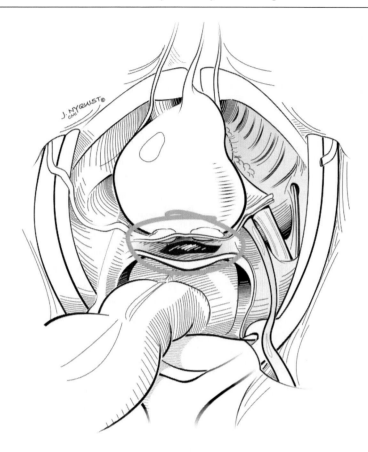

Figure 3. Anterior Rectal Space.

Control of Vascular Pedicles

After development of all three spaces, the vascular pedicles are easily visible juxtaposed to preserved anatomic landmarks. The bladder remains anteriorly suspended as mentioned and further manipulation with a Cobra grasper in the 4th arm provides exposure of the pedicles and ureters. The ureters are ligated close to the ureterovesical junction with hemo-lok clips. Ureteral margins are sent for frozen section analysis. The bladder and prostate pedicles are secured using either hemo-lok clips or an endovascular stapler. In advanced disease we advocate wide excision (non-nerve sparing) through use of the latter. The endopelvic fascia is opened bilaterally and the prostate is completely freed posteriorly. Nerve-sparing can be performed when indicated by releasing the lateral prostatic fascia during the posterior dissection.

Anterior Exposure and Apical Dissection

After completion of the posterior dissection the urachus and medial umbilical ligaments are divided to drop the bladder from the anterior abdominal wall. The superficial dorsal vein is located and ligated following removal of the retropubic fat. The dorsal venous complex is suture-ligated and divided. Any remaining attachments are dissected and the urethra is freed and incised. Frozen section of the urethral margin can be done at this time if orthotopic diversion is considered.

Specimen Removal

The specimen is placed in a large specimen bag brought in through a 15 mm port. The specimen is removed either through an incision made for extra-corporeal diversion or through extension of the supra-pubic port site in the case of intra-corporeal diversion. The pelvic cavity is irrigated with approximately one liter of sterile water and hemostasis is achieved.

Modifications in the Female Patient

Although bladder cancer is three times more common in men, an estimated 17, 700 new female cases and 4,300 female deaths are expected in 2010. [7] Some estimate the incidence in women to be growing out of proportion to the increase in tobacco use in women. [8] Anterior exenteration with or without vaginal, ovarian and/or urethral sparing maneuvers in select cases is the procedure of choice for muscle-invasive bladder cancer. Special considerations and modifications in technique in the female patient are discussed below.

The initial incision of the peritoneum is made overlying the ovarian pedicle which is ligated at this point revealing the ureter beneath. During development of the periureteric space, the plane between the bladder and vagina is developed through blunt separation of the loose areolar tissue, dissection with a cold round tip scissor and precise bipolar cauterization where necessary. The uterine artery isolated and preserved as it courses laterally and crosses anterior to the distal ureter.

As the lateral pelvic space is dissected, the round ligament is encountered and divided (instead of the vas deferens). Development of the pouch of Douglas and vaginal dissection is delayed until after the pedicles are taken because opening the vagina disrupts pneumoperitoneum. The uterine pedicle which was preserved earlier to aid in anatomic dissection is taken along with the bladder pedicles. A vaginal apple is placed in the vagina to facilitate identification of the proper planes and the fourth arm is used to retract the uterus anteriorly. The vagina is entered just distal to the cervix (or at the junction of the bladder and vagina if hysterectomy has been performed previously). The opening is extended anteriorly past the urethra to ensure en bloc removal of an anterior strip of vagina. In cases of vaginal preservation a plane is developed between the vaginal wall and the bladder. Urethrectomy is included in the vaginal dissection. For patients desirous of a neobladder (and without gross disease at the vesicourethral junction), the urethra is divided just distal to the bladder neck. If frozen section analysis of the urethral margin is negative for carcinoma the urethra is preserved.

The specimen is removed en bloc through the vaginal opening if large enough or placed in a specimen bag for removal following lymphadenectomy. The vaginal walls are reapproximated using a running 2-0 Vicryl suture incorporating closure of the urethral defect in cases of anterior exenteration.

Lymphadenectomy

Pelvic lymph node dissection is a crucial step in radical cystectomy. The goal should be removal of all nodal tissue included in a standard lymphadenectomy as outlined by the Mansoura experience and as is identical to open dissection. [9] The boundaries of standard lymphadenectomy are as follows: the mid common-iliac vessels – proximally; the genitofemoral nerve – laterally; the circumflex iliac vein and lymph node of Cloquet – distally; the hypogastric vessels – posteriorly. [10] It is preferable to aim for lymph node yields in excess of 20 which may be facilitated by sending several separate nodal packets. However, removing all tissue in an anatomic fashion is ultimately what is essential.

We prefer performing lymphadenectomy after cystectomy because there is more space to work and tissue planes are not disrupted prior to cystectomy. Pneumoperitoneum pressure may be reduced to 12 mm Hg to allow distention of the iliac veins. Dissection begins caudally and proceeds to the level of aortic bifurcation. Exposure and development of the triangle of Marcille allows separation of the major vessels from the pelvic sidewall thus facilitating maneuverability of the Endowrist. Cold scissor dissection with bipolar point cauterization are preferred for prevention of lymphocele and avoidance of vessel injury. Nodal packets are placed in specimen bags for retrieval to prevent port site recurrence. Aggressive sterile water irrigation is carried out and hemostasis again achieved.

Lymph Node Yield

The incidence of node positive disease at the time of cystectomy is in excess of 20%. [11] Based on the observed therapeutic and prognostic advantages, experts suggest removal of a minimum of 10-15 lymph nodes. [12,13] Adequacy of lymphadenectomy and number of nodes retrieved has been the subject of criticism of minimally invasive cystectomy. The extent of lymph node dissection reported in RARC series is similar to open series, i.e. either to the common iliac bifurcation (termed standard) or the inferior mesenteric artery (extended). Considering all RARC series with more than ten patients, lymph node yields are similar to open series (Table 2).

Table 2. All series with >10 pts and LNY

Series	No. cases	Type LND *	Mean or Median LN yield (range)	No. N+ (%)
Menon et al. (2003) [36]	17	S	12 (4-27)	1 (5.8)
Hemal et al (2004) [37]	24	E	NA (3-27)	1 (4.2)
Abraham et al. (2007) [20]	14	E	23.3 (15-31)	3 (21.4)
Wang et al. (2008) [14]	33	E	17 (6-32)	6 (18.2)
Murphy et al. (2008) [38]	23	S	16 (8-24)	2 (8.7)
Guru et al. (2008) [15]	67	E	18 (6-43)	17 (25.4)
Ng et al (2009) [21]	83	S	17.9 (7.5-28)	13 (15.7)
Pruthi et al. (2009) [62]	50	E	19 (8-37)	8 (16.0)
Nix et al. (2010) [16]_ENREF_16_ENREF_16	21	E	19 (12-30)	NA
Davis et al. (2011) [17]	11	E	43 (19-63)	1 (9.1)

In direct comparison, Wang and colleagues found no difference in the number of lymph nodes retrieved via RARC or ORC (20 vs 17). [14] Guru et al. reported the feasibility and safety of performing adequate robotic extended lymph node dissection where yields improved with increasing case volume. [15] A recent prospective, randomized, non-inferiority study by Nix et al demonstrated a mean lymph node yield of 19 in the RARC group vs. 18 in the ORC group. [16] Second look open lymphadenectomy by a different surgeon showed minimal additional yield (range 0 – 8) to the median 43 nodes removed by RARC. [17] Collaborative evaluation by the International Robotic Cystectomy Consortium (IRCC), consisting of many of the series in Table 2, has demonstrated a mean lymph node yield of 19 with high-volume centers (> 100 cases) having the highest yields and high surgeon volume (>50 cases) independently predicting extended (rather than standard) lymphadenectomy. [18]

The number of lymph nodes retrieved during lymphadenectomy depends on the number of nodes present in a given patient (which may vary), the manner in which the nodes are submitted for evaluation (en bloc or separately), and the pathologic processing technique. Therefore, we advocate thorough anatomical dissection around the pelvic vessels and complete clearance of all nodal tissue within the anatomical boundaries previously discussed rather than dictating dissection by nodal number.

Surgical Margins

The 3-dimensional, high definition, magnified vision of the robotic interface allows for surgical precision in excising localized disease and sparing nerves in select cases of cystectomy. However, the lack of tactile feedback has created concerns about adequacy of excision in advanced disease and positive surgical margin (PSM) rates. PSMs in bladder cancer are associated with high local recurrence and resulting poor overall survival. [11,19] Expert consensus thus recommends < 10% of all cases and < 15% for bulky tumors as acceptable PSM rates in radical cystectomy. [13]

In RARC series PSMs are reported only in patients with advanced pathologic stage (≥pT3) and only in consecutive series. [20-22] In a prospective study of 54 patients (33 robotic and 21 open), Wang and colleagues reported 3 patients with PSMs in the ORC group and 2 patients in the RARC group. [14] Evaluation by the IRCC of 513 patients demonstrated an overall PSM rate of 6.8%. Advanced stage was independently associated with increased likelihood of a PSM while case number and institution volume were not. [23] These findings suggest that PSM is associated more likely with infiltration of the soft tissue boundaries of the bladder rather than surgical error. In patients with large volume tumors and/or suspected extravesical disease, wide dissection of the perivesical tissue is recommended to reduce PSM rates. [22]

Oncologic Outcomes

The long term oncologic efficacy of RARC has yet to be determined however, surrogate markers of oncologic outcomes which include margin status and lymph node yield have been described earlier in this text. Similar to laparoscopic radical cystectomy early studies of RARC suffer from selection bias including younger patients, lower stage and fewer comorbidities than most contemporary open series. [24-26] That selection bias makes interpretation of oncologic outcomes difficult.

Previous open series have reported that patients who experience recurrence after cystectomy do so at a median of 12 months. [27] Martin et al described short term survival of 59 patients undergoing RARC.[28] Patients had at least 6 months follow up with mean follow up of 25 months. Clinical characteristics of these patients appear to be similar to that of open series with 27% of patients having extravesical disease and 34% of patients having lymph node positive disease. [26] Overall survival at 12, 24 and 36 months was 82, 72% and 72%, respectively. Recurrence free survival was 82%, 72% and 72%, respectively. This is comparable to early results of modern open series studies. [27,29] Kaufmann et al. described early oncologic outcomes of 85 patients who under RRC. [30] Two year recurrence free survival, cancer –specific and overall survival rates were 74%, 85% and 79% respectively. These outcomes are similar to those described by Martin. Three patients (4%) in that series had a local recurrence. Recent reports from the International Robotic Cystectomy Consortium of 820 patients revealed overall survival rates 82% and 68% at 1 and 2 years, respectively. Thirty-seven percent (288) of those patients had extravesical disease and 26% (195) had positive lymph nodes. The retrospective nature of these studies with potential selection bias hamper direct comparisons at this time and further non-inferiority studies will need to be performed to evaluate oncologic outcomes.

Complications

Despite advancements in pre- and post-cystectomy patient care, ORC remains a morbid operation with complication rates of 26–64% and mortality rates of 1-7%. [31-34] Readmission rates are high with bowel related and urinary infectious complications being most common. [35] Since the first report of RARC by Menon in 2003 [36], > 500 operations have been performed worldwide. As RARC experience grows, the hope is that the morbidity of cystectomy will be reduced. Estimated blood loss (EBL) reported in robotic series ranges from 100–1100 ml, with most series reporting a mean of <500 ml and transfusion rates below 2%. Reported complication rates following RARC are similar to ORC at 6-65%. [14,15,20, 21,36-40] Two small prospective comparisons of ORC and RARC cases showed similar complication rates between the approaches. [14,16] In a prospective comparison of complication rates in 187 consecutive patients who underwent ORC or RARC, the RARC group experienced significantly fewer total complications and major complications at 30 and 90 days. [21] Moreover, RARC was an independent predictor of fewer total and major complications.

Regardless, published series are limited in patient number and long term follow-up. Reporting of complications following cystectomy is also limited by patient selection bias, possible under-reporting and non-standardized documentation. [41] In an attempt to overcome these biases, we have reported complications on 156 consecutive (non-selected) patients who have undergone RARC at our institution using the standardized Memorial Sloan Kettering methodology and fulfilling the Martin criteria for adequate reporting of adverse events following surgery. [33,42] The 90-day complication rate of 52% and overall complication rate 65% at a median follow-up of 9 months are similar to open series. [40] The 90-day complication-related mortality rate was low at 2.6% and the majority of complications were low grade (63%).

Careful reporting of complications following RARC thus revealed rates similar to ORC, but the rates in RARC are not yet well supported by a large base of literature or level 1 evidence.

Quality of Life

Health related quality of life (HRQoL) outcomes after surgery remain an important consideration for patients and should not be neglected in treatment decisions. Studies investigating health related quality of life (HRQoL) in patients undergoing radical cystectomy and urinary diversion are increasing but are still lacking. [43] Many of the studies are retrospective or cross sectional by design, do not use validated questionnaires, and lack a baseline or preoperative assessment.

The most common tools used to asses HRQoL in bladder cancer patients in previous studies are the FACT-BL, FACT-VCI andEORTC QLQ-BLM30. More recently Gilbert et al. evaluated HRQoL outcomes for patients with bladder cancer using the Bladder Cancer Index (BCI) in 315 patients. [44] Similar to the FACT-VCI, the BCI addresses general post-operative HRQoL measures but also address cystectomy specific outcomes including stomal care and leakage. In that series, patients undergoing open radical cystectomy had lower sexual function scores than patients who kept their native bladder. The difference urinary and bowel domains between cystectomy and non-cystectomy patients differed by type of urinary diversion, ileal conduit or neobladder.

As RARC is an emerging technique, there is a paucity of literature evaluating HRLQoL after surgery. Yuh et al. prospectively evaluated short term HRQoL outcomes after RARC and ileal conduit diversion using the FACT-BL questionnaire. [45] The FACT-BL questionnaire includes 5 domains: well-being, physical, social/family, emotional, and functional as well as 12 additional bladder cancer specific questions. 34 patients were included in the study with follow up questionnaires at 1, 3 and 6 month postoperative time periods. Scores decreased significantly at the initial period with improvement to baseline at the 6 months. Emotional domains improved almost immediately after surgery and exceeded baseline scores at 6 months. It is important to keep in mind that much of the long term morbidity of radical cystectomy is associated with urinary diversion not extirpation. There is currently not enough evidence to support one diversion type over another. [46,47] Further studies evaluating the effect of robot-assisted urinary diversion and associated HRQoL are currently underway.

References

[1]   Sanchez de Badajoz E, Gallego Perales JL, Reche Rosado A, Gutierrez de la Cruz JM, Jimenez Garrido A. Laparoscopic cystectomy and ileal conduit: case report. *J. Endourol.* Feb 1995;9(1):59-62.

[2]   Menon M, Hemal AK, Tewari A, et al. Nerve-sparing robot-assisted radical cystoprostatectomy and urinary diversion. *BJU Int.* Aug 2003;92(3):232-236.

[3]   Chade DC, Laudone VP, Bochner BH, Parra RO. Oncological Outcomes After Radical Cystectomy for Bladder Cancer: Open Versus Minimally Invasive Approaches. *The Journal of Urology.* 2010;183(3):862-870.

[4]   Davis JW, Castle EP, Pruthi RS, Ornstein DK, Guru KA. Robot-assisted radical cystectomy: An expert panel review of the current status and future direction. *Urologic Oncology: Seminars and Original Investigations.* 2010;28(5):480-486.

[5]   Hayn MH, Hussain A, Mansour AM, et al. The learning curve of robot-assisted radical cystectomy: results from the International Robotic Cystectomy Consortium. *Eur Urol.* Aug 2010;58(2):197-202.

[6]   Bhanot N, Sahud AG, Sepkowitz D. Best practice policy statement on urologic surgery antimicrobial prophylaxis. *Urology.* Jul 2009;74(1):236-237.

[7]   Jemal A, Siegel R, Xu J, Ward E. Cancer statistics, 2010. *CA Cancer J Clin.* Sep-Oct 2010;60(5):277-300.

[8]   Malkowicz SB, van Poppel H, Mickisch G, et al. Muscle-Invasive Urothelial Carcinoma of the Bladder. *Urology.* 2007;69(1):3-16.

[9]   Ghoneim MA, Abdel-Latif M, El-Mekresh M, et al. Radical Cystectomy for Carcinoma of the Bladder: 2,720 Consecutive Cases 5 Years Later. *The Journal of Urology.* 2008;180(1):121-127.

[10] Mansour AM, Marshall SJ, Arnone ED, et al. Status of robot-assisted radical cystectomy. *Can J Urol.* Feb 2010;17(1):5002-5011.

[11] Herr HW. Surgical Factors Influence Bladder Cancer Outcomes: A Cooperative Group Report. *J. Clin. Oncol.* 2004;22(14):2781-2789.

[12] Stein JP, Cai J, Groshen S, Skinner DG. Risk factors for patients with pelvic lymph node metastases following radical cystectomy with en bloc pelvic lymphadenectomy: concept of lymph node density. *J. Urol.* Jul 2003;170(1):35-41.

[13] Herr H, Lee C, Chang S, Lerner S. Standardization of radical cystectomy and pelvic lymph node dissection for bladder cancer: a collaborative group report. *J. Urol.* May 2004;171(5):1823-1828; discussion 1827-1828.

[14] Wang GJ, Barocas DA, Raman JD, Scherr DS. Robotic vs open radical cystectomy: prospective comparison of perioperative outcomes and pathological measures of early oncological efficacy. *BJU Int.* 2007;0(0):070921231855002-???

[15] Guru KA, Sternberg K, Wilding GE, et al. The lymph node yield during robot-assisted radical cystectomy. *BJU Int.* Jul 2008;102(2):231-234; discussion 234.

[16] Nix J, Smith A, Kurpad R, Nielsen ME, Wallen EM, Pruthi RS. Prospective Randomized Controlled Trial of Robotic versus Open Radical Cystectomy for Bladder Cancer: Perioperative and Pathologic Results☆. *Eur. Urol.* 2010;57(2):196-201.

[17] Davis JW, Gaston K, Anderson R, et al. Robot assisted extended pelvic lymphadenectomy at radical cystectomy: lymph node yield compared with second look open dissection. *J. Urol.* Jan 2011;185(1):79-83.

[18] Marshall SJ, Hayn MH, Stegemann AP, Argawal PK, Badani KK, Balbay MD. Lymph node yield and predictors of extended lymphadenectomy at the time of robot-assisted radical cystectomy: Results from the International Robotic Cystectomy Consortium. *Presented at the American Urologic Association annual meeting, 2011.*Abstract #1103945.

[19] Dotan ZA, Kavanagh K, Yossepowitch O, et al. Positive surgical margins in soft tissue following radical cystectomy for bladder cancer and cancer specific survival. *J. Urol.* Dec 2007;178(6):2308-2312; discussion 2313.

[20] Abraham JB, Young JL, Box GN, Lee HJ, Deane LA, Ornstein DK. Comparative analysis of laparoscopic and robot-assisted radical cystectomy with ileal conduit urinary diversion. *J. Endourol.* Dec 2007;21(12):1473-1480.

[21] Ng CK, Kauffman EC, Lee MM, et al. A comparison of postoperative complications in open versus robotic cystectomy. *Eur. Urol.* Feb 2010;57(2):274-281.

[22] Yuh B, Padalino J, Butt ZM, et al. Impact of tumour volume on surgical and patho-
      logical outcomes after robot-assisted radical cystectomy. *BJU Int.* Sep
      2008;102(7):840-843.

[23] Hellenthal NJ, Hussain A, Andrews PE, et al. Surgical Margin Status After Robot
      Assisted Radical Cystectomy: Results From the International Robotic Cystectomy
      Consortium. *The Journal of Urology.* 2010;184(1):87-91.

[24] Pruthi RS, Nielsen ME, Nix J, Smith A, Schultz H, Wallen EM. Robotic radical
      cystectomy for bladder cancer: surgical and pathological outcomes in 100 consecutive
      cases. *J. Urol.* Feb 2010;183(2):510-514.

[25] Cha EK, Wiklund NP, Scherr DS. Recent advances in robot-assisted radical
      cystectomy. *Curr. Opin. Urol.* Jan 2011;21(1):65-70.

[26] Hautmann RE. The oncologic results of laparoscopic radical cystectomy are not (yet)
      equivalent to open cystectomy. *Curr. Opin. Urol.* Sep 2009;19(5):522-526.

[27] Stein JP, Lieskovsky G, Cote R, et al. Radical cystectomy in the treatment of invasive
      bladder cancer: long-term results in 1,054 patients. *J. Clin. Oncol.* Feb 1
      2001;19(3):666-675.

[28] Martin AD, Nunez RN, Pacelli A, et al. Robot-assisted radical cystectomy: intermediate
      survival results at a mean follow-up of 25 months. *BJU Int.* Jun 2010;105(12):1706-
      1709.

[29] Stein JP, Skinner DG. Results with radical cystectomy for treating bladder cancer: a
      'reference standard' for high-grade, invasive bladder cancer. *BJU Int.* Jul 2003;92(1):12-
      17.

[30] Kauffman EC, Ng CK, Lee MM, Otto BJ, Wang GJ, Scherr DS. Early oncologic
      outcomes for bladder urothelial carcinoma patients treated with robotic-assisted radical
      cystectomy. *BJU Int.* Sep 30 2010.

[31] Chang SS, Cookson MS, Baumgartner RG, Wells N, Smith JA, Jr. Analysis of early
      complications after radical cystectomy: results of a collaborative care pathway. *J Urol.*
      May 2002;167(5):2012-2016.

[32] Quek ML, Stein JP, Daneshmand S, et al. A critical analysis of perioperative mortality
      from radical cystectomy. *J. Urol.* Mar 2006;175(3 Pt 1):886-889; discussion 889-890.

[33] Shabsigh A, Korets R, Vora KC, et al. Defining early morbidity of radical cystectomy
      for patients with bladder cancer using a standardized reporting methodology. *Eur. Urol.*
      Jan 2009;55(1):164-174.

[34] Novara G, De Marco V, Aragona M, et al. Complications and mortality after radical
      cystectomy for bladder transitional cell cancer. *J. Urol.* Sep 2009;182(3):914-921.

[35] Stimson CJ, Chang SS, Barocas DA, et al. Early and Late Perioperative Outcomes
      Following Radical Cystectomy: 90-Day Readmissions, Morbidity and Mortality in a
      Contemporary Series. *The Journal of Urology.* 2010;184(4):1296-1300.

[36] Menon M, Hemal AK, Tewari A, et al. Nerve-sparing robot-assisted radical
      cystoprostatectomy and urinary diversion. *BJU Int.* Aug 2003;92(3):232-236.

[37] Hemal AK, Abol-Enein H, Tewari A, et al. Robotic radical cystectomy and urinary
      diversion in the management of bladder cancer. *Urol. Clin. North Am.* Nov
      2004;31(4):719-729, viii.

[38] Murphy DG, Challacombe BJ, Elhage O, et al. Robotic-assisted laparoscopic radical
      cystectomy with extracorporeal urinary diversion: initial experience. *Eur. Urol.* Sep
      2008;54(3):570-580.

[39] Pruthi RS, Wallen EM. Is robotic radical cystectomy an appropriate treatment for bladder cancer? Short-term oncologic and clinical follow-up in 50 consecutive patients. *Urology.* Sep 2008;72(3):617-620; discussion 620-612.

[40] Hayn MH, Hellenthal NJ, Hussain A, Stegemann AP, Guru KA. Defining Morbidity of Robot-Assisted Radical Cystectomy Using a Standardized Reporting Methodology. *Eur. Urol.* 2011;59(2):213-218.

[41] Donat SM. Standards for surgical complication reporting in urologic oncology: time for a change. *Urology.* Feb 2007;69(2):221-225.

[42] Martin RC, 2nd, Brennan MF, Jaques DP. Quality of complication reporting in the surgical literature. *Ann. Surg.* Jun 2002;235(6):803-813.

[43] Porter MP, Penson DF. Health related quality of life after radical cystectomy and urinary diversion for bladder cancer: a systematic review and critical analysis of the literature. *J. Urol.* Apr 2005;173(4):1318-1322.

[44] Gilbert SM, Wood DP, Dunn RL, et al. Measuring health-related quality of life outcomes in bladder cancer patients using the Bladder Cancer Index (BCI). *Cancer.* May 1 2007;109(9):1756-1762.

[45] Yuh B, Butt Z, Fazili A, et al. Short-term quality-of-life assessed after robot-assisted radical cystectomy: a prospective analysis. *BJU Int.* Mar 2009;103(6):800-804.

[46] Evans B, Montie JE, Gilbert SM. Incontinent or continent urinary diversion: how to make the right choice. *Curr. Opin. Urol.* Sep 2010;20(5):421-425.

[47] Lee CT, Latini DM. Urinary diversion: evidence-based outcomes assessment and integration into patient decision-making. *BJU Int.* Nov 2008;102(9 Pt B):1326-1333.

[48] Beecken WD, Wolfram M, Engl T, et al. Robotic-assisted laparoscopic radical cystectomy and intra-abdominal formation of an orthotopic ileal neobladder. *Eur. Urol.* Sep 2003;44(3):337-339.

[49] Yohannes P, Puri V, Yi B, Khan AK, Sudan R. Laparoscopy-assisted robotic radical cystoprostatectomy with ileal conduit urinary diversion for muscle-invasive bladder cancer: initial two cases. *J. Endourol.* Nov 2003;17(9):729-732.

[50] Hemal AK, Abol-Enein H, Tewari A, et al. Robotic radical cystectomy and urinary diversion in the management of bladder cancer. *Urol. Clin. North Am.* Nov 2004;31(4):719-729, viii.

[51] Sala LG, Matsunaga GS, Corica FA, Ornstein DK. Robot-assisted laparoscopic radical cystoprostatectomy and totally intracorporeal ileal neobladder. *J. Endourol.* Apr 2006;20(4):233-235; discussion 236.

[52] Rhee JJ, Lebeau S, Smolkin M, Theodorescu D. Radical cystectomy with ileal conduit diversion: early prospective evaluation of the impact of robotic assistance. *BJU Int.* Nov 2006;98(5):1059-1063.

[53] Galich A, Sterrett S, Nazemi T, Pohlman G, Smith L, Balaji KC. Comparative analysis of early perioperative outcomes following radical cystectomy by either the robotic or open method. *JSLS.* Apr-Jun 2006;10(2):145-150.

[54] Lowentritt BH, Castle EP, Woods M, Davis R, Thomas R. Robot-assisted radical cystectomy in women: technique and initial experience. *J. Endourol.* Apr 2008;22(4):709-712.

[55] Dasgupta P, Rimington P, Murphy D, et al. Robotic assisted radical cystectomy: short to medium-term oncologic and functional outcomes. *Int. J. Clin. Pract.* Nov 2008;62(11):1709-1714.

[56] Park SY, Cho KS, Ham WS, Choi HM, Hong SJ, Rha KH. Robot-assisted laparoscopic radical cystoprostatectomy with ileal conduit urinary diversion: initial experience in Korea. *J. Laparoendosc. Adv. Surg. Tech. A.* Jun 2008;18(3):401-404.

[57] Ng CK, Kauffman EC, Lee MM, et al. A comparison of postoperative complications in open versus robotic cystectomy. *Eur. Urol.* Feb 2010;57(2):274-281.

[58] Kasraeian A, Barret E, Cathelineau X, et al. Robot-assisted laparoscopic cystoprostatectomy with extended pelvic lymphadenectomy, extracorporeal enterocystoplasty, and intracorporeal enterourethral anastomosis: initial Montsouris experience. *J. Endourol.* Mar 2010;24(3):409-413.

[59] Josephson DY, Chen JA, Chan KG, Lau CS, Nelson RA, Wilson TG. Robotic-assisted laparoscopic radical cystoprostatectomy and extracorporeal continent urinary diversion: highlight of surgical techniques and outcomes. *Int J Med Robot.* Sep 2010;6(3):315-323.

[60] Manoharan M, Katkoori D, Kishore TA, Antebie E. Robotic-assisted Radical Cystectomy and Orthotopic Ileal Neobladder Using a Modified Pfannenstiel Incision. *Urology.* Aug 4 2010.

[61] Hayn MH, Hellenthal NJ, Seixas-Mikelus SA, et al. Is patient outcome compromised during the initial experience with robot-assisted radical cystectomy? Results of 164 consecutive cases. *BJU Int.* Dec 16 2010.

[62] Pruthi RS, Stefaniak H, Hubbard JS, Wallen EM. Robotic anterior pelvic exenteration for bladder cancer in the female: outcomes and comparisons to their male counterparts. *J. Laparoendosc. Adv. Surg. Tech. A.* Feb 2009;19(1):23-27.

In: Essentials and Updates in Urologic Oncology
Editor: Philippe E. Spiess

ISBN: 978-1-62081-494-9
© 2013 Nova Science Publishers, Inc.

Chapter XXXVI

Robotic Retroperitoneal Lymph Node Dissection for Testis Cancer

Sandhya Rao and Julio Powsang

Moffitt Cancer Center, Department of Genitourinary Oncology
Tampa, Florida, US

Abstract

Testis cancer is rare accounting for only a small percentage of all cancers in men. However it is the most common solid malignancy in men 20 to 35 years of age and the incidence is increasing. Open retroperitoneal lymph node dissection (O-RPLND) remains the current standard when surgery is required for stage I non-seminomatous germ cell cancer or post-chemotherapy residual masses but is associated with significant morbidity and a lengthy convalescence. In a continued effort to reduce the morbidity of this procedure, minimally invasive techniques have been applied to the surgical management of testis cancer. Laparoscopic retroperitoneal lymph-node dissection (L-RPLND) was first reported in the early 90s and more recently, robotic technology (R-RPLND) incorporated to this very challenging surgical procedure. We discussed the surgical technique and recent series in the medical literature reporting their early outcomes with this procedure.

Introduction

Testis cancer is rare accounting for only a small percentage of all cancers in men. However it is the most common solid malignancy in men 20 to 35 years of age and the incidence is increasing. [1] The multimodal management of testis cancer has yielded impressive cure rates and the challenge now is to reduce treatment related morbidity without jeopardizing effectiveness. Open retroperitoneal lymph node dissection (O-RPLND) remains the current standard when surgery is required for stage I non-seminomatous germ cell cancer or post-chemotherapy residual masses but is associated with significant morbidity and a lengthy convalescence. [2] In a continued effort to reduce the morbidity of this procedure, minimally invasive techniques have been applied to the surgical management of testis cancer. Laparoscopic retroperitoneal lymph-node dissection (L-RPLND) was first reported in 1992 by Rukstalis and Chodak for a patient with Stage I testis cancer. [3] The technique has evolved over the years so that it now more readily duplicates open RPLND. [4,5] Over the years, the staging accuracy and low morbidity of L- RPLND have been well documented in different series and it is now considered a viable approach. [6,7,8,9] Currently, L-RPLND in the hands of dedicated experts is safe, with decreased postoperative morbidity, quicker convalescence, better cosmetic results, higher patient satisfaction and better QOL scores than open RPLND. [10-14] The procedure has demonstrated inferiority only in terms of increased operative time and overall costs. [15,16] Despite these demonstrated advantages, the long term therapeutic efficacy of L-RPLND is unknown as the majority of patients with positive nodes receive adjuvant chemotherapy. In a comprehensive review of the current status of L-RPLND, Finelli and Hamilton concluded that although LRPLND holds much future promise, a longer follow-up of the limited numbers of patients forgoing chemotherapy in the setting of positive lymph nodes needs to be conducted to assess the oncologic efficacy of L_RPLND. [17]. Despite its advantages, laparoscopic RPLND is a technically challenging and difficult procedure with a long and steep learning curve that can be undertaken only by very experienced laparoscopic surgeons at high volume centers. [18] More recently, robotic RPLND (R-RPLND) was demonstrated to be a feasible minimally invasive approach. Robotic RPLND was first reported by Davol et al in 2006 in an 18 year male with a clinical Stage I mixed germ cell tumor. [19] Subsequently, other groups have demonstrated robotic RPLND to be a safe and effective approach. Annerstedt et al reported robotic RPLND in three patients after chemotherapy for clinical stage II testicular cancer and Correa et al reported post chemotherapy robotic RPLND in a 27 year old man with Stage II NSGCT. [20,21] The six-degrees of freedom in movement, fine-scaling, and superb 3-D optics offered by the da Vinci system are of benefit during the meticulous dissection around the great vessels and viscera that is required during RPLND. Ahlering demonstrated that using a robotic interface, a laparoscopically naive yet well trained open surgeon can successfully transfer open surgical skills to a laparoscopic environment. [22]

Indications for Robotic RPLND in Testis Cancer

The indications for R-RPLND in low stage NSCGT are the same as those for O-RPLND or L-RPLND and include all men with high-risk testis cancer after orchiectomy and selected men with post-chemotherapy residual masses.

Low Stage Nonseminomatous Germ Cell Tumors (NSGCT)

There are three management options after radical orchidectomy for patients who have low stage NSGCT. These include primary retroperitoneal lymph node dissection RPLND,

[23] close surveillance with combination chemotherapy at relapse [24,25] or primary chemotherapy. [26,27] All three options result in excellent outcomes and differ only in treatment related morbidities and complications and the current recommendation for high-risk men is to consider chemotherapy instead of primary RPLND. Nevertheless, decision recommendations should be individualized depend on many factors including access to health care and patient compliance.

In the US, primary RPLND is the conventional therapeutic option for low stage NSGCT because of multiple factors which include its accuracy of pathological staging as compared to current imaging techniques, its curative potential in selective patients with microscopic lymph node metastases, the difficult rigor of surveillance protocols, and the toxicity of chemotherapy. [28,29]

Clinical Stage II Low Volume NSGCT

RPLND is also the preferred modality in lower volume clinical stage II NSGCT with normal postorchiectomy serum tumor markers, absence of tumor related back pain. unifocal retroperitoneal disease that is 3 cm in diameter or less, and confined to the region below the renal vessels and above the aortic bifurcation. [28] It is generally accepted that stage II bulky disease receives primary chemotherapy. [29] In most LRPLND series, stage II patients receive adjuvant chemotherapy consisting of two cycles of bleomycin, etoposide, and cisplatin.

Postchemotherapy

Post-chemotherapy RPLND is the indicated treatment for persistent radiographic masses in the retroperitoneum after chemotherapy, elevated tumor markers after chemotherapy in tumors which had clinically localized retroperitoneal disease, and persistent tumors after incomplete previous RPLND. [29] Post chemotherapy L-RPLND (PC-RPLND)for uni- or multifocal low-volume residual masses has been limited to a very few centers, due to significant perioperative morbidity and high conversion rates. The main limitation is the intense desmoplastic reaction. [30] Hemorrhage and vascular injury are the most commonly reported complications in PC-LRPLND. [31] However it has been shown to be technically feasible by the robotic approach. [20]

Templates for RPLND

In the past 30 years there has been a considerable modification of the traditional RPLND templates. Historically RPLND included bilateral suprahilar dissections with removal of all nodal tissue between the 2 ureters upto the common iliac bifurcation. This was replaced with bilateral infrahilar dissections to reduce surgical morbidity. The most consistent long tem morbidity is loss of antegrade ejaculation and therefore infertility. A better understanding of the neuroanatomy of seminal emission and the distribution of metastatic disease has led to modified RPLND templates and nerve sparing dissections.

Many templates have been proposed by different investigators both open and laparoscopic. European and South American L-RPLND centers [7,12,14,32,33[follow the template of Weissbach et al [34] including on the left side the upper preaortic, para-aortic nodes and on the right side the paracaval, precaval, interaortocaval upper preaortic and right iliac nodes. Left iliac and suprahilar nodes are not included. North American L-RPLND centers [6,35,36] follow the template proposed by Donohue and Foster [37] including on the left side the upper interaortocaval ,left para-aortic, and left iliac groups and on the right side the paracaval, precaval, interaortocaval and right iliac groups but not the preaortic group. The goal is to thoroughly resect all interaortocaval and ipsilateral nodes between the renal hilum superiorly and the common iliac inferiorly and to minimize contralateral dissections below the level of the IMA. Surgical margins should not be compromised to minimize morbidity, preserve ejaculation or due to technical constraints. [18] When positive nodes are found on frozen sections at the time of surgery, a complete bilateral RPLND to the inferior mesenteric artery should be performed.

The extent of dissection also varies among the various investigators depending upon the intent of laparoscopy. Some consider RPLND primarily to be a diagnostic procedure to confirm lymph-node involvement before delivering chemotherapy. Their templates are more restricted and they omit dissection dorsal to the great vessels. [7] Other investigators have changed from a diagnostic to therapeutic intent and perform a complete bilateral RPLND with dissection dorsal to the great vessels to duplicate the open technique. [4,18] The group from Innsbruck initially reported that laparoscopic RPLND for diagnostic purposes only and patients with node positive patients were treated with adjuvant chemotherapy. [9] However since 2004 they do not add chemotherapy in patients with positive nodes and a full bilateral template is cleared to exactly duplicate the field of an open RPLND. [18]

Surgical Technique

All procedures are performed with the patient in the flank position. A transperitoneal approach is used. A total of six ports are used. A 12-mm camera port is placed off the midline into the peritoneum to either the right or the left, depending on the required template and two robotic 8mm ports are placed lateral to the rectus muscle and approximately 10-cm caudad and cephalad to the first one. A 12 mm port is placed in the midline and approximately 5 cm cephalad to the umbilicus to be used by the assistant.

The robot is docked from the ipsilateral side with the robotic arms reaching over the turned flank. The assistant stands on the opposite side of the table, facing the patient.

The intra abdominal contents are inspected and the colon is mobilized on either side by incision along the line of Toldt. The retroperitoneum is fully exposed and a right, left, or full template dissection performed. For a right-sided dissection, the boundaries include the ipsilateral ureter laterally, the take-off of the renal vessels superiorly, and the bifurcation of the right common iliac artery inferiorly. Medially,the dissection is carried to the midpoint of the anterior aorta, above the take-off of the inferior mesenteric artery. For a left-sided dissection, the boundaries include the ipsilateral ureter laterally, the renal vessels superiorly, and the bifurcation of the left common iliac inferiorly. The Lymph node dissection should not extend below the take-off of the inferior mesentery artery but should extend medially to remove the interaortocaval lymph nodes above this anatomic landmark. In both sides, the gonadal vein is taken from its origin and dissected down to the internal ring where it can be taken out with the reminder of the stump of the specimen cord that was left at the time of the previous radical orchiectomy. The specimens are progressively retrieved in an entrapment bag throughout the dissection and sent for frozen section and lymph node count.

On either side the sympathetic chains and postganglionic fibers are identified and dissected free. The anterior aspect of the aorta below the take-off of the inferior mesenteric artery is not dissected to prevent damage to the superior hypogastric plexus. In post-chemotherapy cases, a full RPLND is performed.

Lymphocele formation is minimized clipping the lymphatic channels. At the completion of the lymph node dissection, the robot is un-docked. The anterior rectus fascia of the 12 mm trocar sites is closed with running 0-vycril and all incision sites with a sub-cuticular 4-0 monocryl.

A nasogastric tube is placed at the beginning of the procedure and removed at the end of surgery. A Foley catheter is left indwelling overnight. Patients are started on clear liquids the evening of the surgery and advanced to a full diet by the first postoperative day and are usually discharged the third post-operative day.

Technical Aspects and Results from Reported Cases

Davol et al reported the first case of robotic RPLND as a staging procedure in an 18 year old man with right sided mixed germ tumor, predominately mature teratoma with focal seminoma. [19] They used a total of 5 ports. A modified RPLND was planned but after identification of an enlarged lymph node anterior to the IVC the procedure was converted to a full bilateral RPLND sparing only the contralateral tissue below the inferior mesenteric artery. They noted that the robotic arms retracted the bowel away from the region of dissection so that the bilateral procedure was completed without repositioning the patient. There was minimal conflict between the robot arms. The total operating time was 235 minutes with the robot docked for 169 minutes. Five robotic instruments were used, including hook cautery, harmonic scalpel, Prograsp forceps, and scissors. Laparoscopic clip appliers and a suction irrigator were used through the assistant port. No intraoperative complications occurred; the blood loss was 125 mL. Final histopathology revealed metastatic teratoma in 2 of 21 lymph nodes with no seminoma detected. At five month of follow-up the patient remained disease free with preserved anterior ejaculation.

Annerstedt et al reported three cases of robotic RPLND following 4 cycles of BEP for clinical Stage II disease. [20] Two were right sided, one was left sided. The exact extent of lymphadenectomy is not described. Five ports were used and three robotic instruments including the Maryland bipolar forceps, monopolar scissors and the Prograsp forceps. A laparoscopic suction irrigator was used through the assistant port. In all patients they reported conflicts between the cranial robot arm and the cranial assistant port instruments.

Operative times were 144mins, 129 mins and 155 mins respectively for the three cases and blood loss was 30ml, 50ml and 50ml. There were no intraoperative complications. Final histopathology revealed 2, 1 and 6 benign lymph nodes in the three cases respectively.

Conclusions

The technical feasibility and safety of robotic RPLND in both primary and the post chemotherapy have been reported in recent series. The robotic approach has all the benefits of minimally invasive surgery with easy transition from an open experience to the robotic environment. The steep learning curve of laparoscopic RPLND is avoided. Robotic assisted surgery provides high definition vision with depth perception, wristed instrumentation, six degrees of freedom, intuitive finger controlled movements and an ergonomic position for the surgeon. Preliminary results support the concept that robotic RPLND provides results equivalent to the open approach. Further experience in larger series of patients with longer follow-up is required to determine the definitive role of robotics in men requiring a retroperineal lymph node dissection.

References

[1]   Huyghe E, Matsuda T, Thonneau P. Increasing incidence of testicular cancer worldwide: a review. *J Urol.* 2003 Jul;170(1):5-11. Review.

[2]   Foster RS, Donohue JP. Retroperitoneal lymph node dissection for the maagement of clinical stage I nonseminoma. *J Urol* 2000;163:1788–1792.

[3]   Rukstalis DB, Chodak GW. Laparoscopic retroperitoneal lymph node dissection in a patient with stage 1 testicular carcinoma. *J Urol.* 1992;148: 1907-1910.

[4]   Allaf ME, Bhayani SB, Link RE, Schaeffer EM, Varkarakis JM, Shadpour P, Lima G, Kavoussi LR. Laparoscopic retroperitoneal lymph node dissection: Duplication of open technique. *Urology* 2005;65:575–577.

[5]   Bhayani SB, Allaf ME, Kavoussi LR. Laparoscopic RPLND for clinical stage I nonseminomatous germ cell testicular cancer: Current status. *Urol Oncol* 2004;22:145–148.

[6]   Nielsen ME, Lima G, Schaeffer EM, Porter J, Cadeddu JA, Tuerk I, Kavoussi LR. Oncologic efficacy of laparoscopic RPLND in treatment of clinical stage I nonseminomatous germ cell testicular cancer. *Urology* 2007;70:1168–1172.

[7]   Albqami N, Janetschek G. Laparoscopic retroperitoneal lymph-node dissection in the management of clinical stage I and II testicular cancer. *J Endourol* 2005;19:683–692.

[8]   Bhayani SB, Ong A, Oh WK, Kantoff PW, Kavoussi LR. Laparoscopic retroperitoneal lymph node dissection for clinical stage I nonseminomatous germ cell testicular cancer: A long-term update. *Urology* 2003;62:324–327.

[9]   Janetschek G, Hobisch A, Holtl L, Bartsch G. Retroperitoneal lymphadenectomy for clinical stage I nonseminomatous testicular tumor: laparoscopy versus open surgery and impact of learning curve. *J Urol* 1996; 156 : 89–93

[10] Steiner H, Peschel R, Janetschek G, Ho¨ ltl L, Berger AP, Bartsch G, Hobisch A. Long-term results of laparoscopic retroperitoneal lymph node dissection: A single-center 10-year experience. *Urology* 2004;63:550–555.

[11] Skolarus TA, Bhayani SB, Chiang HC, Brandes SB, Kibel AS, Landman J, Figenshau RS. Laparoscopic retroperitoneal lymph node dissection for low-stage testicular cancer. *J Endourol* 2008;22;1485–1489.

[12] Neyer M, Peschel R, Akkad T, Springer-Sto¨hr B, Berger A, Bartsch G, Steiner H. Long-term results of laparoscopic retroperitoneal lymph-node dissection for clinical stage I nonseminomatous germ-cell testicular cancer. *J Endourol* 2007; 21:180–183.

[13] Hobisch A, Tönnemann J, Janetschek G. Morbidity and quality of life after open versus laparoscopic retroperitoneal lymphadenectomy for testicular tumour: The patient's view. In: Jones WG, Appleyard 1, Harnden P, Joffe JK (eds): *Germ Cell Tumours VI.* London: John Libbey, 1998, p 277.

[14] Poulakis V, Skriapas K, de Vries R, et al. Quality of life after laparoscopic and open retroperitoneal lymph node dissection in clinical stage I nonseminomatous germ cell tumor: a comparison study. *Urology* 2006;68:154–60.

[15] Ogan K, Lotan Y, Koeneman K, Pearle MS, Cadeddu JA, Rassweiler J. Laparoscopic versus open retroperitoneal lymph node dissection: A cost analysis. *J Urol* 2002; 168: 1945–1949.

[16] Rassweiler JJ, Scheitlin W, Heidenrich A, Laguna MP, Janetschek G. Laparoscopic retroperitoneal lymph node dissection: Does it still have a role in the management of clinical stage I nonseminomatous testis cancer? A European perspective. *Eur Urol* 2008;54:1004–1015.

[17] Hamilton RJ, Finelli A. Laparoscopic retroperitoneal lymph node dissection for nonseminomatous germ-cell tumors: Current status. *Urol Clin North Am* 2007;34:159–169.

[18] Steiner H, Peschel R, Bartsch G Laparoscopic retroperitoneal lymph node dissection: current concepts and limitations.. *BJU Int.* 2009 Nov;104(9 Pt B):1376-80. Review.

[19] Davol P, Sumfest J, Rukstalis D. Robotic-assisted laparoscopic retroperitoneal lymph node dissection. *Urology* 2006;67:199.

[20] Magnus Annerstedt · Sigurdur Gudjonsson · Björn Wullt · Bengt Uvelius Robot-assisted laparoscopic retroperitoneal lymph node dissection in clinical stage II testicular cancer. *J Robotic Surg* (2008) 2:189–191

[21] Jose Correa, Lucas Wiegand, Alexander Grieco, Tariq Hakky, Julio Pow-Sang Post chemotherapy robotic assisted retroperitoneal lymph node dissection.*J Urol* 2009;181:4,Suppl 1: 604.

[22] Ahlering TE, Skarecky D, Lee D, *et al:* Successful transfer of open surgical skills to a laparoscopic environment using a robotic interface: initial experience with laparoscopic radical prostatectomy. *J Urol* 170: 1738–1741, 2003.

[23] Donohue JP, Thornhill JA, Foster RS, Rowland RG, Bihrle R. Stage I nonseminomatous germ-cell testicular cancer – management options and risk-benefit considerations. *World J Urol* 1994;12:170–7

[24] Read G, Stenning SP, Cullen MH, et al. Medical Research Council prospective study of surveillance for stage I testicular teratoma. *J Clin Oncol* 1992;10:1762–8.

[25] Nicolai N, Pizzocaro G. A surveillance study of clinical stage I nonseminomatous germ cell tumors of the testis: 10-year followup. *J Urol* 1995;154:1045–9.

[26] Oliver RT, Raja MA, Ong J, Gallagher CJ. Pilot study to evaluate impact of a policy of adjuvant chemotherapy for high risk stage I malignant teratoma on overall relapse rate of stage I cancer patients. *J Urol* 1992;148:1453–6.

[27] Bohlen D, Borner M, Sonntag RW, Fey MF, Studer UE. Long-term results following adjuvant chemotherapy in patients with clinical stage I testicular nonseminomatous malignant germ cell tumors with high risk factors. *J Urol* 1999;161:1148–52.

[28] Stephenson AJ, Sheinfeld J The role of retroperitoneal lymph node dissection in the management of testicular cancer..*Urol Oncol.* 2004 May-Jun;22(3):225-33. Review

[29] Leisinger HJ, and Donohue JP: The role of retroperitoneal surgery in testis cancer. *Crit Rev Oncol Hematol* 44: 71–80, 2002.

[30] Rassweiler JJ, Seemann O, Henkel TO, Stock C, Frede T, Alken P. Laparoscopic retroperitoneal lymph node dissection for nonseminomatous germ cell tumors: Indications and limitations. *J Urol* 1996;156:1108–1113.

[31] Kenney PA, Tuerk IA. Complications of laparoscopic retroperitoneal lymph node dissection in testicular cancer.*World J Urol.* 2008 Dec;26(6):561-9. Epub 2008 Jul 2.

[32] Janetschek G, Reissigl A, Peschel R, Hobisch A, Bartsch G.Laparoscopic retro-peritoneal lymphadenectomy for clinical stage I nonseminmatous testicular tumor. *Urology* 1994;44:382–91.

[33] Corvin S, Kuczyk M, Anastasiadis A, Stenzl A. Laparoscopic retroperitoneal lymph node dissection for nonseminomous testicular carcinoma. *World J Urol* 2004;22: 33–6.

[34] Weissbach L, Boedefeld EA, Horstmann-Dubral B. Surgical treatment of stage-I non-seminomatous germ cell testis tumor. Final results of a prospectivemulticenter trial 1982– 1987. Testicular Tumor Study Group. *Eur Urol* 1990;17: 97–106.

[35] Nelson JB, Chen RN, Bishoff JT, et al. Laparoscopic retroperitoneal lymph node dissection for clinical stage I nonseminomatous germ cell testicular tumors. *Urology* 1999; 54:1064–7.

[36] Gerber GS, Bissada NK, Hulbert JC, et al. Laparoscopic retroperitoneal lymphadenec-tomy: a multi-institutional analysis. *J Urol* 1994;152:1188–92.

[37] Donohue JP, Foster RS. Retroperitoneal lymphadenectomy in staging and treatment. The development of nervesparing techniques. *Urol Clin N Amer* 1998;25:461–8.

Section 10. Geriatric Oncology

Lodovico Balducci
Section Editor

In: Essentials and Updates in Urologic Oncology
Editor: Philippe E. Spiess

ISBN: 978-1-62081-494-9
© 2013 Nova Science Publishers, Inc.

Chapter XXXVII

Fundaments of Geriatric Oncology

Lodovico Balducci

Moffitt Cancer Center, Department of Geriatric Oncology
Tampa, Florida, US

Abstract

Cancer is a disease of aging. The interactions of cancer and aging encompass biological and clinical factors which include: [1] age as a risk factor for carcinogenesis, [2] aging and tumor growth, and [3] benefit and risks of antineoplastic treatment in the older person.

Cancer is more common in older individuals for three essential reasons: duration of carcinogenesis, increased susceptibility to environmental carcinogens, and changes in the body environment that may favor cancer growth.

The prognosis of some tumors becomes more favorable (breast cancer), whereas that of other tumors (acute leukemia, lymphoma) worsen with increasing age.

In the management of an older person with cancer, the basic questions include: is the patient going to die of cancer or with cancer? Is the patient able to tolerate cancer treatment? Are there social and economic issues that prevent effective cancer treatment in the older aged person? The only validated instrument to answer these questions is a comprehensive geriatric assessment tool. Laboratory and functional markers of functional aging are undergoing current investigation.

Introduction

Cancer is a disease of aging [1[. It is currently estimated 50% of all malignancies occur in individuals 65 and over [1] and by the year 2030 older individuals will likely account 70% of afflicted patients with cancer. This increase is premised to result from our aging population, a phenomenon described as the "squaring of the pyramids." [2]. In 1900, the age-weighted profile of the US population looked like a pyramid with a large bottom of individuals under 20 years of age and a very small top of the pyramid representing those 65 years and older. By the year 2000, the base of the pyramid had become shorter and the top larger with the resulting age pyramid now appearing as a square. Both decreased mortality and decreased birth rate contributed to this change.

The issues of geriatric oncology are both biological and clinical. The questions include: why does cancer become more common with advanced age? Does the prognosis of cancer change with age? What are the benefits of cancer prevention and cancer treatment in the older aged person?

In this chapter, we will address in detail the clinical issues after a brief outline of the biological interfaces of cancer and age. In particular, we will discuss the definition and clinical assessment of aging and the influence of aging on cancer prevention and treatment.

Cancer and Age: Biological Issues

We will discuss separately the interaction of aging with carcinogenesis and tumor growth.

Carcinogenesis and Age

The association of cancer and age may be explained by three non-mutually exclusive mechanisms:

- Duration of carcinogenesis. This process may take decades and consequently cancer develops more frequently in older individuals. The changing epidemiology of lung cancer exemplifies this phenomenon. Currently, the median age of lung cancer patients at time of diagnosis is 71 years [3] up from the late fifties which we observed two decade ago. The increased incidence of lung cancer in ex-smokers accounts largely for this finding. Upon smoking cessation, the risk of cardiovascular death drops dramatically and smokers live long enough to develop lung cancer.
- Increased susceptibility of aging tissues to environmental carcinogens [4]. This event has been documented repeatedly in experimental animals, in whom many, albeit not all aging tissues are primed to the action of environmental carcinogens. Aging is associated with a number of genomic and molecular changes (DNA hyper- and hypomethylation, point mutations, chromosomal breakage) that mimic carcinogenic changes. Of special interest is the suppression of two groups of genes: the caretaker and the gatekeeper genes [5 -6]. The caretaker genes are needed to repair DNA damage, and the gatekeeper ones required to stop the proliferation of the damaged cell until the DNA damage has been repaired. The best known example of a gatekeeper gene is the one that encodes the P53 glycoprotein [7]. When the influence of one or both groups of genes is weakened or abolished, the body is flooded with cells in advanced carcinogenesis. Circumstantial evidence intimates that this may be the case in humans as well. The incidence of prostate and colon cancer in humans increase geometrically with age, suggesting accelerated carcinogenesis in these organs during the last years of life.[8] Between 1970 and 1990, the incidence of

lymphomas and malignant brain tumors has increased in older individuals, suggesting that the older tissues were primed for the action of some new and yet unidentified environmental carcinogen(s). [9-10]. Age is a risk factor for secondary acute leukemia and myelodysplasia induced by cytotoxic chemotherapy [11]. A recent longitudinal study found that the incidence of cancer over a 10 year period was fourfold increased in individuals with shorter leukocyte telomeres [12]. As the telomere length is a marker of biological aging, these findings suggest that age is a risk factor for carcinogenesis

- Changes in the corporeal environment that may favor the development of certain cancers. These include senescence of the immunological and endocrine systems, proliferative senescence and chronic inflammation. Aging is associated with increased prevalence of insulin resistance that leads to increased circulating concentration of insulin and insulin-like growth factor 1 (IGF-1), a powerful stimulator of cancer growth [13]. The importance of this finding has been underlined by recent studies demonstrating that metformin, that restores insulin sensitivity prolongs the lifespan and delays, albeit does not abolish the development of cancer in experimental mice [14]. Proliferative senescence of the fibroblasts has been associated with over-expression of the so called "senescence associated genes" that encode tumor growth factors and inflammatory cytokines [15]. In addition, aging fibroblasts (and possibly other aging cells) release lytic enzymes that favor metastases [16]. Aging is associated with a chronic and progressive inflammation that may favor the development of cancer [16-17] For example, the inflammation of the bone marrow micro-environment has been associated with myelodysplasia [18]. One of the proposed mechanisms of action of thalidomide and lenalidomide for the treatment of myelodysplasia and multiple myeloma is the suppression of marrow inflammation [19].

These general insights of the association of aging and carcinogenesis may have important clinical implications. In particular, they suggest that cancer prevention may be effective in older individuals both in the form of chemoprevention and in the elimination of environmental carcinogens.

Aging and Tumor Growth

The growth of a plant is conditioned by two factors: the seed and soil. Likewise, the growth of a tumor may be determined by the nature of the neoplastic cell and by the tumor host. The importance of the tumor host has been established in elegant experimental studies by Ershler et al. [20] over two decades ago. These investigators injected the same load of Lewis Lung carcinoma and B16 melanoma in C57 black mice of different ages. The death was delayed and the number of metastases reduced in the older animals.

In humans, several examples of cancers whose prognosis changes with age are found. Acute myelogenous leukemia is more frequently lethal in older than in younger individuals because of a seed effect which includes higher prevalence of mutlidrug resistance and of unfavorable cytogenetics and molecular markers [21]. Breast cancer may become more indolent with age due to a combination of "seed" and "soil" effect [22]. The prevalence of hormone receptor positive and well differentiated tumors increases with age. It is suspected a decreased production of sexual hormones disfavor the growth of these endocrine sensitive tumors. The same process may effect the growth of prostate cancer.

Tumor genomics and proteomics have important clinical implications. They may be used to predict the tumor response to cytotoxic chemotherapy or radiation as well as the risk of tumor recurrence and progression [23]. Our insights in the biology of the tumor host lag well behind. In any case, it is important to recognize that tumor biology may change with age and these changes may impact whether an indolent or aggressive tumor behavior ensues.

Age And Cancer Management

Aging is associated with a decline in life expectancy and tolerance of stress, increased risk of functional dependence/comorbidity, and reduced social support [24]. These changes occur at different rates in different persons and are only partly reflected in chronologic age. A clinical definition of age apart from chronologic age is then necessary to address the questions implied in the management of cancer in the aging patient. These questions include: :

- Is the patient going to die of cancer or with cancer? Does the cancer reduce the life expectancy of the patient?
- Is the patient able to tolerate the treatment? That is to say, what capacity does the patient stand to endure physiological stress? Is the patient's functional reserve so reduced that even a minimal stress can cause functional dependence? Is the patient frail?
- What are the treatment goals? In addition to prolongation of survival and symptom palliation, an important goal of medical treatment in older patients include prolongation of the so called "active life expectancy" which is the preservation of the ability to take care of oneself and to enjoy life.

Clinical Definition of Aging

Aging has been defined as loss of entropy and fractality [25] as well as loss of homeostasis [13]. Entropy is the degree of disorder of a system and is related to the ability of the system to produce and waste energy. Loss of entropy entails the need of saving energy, which leads to a progressive limitation of a person's activity and ability to withstand stress. A fractal is a unit subdividing into subunits of the same type, but whose number and length are unpredictable. The branch of a tree is a good example of a fractal. It predictably subdivides into more branches whose number and length are impossible to predict. The function of the mammalian body is maintained by a number of structural fractals such as the respiratory, circulatory, and nervous systems. In addition, the process of cell generation may also be considered a dynamic fractal. Taking as an example the hemopoietic system, few pluripotent stem cells give origin to a number of committed progenitors from which the differentiated precursors of the circulating blood cells are derived. Commitment and differentiation involve the branching of the pluripotent stem cell into progressively larger cell populations. The mechanisms by which the loss of entropy and fractality occurs involve cellular, stromal, and systemic damages [26-27]. Neither entropy nor fractality can be assessed by clinical means. Their definition constitute a theoretical frame of reference to study the clinical aspects of aging. A number of recent studies suggested that a number of aging manisfestations, including cancer, were associated with a shortening of the leukocyte telomeres [12, 28-32]. The shortennig of the telomeres reflects the loss of cellular self reproductive ability and it could be considered as an indirect estimate of fractality. This data at the present time remains controversial [33].

Homeostasis is the self regulatory ability of a system, that is the ability to restore basic conditions after stress imposed by environmental interactions. A number of parameters become dysregulated with aging including blood pressure, circulating concentrations of sugar, cortisol, and cathecholamines. The so called "allostatic load" assesses the dysregulation of 12 different parameters and is being used for estimating the physiologic age of a person in the research arena [13]. Among the manifestations of allostasis, chronic and progressive inflammation are of special interest. Aging is associated with increased concentration of circulating inflammatory markers, including inflammatory cytokines and fibrinolytic products. The concentration of some of these substances is associated with increased risk of death, functional dependence and geriatric syndromes [34- 37] and may mirror the functional age of a person.

Except for some inflammatory markers and possibly for the shortening of leukocyte telomeres, there are no laboratory tests that establish the physiologic age of a person. This determination is largely clinically based and is assessed by a "Comprehensive Geriatric Assessment" (CGA) [38-40]. The basic elements of the CGA are illustrated in table 1.

Dependence in one or more activities of daily living (ADLs) implies minimal functional reserve, very limited tolerance of stress and the need of a full time home caregiver, or admission to an adult living facility. Dependence in one or more instrumental activities of daily living (IADLs) heralds increased risk of mortality [41-44], dementia, and chemotherapy-induced toxicity [43-44]. These individuals require the help of a caregiver to negotiate the outside world. Dependence in ADLs or IADLs may be in part reversible with proper rehabilitation and environmental adjustments. For example, a car with only manual commands may render a person unable to drive because they are paraplegic.

Comorbidity is associated with reduced life-expectancy and increased risk of treatment complications [45-48]. In addition, comorbidity may affect the natural history of cancer: diabetes has been associated with a worsened prognosis for most common neoplasms including cancer of the large bowel, prostate and breast [45,47]. Anemia is particularly important because it is associated with an increased risk of overall mortality in older individuals and of chemotherapy-induced myelotoxicity [49]. In about 50% of cases, anemia can be accounted for by reversible causes, such as iron or cobalamin deficiency, or chronic renal insufficiency. Another common mechanism of anemia in older cancer patients is inflammation, that causes a condition of relative erythropoietin insufficiency. Comorbidity is also a cause of polypharmacy that may interact with anti-neoplastic drugs and alters both the effectiveness and safety of these agents [50-51]. In addition, drug interactions are a major cause of iatrogenic morbidity.

Though not unique to aging, geriatric syndromes become more prevalent with advanced age [52] and are harbingers of critically reduced functional reserve. The practitioner needs particular caution in labeling a condition a geriatric syndrome. Dementia may span from mild memory disorder, without effect on a person's health and independence to a complete loss of orientation in time and space, associated with immediate risk of mortality and harm. Likewise, delirium should be considered a geriatric syndrome only when it is not caused by primary acute diseases of the central nervous system or by the administration of drugs known to cause delirium [53[. Indeed delirium is a common presentation of a number of diseases in older individuals including respiratory and urinary tract infections, anti-cholinergic medications, and cardiac ischemia. Depression is considered a geriatric syndrome only when it is unresponsive to treatment.

Table 1. Comprehensive Geriatric Assessment (CGA)

Domain	Assessment
Function	<ul><li>Performance Status (PS)</li><li>ADL</li></ul> Continence, transferring, grooming, dressing, feeding, utilization of the bathroom. <ul><li>IADL</li></ul> Use of transportation, ability to take medications, to use the telephone, to go shopping, to take care of finances, to provide to one's meals <ul><li>Advanced activities of daily living.</li></ul> These include all activities that make the patient's life enjoyable. <ul><li>Number of comorbid conditions</li><li>Comorbidity scales (assessing the seriousness of each condition)</li></ul>
Comorbidity	<ul><li>Dementia (cognitive evaluation)</li><li>Depression (screening tests, such as the geriatric depression scale)</li><li>Delirium</li><li>Falls (risk of falls assessment)</li><li>Vertigo</li></ul>
Presence of Geriatric Syndromes	<ul><li>Spontaneous fractures</li><li>Failure to thrive (weigh loss in face of normal food intake)</li><li>Neglect and abuse</li></ul> <ul><li>Living conditions</li><li>Presence and reliability of the caregiver</li><li>Economical resources</li></ul> <ul><li>Nutritional status</li><li>Nutritional risk (typical meals, access to food, etc)</li><li>Number of medications</li><li>Risk of drug interactions</li></ul>
Social support	
Nutrition	
Polypharmacy	

The CGA provides an estimate of a person's mortality risk over four years [54-56)] (Figure 1), and may be utilized to predict the risk of chemotherapy induced toxicity [43-44]. The CGA may also discover reversible conditions liable to interfere with cancer treatment, including comorbidity, malnutrition, absence of a reliable caregiver [57-59]. A number of studies also demonstrated that the CGA may help predict the risk of postoperative morbidity in older cancer patients undergoing surgery [60]. The Preoperative Assessment of in Elderly Cancer Patients (PACE) demonstrated that dependence in IADLs and abnormal Mini-mental status assessments were associated with an increased risk of post-surgical morbidity and duration of hospitalization.

Clinical definition frailty assessment. A discussion of physiologic age is not complete without mentioning the concept of frailty. The frail person has a critically reduced physiologic reserve such that a minimal stress may cause loss of independence and start a sequence of events that can lead to a patient 's death [25]. Seemingly, cancer chemotherapy or cancer surgery may represent the stress that precipitates functional dependence and death in older patients.

While frailty is very real, the clinical definition of frailty has remained elusive, until the Cardiovascular Health Study (CHS) investigators provided a well validated operational definition of this syndrome [61]. Eighty-five hundred individuals 65 years and over were followed for a mean of 11 years. Based on five simple parameters, they could be divided into three groups with a different risk of mortality, disability, and admission to adult living facilities. The parameters of interest included:

- Involuntary weight loss of 10 lbs or more over a 6 months period;
- Decreased grip strength;
- Difficulty in starting movements;
- Reduced walk speed;
- Exhaustion.

Three groups of individuals were categorized: non-frail (no abnormalities); pre-frail (up to two abnormalities), and frail (three or more abnormalities).

The definition of frailty by the CHS is operational and well validated. As such, it provides a useful frame of reference for further studies on frailty. Recently, the CHS definition of frailty has been debated and other frailty indices have been proposed. The Study of Osteoporotic Fracture (SOF) index has been validated both in older women [62] and older men [63]. It involves the performance of simple exercises (rising five times from a chair) and appears as accurate a predictor of falls, death, fractures and disability as the CHS instrument. The SOF index has a much shorter follow up than the CHS study and has not been validated for risk of hospitalization and institutionalization. The frailty index developed by the Canadian investigators [64] is very sensitive in predicting mortality and quite comprehensive as it involves the accumulation of 40 functional deficits, but it is too cumbersome for use in clinical practice. While the detection of frailty is evolving, the CHS classification represents the "gold standard" for ongoing studies. Of special interest, fatigue heralded about 73% of the cases of frailty detected in the CHS (65). Early detection of frailty appears as one of the most urgent issue in geriatrics, because a number of interventions may prevent or delay its development [66]. Several questions pertain to frailty and cancer: is cancer a cause of frailty?

Is frailty reversible with the treatment of cancer? Is frailty a complication of cancer treatment?

Conclusions related to the clinical assessment of age. In conclusion, physiologic age is poorly reflected in chronologic age. Chronologic age is at most a landmark (established at age 70) beyond which most physiologically old individuals are seen. The older population is highly diverse and clinical trials should consider the influence of physiologic rather than chronologic age on treatment outcome. A number of studies have established that the CGA is currently the most reliable way top predict the patient's risk of mortality and treatment complications. In addition, the CGA allows the practitioner to optimize other conditions that may compromise the patient's treatment including comorbidity, malnutrition, and inadequate social support.

Aging and Cancer Prevention

Primary prevention of cancer involves the avoidance of exposure to carcinogens or administration of substances that offset carcinogenesis (chemoprevention). In addition, vaccines for viral-induced cancers, such as cancer of the cervix, penis, and anus appear promising, but they are mainly of interest for younger individuals [67].

Secondary prevention involves prevention of cancer death by early detection of common cancers through screening asymptomatic individuals at risk.

Chemoprevention and age. A number of substances are able to prevent common cancers (Table 2), but they for the most part have limited clinical use.

Table 2. Substances with Demonstrated Value in the Chemoprevention of Cancer

Chemopreventative agents	Cancer
Selective Estrogen Receptor Modulators (SERMs) • Tamoxifen • Toremifene • Raloxifen	Breast Possibly prostate
Retinoids	Cancer of the upper airways
5-α Reductase inhibitors Finasteride Dutasteride	Cancer of the prostate
Aspirin and other non-steroidal agents	Cancer of the large bowel

In a randomized controlled study, tamoxifen was shown to prevent hormone receptor rich breast cancer and a subsequent study demonstrated that raloxifene was as effective as tamoxifen (68). Unlike tamoxifen, raloxifene does not cause endometrial cancer. The benefits of the SERM are tempered by several considerations including lack of survival advantage, cost, and complications including hot flashes and deep vein thrombosis whose risk increases with age. Over the age of 70, the benefits of chemoprevention in breast cancer are at best marginal and limited to women at very high risk. The suggestion that toremifene may prevent prostate cancer has not been documented in a randomized placebo controlled study [69].

While retinoic acid prevents the development of a second cancer of the upper airways, the toxicity of this compound is prohibitive [70]. Furthermore, it has been demonstrated that retinoic acid does not reverse the molecular changes that lead to cancer.

The 5-α reductase inhibitors finasteride an dutasteride reduce the risk of prostate cancer, but they cause substantial side effects including gynecomastia, hot flushes, and loss of libido and are not associated with a decreased risk of prostate cancer related deaths [71]. There has as well been some controversies regarding their potential of inducing higher grade tumors.

A number of retrospective case control studies suggests that aspirin reduces the risk of colorectal cancer and possibly other malignancies, but it is not clear what the optimal dose or the optimal treatment duration of use should be [72].

In conclusion, cancer chemoprevention is possible, but its clinical benefits are marginal at best. Theoretically, older individuals are ideal candidates for chemoprevention due to their increased susceptibility to environmental carcinogens, but the potential benefits are counterbalanced by their increased risk of treatment complications. A number of experimental studies suggest that some substances may prolong an animal life span and at the same time delay the manifestations of aging such as cancer. The mechanisms of action of these protective agents involves mostly prevention of oxidative damage, or reinstitution of homeostasis (example metformin that reinstitutes sensitivity to insulin) [73-74]

Secondary prevention of cancer. The benefits of early cancer diagnosis are based on the construct that cancer undergoes a pre-clinical phase and that it is more curable when diagnosed and treated at an early stage. To prove this hypothesis, randomized controlled studies of cancer screening need to demonstrate that screening is associated with a reduced incidence of cancer-related deaths [75]. Intermediate end-points such as more prolonged survival of patients undergoing screening or earlier stage of cancers diagnosed through screening are inadequate as they are subject to three type of potential biases:

- Lead time bias (individuals diagnosed through screening seem to live longer simply because one has been aware of their cancer diagnosis for a longer time);
- Length time bias (only slow growing cancers are diagnosed through screening while the most rapidly growing ones, that are also the most lethal, escape screening);
- Over-detection bias (diagnosis of a number of cancers that would have never become clinically relevant).

Only screening mammography for women aged 50-69 and yearly examination of stools for fecal occult blood in individuals 50 and above proved to reduce the mortality rate from breast and colon cancer, respectively [75]. The screening of sexually active women for cervical cancer is also a generally accepted practice though its value was never proven in randomized prospective studies. In a retrospective study, it reduced the mortality of cervical cancer in women younger than 40 by 75% [76].

The benefits of any form of cancer screening in individuals 70 and older is controversial (77-79). On one side, the predictive positive value of a screening test increases with age due to the increasing prevalence of cancer. On the other side, the benefits are lessened by a reduced life expectancy and an increased risk of treatment related complications. Also, after multiple screening interventions, all so called "prevalence cases" (that is cases present at the time screening was initiated) have been detected. The yield of successive screening sessions seemingly becomes progressively lower. In addition to cost, the drawbacks of screening include anxiety, complications of the screening and treatment procedures, and overtreatment due to over-detection. A common practice is to recommend screening for breast and large bowel neoplasms to individuals with a life-expectancy of five years and longer, because the initial benefits of early detection are typically seen five years or more after the institution of this screening test.

Aging and Cancer Treatment

The treatment of cancer may be either local (surgery, radiation therapy) and/or systemic (hormonal therapy, cytotoxic chemotherapy, targeted therapy).

Surgery. The risk of surgical complications increases with age, especially for emergency surgery, which is associated with a substantial risk of death [80]. The Preoperative Assessment of Cancer in the Elderly (PACE) index, that combines elements of the CGA with more traditional surgical parameters may be used to predict the benefits and risks of surgery in the older aged person [60] (Table 3) In a prospective study of 460 patients 70 and over undergoing different types of surgery, the authors demonstrated IADL dependence, BFI and PS predicted major surgical complications, whereas ADL, IADL and PS predicted prolonged hospitalization. These data were confirmed in older patients undergoing colorectal cancer surgery by Swedish investigators [81] Recent advances in surgery and anesthesiology have resulted in progressively improved outcomes in this cohort with surgical intervention.

Table 3. Preoperative Assessment in Elderly Cancer Patients (PACE)

Instrument	Score
Mini-Mental Status (MMS)	10-30 - Increasing score = increasing cognitive capacity
Activities of daily living (ADL)	0-6 - Increasing score =increasing dependence
	40-8 - Increasing score = increasing dependence
Instrumental Activities of Daily Living (IADL)	0-15 - Increasing score = increasing depression
Geriatric depression scale (GDS)	0-90 - Increasing score = increasing level of fatigue
Brief fatigue Inventory (BFI)	0-4 - Increasing score = increasing dependence
	1-4 - Increasing score = increase risk of death
ECOG performance Status (PS)	0-6 - Increasing score = Increased number of comorbidities
American Society of Anesthesiology Scale (ASA)	
Satariano Index of Comorbidity (SIC)	

Radiation Therapy. Several older studies showed that external beam irradiation could be safely administered to older cancer patients even beyond the age of 80 years (82-84). New radiation techniques, including Intensity Modulated Radiation (IMR), proton beam therapy, brachytherapy, and radiosurgery have resulted in reduced complications of radiation therapy by sparing treatment to surrounding normal tissue.

An issue of special concern in the management of older patients is the safety of the combination of chemotherapy and radiotherapy, which is commonly used in the management of locally advanced cancer of the upper airway, lung, esophagus, bladder, cervix, and anal canal. The data in older individuals are limited. In a retrospective analysis of patients with locally advanced non-small cell lung cancer the combination of chemoradiation was not superior to radiation alone in individuals 70 years and older, while it was in younger individuals [85]. Combined modality treatment has two substantial benefits which include potential increased cure rates and increased rates of organ preservation. Older individuals should not be excluded from this form of treatment on the account of their age. It appears important to develop instruments that can predict which older patients are more likely to benefit from a combined multimodality treatment approach.

Hormonal treatment of cancer. Hormonal compounds commonly used in the treatment of cancer are listed in table 4. Though hormonal treatment has been used also in the management of endometrial and ovarian cancer, breast and prostate cancer are the tumors for which this treatment approach is most commonly employed.

Table 4. Hormonal Treatment of Cancer

Cancer	Hormonal Treatment	Complications
Breast	Selective Estrogen Receptors Modulators (SERM). Tamoxifen Toremifene	Hot flushes, vaginal secretions, thrombo-embolism, Endometrial Cancer
	Pure anti-estrogens Faslodex	Hot flushes, osteoporosis
	Aromatase Inhibitors Anastrozole Letrozol	Hot flushes, vaginal dryness, osteoporosis
	Examesthane	Thrombo-embolism, endometrial cancer, fluid retention
	Estrogen	Fluid retention, thrombo-embolism Virilism, hepatitis
	Progestins	
	Androgens	
Prostate	Androgen deprivation Orchiectomy LHRH analogs LHRH antagonist	Hot flushes, osteoporosis, diabetes, myocardial infarction
	Antiandrogens	Gynecomastia, hepatitis, diarrhea, nausea
	CPY inhibitors	Thrombo-embolism, congestive heart failure, fluid retention
	Estrogen	

The risk of SERM complications, especially endometrial cancer and deep vein thrombosis increase with age (86). These medications have more limited use today than they did a decade ago. The main indications include adjuvant treatment of breast ductal carcinoma *in situ*, adjuvant treatment of breast cancer in patients who cannot tolerate aromatase inhibitors, as well as treatment of hormone responsive male breast cancer both in the adjuvant and metastatic setting. In the management of metastatic breast cancer, faslodex has largely superseded the SERMs. Raloxifene is preferred to tamoxifen for the chemoprevention of breast cancer as it does not cause endometrial cancer, but it still can cause thrombo-embolisms.

Osteoporosis is the main complication of both aromatase inhibitors and androgen deprivation. In patients with prostate cancer, the risk of bone fractures increases with the duration of treatment [54, 86-87]. This complication may be ameliorated by:

- Vitamin D and calcium supplementation. Vitamin D supplementation is mandatory for patients with circulating levels of 25 OH vitamin D lower than 40nm/ml [88-89].
- Use of bisphosphonates in patients with evidence of osteopenia undergoing treatment with aromatase inhibitors or androgen deprivation. In prostate cancer patients, zolendronic acid every three months in combination with androgen deprivation has prevented bone loss related to androgen deprivation, according to a number of randomized controlled studies. (90). So far this practice has not reduced the fracture rates. The RANK ligand denosumab has recently been approved for the management of osteoporosis in postmenopausal women and holds promise for the prevention of bone loss during androgen deprivation (91). It is important to remember that these treatments are not without their potential complications. A rare but devastating side effect of such therapy is osteonecrosis of the jaw, observed after oral surgery in patients treated either with bisphosphonates or denosumab.
- Use of estrogen "in lieu' of androgen deprivation in the management of prostate cancer. This treatment which is as effective as androgen deprivation does not cause osteoporosis, loss of libido, or hot flushes. Unfortunately, it has been prematurely abandoned for the most part because of its increased risk of cardiovascular complications [92].

Other complications of LHRH deprivation include diabetes and myocardial infarction in patients with pre-existing coronary artery disease [93]

Cytotoxic chemotherapy. Cytotoxic chemotherapy has been the mainstay systemic treatment of most cancers for the past four decades.

Aging is associated with pharmacokinetic and pharmacodynamic changes that generally potentiate the toxicity of these agents (Table 5). [94]

The most consistent pharmacokinetic changes include reduced renal excretion and reduced volume of distribution (Vd) of water-soluble agents that may lead to a prolongation of the serum concentrations of active and toxic drug metabolites. A progressive decline in glomerular filtration rate occurs in the majority of aging individuals. The volume of distribution is determined by body composition, serum albumin, and hemoglobin concentration. With increasing age, there is a progressive decline in the total body water and a progressive increase in body fat composition. It is important to remember that drugs excreted from the biliary tract, such as the anthracyclines or morphine, result in active and toxic metabolites excreted through the kidneys. Thus, renal insufficiency may be associated with enhanced toxicity of these drugs.

Table 5A. Pharmacokinetic Changes of Aging

Parameter	Age-related change
Absorption and bioavailability	Probably decreased
Vd	Decreased for water-soluble agents ---→ increased plasma concentrations Increased for lipid-soluble agents
Metabolism	Decreased hepatic metabolism
Excretion	Renal: deacreased Biliary: not affected

Tabel 5B. Common Complications of Cytotoxic Chemotherapy

Universal complications
• Myelosuppression
• Nausea and vomiting
• Mucositis
• Fatigue
Complications specific of certain agents
• Cardiotoxicity: anthracyclines
• Neurotoxicity (peripheral): alkaloids, taxanes, epothlilones, platinum derivatives
• Neurotoxicity (central): cytarabin in high doses, methotrexate in high doses; ifosphamide; gemcitabine
• Pulmonary fibrosis: bleomycin, methotrexate
• Renal insufficiency: cisplatin

With aging, there is a progressive decline in the absorption of food due to decreased gastro-intestinal secretions, decreased intestinal mucosal surface, and decreased splanchnic circulation. How these changes affect the absorption of medications is unknown at the present time.

Decreased splanchnic circulation and decreased hepatocyte mass lead to a reduction in drug metabolism, especially when the cytochrome P450 pathway is involved. These are mostly oxido-reductive reactions responsible for activation and deactivation of a number of agents. In addition, the cytochrome P450 system is inhibited by a number of drugs. Polypharmacy of aging further complicates the issue of drug metabolism.

Some complications of cytotoxic chemotherapy become more common with aging.

The risk of neutropenia, neutropenic infections, and death from neutropenic infections increase with the age of the patient [95]. Fortunately, the Granulocyte Colony Stimulating Factors (G-CSF) filgrastim, pegfilgrastim and lenograstim are effective in older individuals and reduce by more than 50% the risk of infections [96-97].

The risk of thrombocytopenia and anemia also increase in older individuals. Erythropoietic stimulating agents reverse the majority of chemotherapy-related anemias, but the use of these compounds is currently limited out of concern for hypertension, thrombosis, and enhanced tumor growth [98].

Age is a risk factor for mucositis. This complication may cause dysphagia, diarrhea, and rapid volume depletion in older individuals. Aggressive fluid resuscitation should be initiated in patients unable to ingest fluids. The prevention of mucositis has limited effectiveness and may include solutions containing glutamine, supersaturated solutions of calcium phosphate, and keratinocyte growth factor [99].

Fatigue is a condition of tiredness that is not relived by rest and is the most common long term complication of systemic chemotherapy [100-101]. The pathogenesis of chemotherapy induced fatigue is poorly understood. Correction of anemia may improve fatigue in some patients. While it is not clear whether it is more common in the aging patient, fatigue is particularly threatening in older individuals as it is a harbinger of frailty [65].

Age is also a risk factor for anthracycline induced cardiomyopathy and peripheral neuropathy [94]. The risk of cardiomyopathy may be reduced by the administration of doxorubicin as a continuous infusion, by the concomitant administration of doxorubicin and the antidote desrazoxan, or by the use of pegylated liposomal doxorubicin "in lieu" of doxorubicin. None of these approaches is routinely used in older individuals, because of cost, alternative toxicity, and also because the dose of doxorubicin employed is rarely associated with cardiotoxic complications.

No antidote for peripheral neurotoxiciy currently exists. This complication may impair the independence of older individuals by impeding both their walking and fine hand movements. The only prevention consists of trying to avoid a combination of neurotoxic drugs (example cisplatin and paclitaxel) and by the early interruption of treatment when the neuropathy may interfere with an individual's activity.

An important and unanswered question is whether age is a risk factor for more frequent and more severe manifestations of "chemobrain" that is a cognitive dysfunction caused by chemotherapy?

Recently, it was found that age is a risk factor for delayed complications of chemotherapy. Myelodysplasia and acute myeloid leukemia may develop in 1-2% of women 65 years and over who had received adjuvant breast cancer treatment containing an anthraxcycline, and the risk of this complications is enhanced by myelopoietic growth factors [11]. The incidence of a chronic cardiomyopathy, manifested by a progressive decline in the ejection fraction, is seen in approximately 19% of individuals 65 years or older, 5 years or longer following treatment with an anthracycline [102].

As mentioned earlier, elements of the CGA may be integrated into formulas that predict the risk of chemotherapy-related complications in older individuals [43-44].These models will help determining which patients are more likely to benefit from therapy and which ones are more likely to be adversely impacted by this form of treatment

Targeted agents. This term is an umbrella for newly developed cancer treatment compounds that target a specific component of a neoplasm or a specific molecular pathway pivotal to its growth/progression. A systematic classification of these agents is still needed [103]. In table 6, a provisional classification is proposed based on their resulting mechanisms of action. It should be remembered that compounds of different natures, such as the monoclonal antibody bevacizumab and the small molecule tyrosine kinase inhibitors such as sorafenib, sunitinib, and pazopanib function essentially in the same manner i.e. inhibition of neoangiogenesis through different molecular pathways/targets. Likewise cetuximab, panitumumab, and erlotinib lead to inhibition of signal transduction. Furthermore, most of these compounds may have multiple and yet undiscovered mechanisms of action.

Table 6. Classification of Targeted Agents based on Mechanism(s) of Action

Mechanism of action	Agents	Disease for which they are indicated
Monoclonal antibodies targeting a tumor components	Rituximab (CD20) Ofatumumab (CD20) Alentuzumab (CD52)	B cell malignancies
Monoclonal antibodies used as carrier of a radioiosotope	Ibritumumab Tiuxetan (CD20) Tositumomab (CD20)	B cell Malignancies
Monoclonal antibodies targeting growth factors or growth factor receptors (GFR)	Trastuzumab (Her2neu)	Breast cancer
	Cetuximab (EGFR1) Panitumumab (Multiple Receptors)	Cancer of the large bowel, of the head and neck and of the lung
	Bevacizumab (VEGF)	Multiple cancers (colorectal, lung, breast, kidney, glioblastoma multiformis)
Monoclonal antibodies modulating the immune response	Ipilumimab	Melanoma
Inhibitors of free Tyrosine Kinase	Imatinib Nilotinib Desatinib	Chronic Myelogenous Leukemia Gastro-Intestinal Stromal Tumors (GIST)
Inhibitors of receptor bound tyrosine Kinase	Erlotinib	Lung cancer Pancreatic cancer
	Lapatinib	Breast cancer
	Sunitinib Pazopanib	Renal cell
	Sorafenib	Renal cell Hepatocellular carcinoma
mTOR inhibitors	Temsirolimus Everolimus	Renal cell Carcinoma Mantle cell lymphomas
Small Molecule Immune modulators	Thalidomide Lenalidomide	Myelodysplasia Multiple myeloma
Proteosome inhibitors	Bortezomib	Multiple myeloma Lymphoma
Hypomethylating agents	Azacitidine Decitabine	Myelodysplasia
Histonedeacetylase inhibitors	Vorinostat	Cutaneous T cell lymphoma

In theory, targeted agents should have a better toxicity profile than cytotoxic chemotherapy, due to a more specific mechanism of action which would spare normal tissues from potential toxicity. This is however not necessarily always the case. For example, alentuzumab may cause severe and protracted myelosuppression and immunosuppression and should only be administered in combination with antibiotic, antifungal, and antiviral prophylaxis. In addition, a number of new complications have emerged with the use of these agents. Those of major concern to older individuals include:

- Myocardial depression with trastuzumab, which is due to a "stunned myocardium." It is more common in older individuals. It is generally reversible upon discontinuation of the drug, at least after a short treatment duration (1-2 years)
- Hypertension and thrombo-embolism may complicate the treatment with angiogenesis inhibitors, such as bevacizumab, sunitinib, sorafenib, pazopanib
- A maculo-papular rash is a common complication of treatment with signal transduction inhibitors (such as cetuximab, panitumumab, and erlotinib). In some cases, this rash may cause severe dehydration.

Though the studies are limited, the risk of complications from targeted agents seem to be increased with increasing age [104].

Supportive care of the aged patient with cancer. The main issues include pain management, function and nutrition preservation, as well as prevention of delirium.

Pain management in older individuals entails the following problems [105]:
- Patients are at increased risk of gastrointestinal bleeding and renal insufficiency from non-steroidal anti-inflammatory drugs (NSAID). In general, these medications should not be used in the elderly.
- Older individuals are at increased risk of complications from opioids [105]. This is due to the imbalance of μ and δ receptor concentrations in the brain as well as to the pharmacokinetic changes of aging. While morphine and its congeners are excreted through the biliary tract, 6-glucoronide which is responsible in part for the analgesic effect and 3-glucoronide which is responsible for the toxic effects, are excreted through the kidneys. In the presence of renal insufficiency, the resulting effects of these compounds are prolonged. It is advisable to titrate very slowly the doses of opioids in the aged and institute treatment with long acting agents only when the titration process has been completed. Also, the use of intrathecal opioids, may be indicated in older individuals to minimize the systemic complications of these compounds

Patients at risk of malnutrition should be identified by a dietitian at the initial clinic visit and followed very closely to establish whether they have access to an appropriate diet and the similarly that this can be followed. Likewise, patients should be encouraged to perform daily simple exercises and avoid bed rest for most of the daytime period.

Delirium is a geriatric syndrome that may be triggered by a number of conditions including medications, infections, electrolyte imbalance, anesthesia, and hospitalization [106]. The management of delirium includes prompt recognition and management of the underlying cause, as well as proper environmental conditions during hospitalization. These may include the consistent presence of a caregiver well known to the patient and avoidance of medications more likely to result in delirium.

It is well known that caregivers of the older individuals with chronic diseases are subjected to a number of social and medical problems [107]. Since a functional caregiver may represent the only way to access treatment for an older patient, it behooves the practitioner to investigate the emotional and physical health of the caregiver and to support the caregiver with encouragement and recommendations when deemed appropriate. Two typical caregiver profiles are common. In one case, the caregiver is an older spouse with medical and social problems of his her own. In the other, the caregiver is a married child that needs to keep working and support his or her family while taking care of their older parent (the so called Aenea's syndrome).[108]

Treatment goals. Cure, prolongation of survival, and symptom palliation are universal goals of medical treatment. In the management of the older aged person, it is very important to attempt to maintain an active life expectancy. For this purpose, it is very important to balance the benefits and the risks of treatment, especially those treatment whose benefits may only be seen late in the future. These include adjuvant chemotherapy for breast, colon, lung cancer, or prolonged androgen suppression in individuals experiencing a biochemical recurrence several years after the local treatment of prostate cancer .

The construct of an active life expectancy [109] includes the preservation of functional independence (that is the ability to carry on ADLs and IADLs) as well as the preservation of the ability to perform activities that are pleasurable and fulfilling (the so-called advanced activities of daily living). For this purpose, it is important to obtain a so called "value history" at the beginning of a treatment to detect what are the patients main objectives in the lasting years of his/her life and to make sure that the treatment is aimed to achieve/preserve these objectives.

Conclusions

Age is a risk factor for cancer. With the aging of our population, cancer in the elderly is becoming the most common presentation of cancer. The biologic interactions of cancer and age include carcinogenesis and tumor behavior. Some cancers, including breast and lung cancer, may become more indolent with age, while others including acute leukemia, lymphoma, and ovarian cancer may become more aggressive. The management of cancer in the older person implies an estimate of life expectancy and treatment tolerance. At the present time, this estimate is best provided by the CGA.

The role of primary or secondary cancer prevention in reducing the risk of cancer-related deaths is not currently well established. Screening for breast and colorectal cancer may be recommended to individuals with a life expectancy of at least five years. Chronologic age should not prevent effective cancer treatment. This should be provided irrespective of chronologic age, to all individuals who are deemed to benefit from treatment due to an adequate life expectancy and tolerance of the ensuing stress imparted by the treatment of the underlying malignancy.

References

[1]   Yancik R; Ries LA: Cancer in the Older Person: an International issue in an aging world. *Sem Oncol*, 2004, 31, 128-136

[2]   Olshansky SJ, Goldman DP, Zheng Y et al *Aging in America in the twenty-first century: demographic forecasts from the MacArthur Foundation Research Network on an Aging Society Milbank Q*. 2009 Dec;87(4):842-62. Review.

[3]   Jemal A, Thun MJ, Ries LA, et al: Annual report to the nation on the status of cancer, 1975-2005, featuring trends in lung cancer, tobacco use, and tobacco control. *J Natl Cancer Inst*. 2008 Dec 3;100(23):1672-94

[4]   Anisimov VN, Sikora E, Pawelec G.: Relationship between cancer and aging a multilevel approach. *Biogerontology*. 2009 Aug;10(4):323-38. Epub 2009 Jan 21. Review

[5]   van Heemst D, den Reijer PM, Westendorp RG.: Ageing and Cancer: a review on the role of caretakers and gatekeepers. *Eur J Cancer*. 2007 Oct;43(15):2144-52. Epub 2007 Aug 30. Review.

[6]   Campisi J, Sedivy J. How does proliferative homeostasis change with age? What causes it and how does it contribute to aging. *J Gerontol A Biol Sci Med Sci*. 2009 Feb;64(2):164-6.

[7]   Papazoglu C, Mills AA.: P53 at the crossroad between cancer and aging. *J Pathol*. 2007 Jan;211(2):124-33

[8]   Edwards BK, Brown ML, Wingo PA, et al: Annual report to the nation on the status of cancer, 1975-2002, featuring population-based trends in cancer treatment. *J Natl Cancer Inst*. 2005 Oct 5;97(19):1407-27.

[9]   Morrison VA: non-Hodgkin's Lymphoma in the elderly: overview and treatment of follicular lymphoma. *Oncology*, 2007, 1104-1110.

[10] Nayak L, Iwamoto FM. Primary Brain Tumors in the Elderly. *Curr Neurol Neurosci Rep*. 2010 Jul;10(4):252-8.

[11] Lyman GH, Dale DC, Wolff DA, et al: Acute myeloid leukemia or myelodysplastic syndrome in randomized controlled clinical trials of cancer chemotherapy with granulocyte colony-stimulating factor: a systematic review. *J Clin Oncol*. 2010 Jun 10;28(17):2914-24. Epub 2010 Apr 12.

[12] Willeit P; Willeit J; Mayr A et al: Telomere length and incident cancer and Cancer Mortality. *JAMA*, 2010, 304, 69-75

[13] Gruenewald TL, Seeman TE, Karlamangla AS, et al: Allostatic Load and frailty in older individuals. *J Am Geriatr Soc*. 2009 Sep;57(9):1525-31. Epub 2009 Jul 21

[14] Anisimov VN, Egormin PA, Piskunova TS, et al Metformin extends life span of HER-2/neu transgenic mice and in combination with melatonin inhibits growth of transplantable tumors in vivo. *Cell Cycle*. 2010 Jan 1;9(1):188-97. Epub 2010 Jan 22.

[15] Coppé JP, Desprez PY, Krtolica A et al: The senescence-associated secretory phenotype: the dark side of tumor suppression. *Annu Rev Pathol*. 2010;5:99-118. Review.

[16] Davalos AR, Coppe JP, Campisi J, et al: Senescent cells as a source of inflammatory factors for tumor progression. *Cancer Metastasis Rev*. 2010 Jun;29(2):273-83.

[17] Freund A, Orjalo AV, Desprez PY, et al: Inflammatory network during senescence: causes and consequences. *Trends Mol Med.* 2010 May;16(5):238-46.

[18] Stirewalt DL, Mhyre AJ, Marcondes M, et al: Tumour necrosis factor-induced gene expression in human marrow stroma: clues to the pathophysiology of MDS. *Br J Haematol.* 2008 Feb;140(4):444-53.

[19] Komrokji RS, List AF.: lenalidomide in the treatment of myelodysplastic syndromes: current status and future directions. *Hematol Oncol Clin North Am.* 2010 Apr;24(2):377-88.

[20] Kaesberg PR, Ershler WB.: the change in tumor aggressiveness with age: lessons from experimental animals. *Semin Oncol.* 1989 Feb;16(1):28-33

[21] Dombret H, Raffoux E, Gardin C.: Acute Myelogenous Leukemia in the Elderly. *Semin Oncol.* 2008 Aug;35(4):430-8.

[22] Balducci L.: treating Elderly patients with hormone sensitive Breast cancer. What do the data show? *Cancer Treat Rev.* 2009 Feb;35(1):47-56.

[23] Dowsett M, Dunbier AK. Emerging biomarkers and new understanding of traditional markers in personalized therapy for breast cancer. *Clin Cancer Res.* 2008

[24] Balducci L, Colloca G, Cesari M, et al: assessment and treatment of elderly patients with cancer. *Surg Oncol*, 2010, in press

[25] Walston J, Hadley EC, Ferrucci L,et al.: Research Agenda for frailty in Older Adults. *J Am Ger Soc*, 2006 54, 991-2001

[26] Campisi J; dAdda di Fagnana F: Cellular senescence: when bad things happen to good cells. *Nature Rev* 2007, 8, 729-740

[27] ViJg J; Campisi J: Puzzles, promises and a cure for ageing. *Nature*, 2008, 454, 1065-1071

[28] Wong LS, van der Harst P, de Boer RA, et al: Aging, telomeres, and heart failure. *Heart Fail Rev.* 2010 in press

[29] Willeit P, Willeit J, Brandstätter A, et al Cellular aging reflected by leukocyte telomere length predicts advanced atherosclerosis and cardiovascular disease risk.,*Arterioscler Thromb Vasc Biol.* 2010 30(8):1649-56.

[30] Sahin E, Depinho RA. Linking functional decline of telomeres, mitochondria and stem cells during ageing. *Nature.* 2010 Mar 25;464(7288):520-8

[31] Babizhayev MA, Savel' yeva EL, Moskvina SN, et al: Telomere Length is a Biomarker of Cumulative Oxidative Stress, Biologic Age, and an Independent Predictor of Survival and Therapeutic Treatment Requirement Associated With Smoking Behavior. *Am J Ther.* 2010 in press

[32] Risques RA; Arbeev KG; Yashin AI et al: Leukocyte Telomere Length is associated with disability in the older USA population. *J Am Ger Soc*, 2010, 58, 1289-1298

[33] Shiels PG: Improves Precision in Investigating Aging: why telomeres can cause problems. *J Gerontol Biol Sc*, 2010, 65A, 789-791

[34] Ferrucci L, Corsi A, Lauretani F, et al.: The origin of Age-related pro-inflammatory state. *Blood*, 2005, 105, 2294-2299

[35] Maggio M, Guralnik JM, Longo DL, et al.: Interleukin-6 in aging and chronic disease: a magnificent pathway. *J Gerontol A Biol Sci Med Sci.* 2006 Jun;61(6):575-84

[36] Crimmins E, Vasunilashorn S, Kim JK, et al.: biomarkers related to aging in the human population. *Adv Clin Chem.* 2008; 46, 161-216

[37] Gurven M, Kaplan H, Winking J, Finch C, Crimmins EM. aging and inflammation in two epidemiological worlds. *J Gerontol A Biol Sci Med Sci.* 2008 Feb;63(2):196-201

[38] Extermann M; Hurria A: Comprehensive Geriatric Assessment in older patients with cancer. *J Clin Oncol,* 2007, 25, 1824-1831

[39] Luciani A, Ascione G, Bertuzzi C, et al Detecting disabilities in older patients with cancer: comparison between comprehensive geriatric assessment and vulnerable elders survey-13. *J Clin Oncol.* 2010 Apr 20;28(12):2046-50

[40] Brunello A, Sandri R, Extermann M.: Multidimensional geriatric evaluation of the older cancer patient as a clinical and a research tool. *Cancer Treat Rev.* 2009 Oct;35(6):487-92.

[41] Störk S, Feelders RA, van den Beld AW, et al.: Prediction of mortality risk in the elderly. *Am J Med.* 2006 Jun;119(6):519-25

[42] Carey EC, Covinsky KE, Lui LY, et al: Prediction of mortality in community-living frail elderly people with long-term care needs. *J Am Geriatr Soc.* 2008 Jan;56(1):68

[43] . M. Extermann, I. Boler, R. Reich, et al: The Chemotherapy Risk Assessment Scale for High-Age Patients (CRASH) score: Design and validation.. *ASCO national conference 2010,* Abstr 9000

[44] . A. Hurria, K. Togawa, S. G. Mohile, et al.: Predicting chemotherapy toxicity in older adults with cancer: A prospective 500 patient multicenter study. *ASCO Proc,* 2010, Abstr 9001

[45] Extermann M: Interactions of Cancer and Comorbidity. *Cancer Control,* 2007, 14, 13-22

[46] Kulminski AM, Ukraintseva SV, Kulminskaya IV,et al.: Cumulative deficits better characterizes susceptibility to death in elderly people than phenotypic frailty. Lessons from the Cardiovascular Health Study. *J Am Ger Soc,* 2008, 56, 898-903

[47] Pal SK, Hurria A.: Impact of age, sex, and comorbidity on cancer treatment and disease progression *J Clin Oncol.* 2010 Jul 19.

[48] Klepin H, Mohile S, Hurria A.: Geriatric assessment in Older patients with Breast Cancer .*J Natl Compr Canc Netw.* 2009 Feb;7(2):226-36

[49] Ferrucci L and Balducci L: Anemia of aging: role of chronic inflammation and cancer. *Semin Hematol,* 2008, 45, 242-249

[50] Haider SI, Johnell K, Weitoft GR et al : The influence of educational level on polypharmacyand inappropriate drug use. A register based study of more than 600000 older people. *J Am Ger Soc,* 2009, 57, 62-69

[51] Maggiore RJ, Gross CP, Hurria A.: Polypharmacy in older Adults with Cancer. *Oncologist.* 2010;15(5):507-22

[52] Inouye SK, Studenski S, Tinetti ME,: Geriatric syndromes: clinical, research, and policy implications of a core geriatric concept. *J Am Geriatr Soc.* 2007 May;55(5):780-91

[53] Fong TG, Tulebaev SR, Inouye SK.: Delirium in elderly adults: diagnosis, prevention and treatment. *Nat Rev Neurol.* 2009 Apr;5(4):210-20.

[54] Lee SJ, Lindquist K, Segal MRet al: Development and validation of a prognostic index for 4-year mortality in older adults. *JAMA.* 2006 Feb 15;295(7):801-8.

[55] Carey EC, Covinsky KE, Lui LY, et al: Prediction of mortality in community-living frail elderly people with long-term care needs. *J Am Geriatr Soc.* 2008 Jan;56(1):68-75

[56] Schonberg MA, Davis RB, McCarthy EP, et al: Index to predict 5-year mortality of community-dwelling adults aged 65 and older using data from the National Health Interview Survey. *J Gen Intern Med.* 2009 Oct;24(10):1115-22

[57] Extermann M; Overcash J; Lyman GH; et al Comorbidity and performance status are independent in older cancer patients. *J Cin Oncol*, 1998, 16, 1582-1587

[58] Ingram SS, Seo PH, Martell RE, et al l: Comprehensive assessment of elderly Cancer patients: the feasiblility of self-report methodology. *J Clin Oncol*, 2002, 20, 770-775

[59] Repetto L, Fratino L, Audisio RA, et al: Comprehensive Geriatric assessment adds information to Eastern Cooperative Group Performance Status in Elderly Cancer Patients: an Italian Group for geriatric Oncology Study. *J Clin Oncol*, 2002, 15, 494-502

[60] PACE participants, Shall we operate? Preoperative assessment of elderly cancer patietiens (PACE) can help. A SIOG surgical taskforce prospective Study. *Crit Rev Oncol Hematol*,2008, 65, 156-163.

[61] Fried LP, Tangen CM, Walston J, et al : Frailty in older adults: evidence for a phenotype. *J Gerontol A Biol Sci Med Sci.* 2001 Mar;56(3):M146-56

[62] Ensrud KE, Ewing SK, Taylor BC, et al. (2008); Comparison of two frailty indices for prediction of falls, disability, fractures, and death in older women. *Arch Intern Med,* 168, 382-389.

[63] Ensrud KE, Ewing SK, Cawthon PM, et al, Cummings SR; Osteoporotic Fractures in Men Research Group (2009): A comparison of two frailty indices for prediciton of falls, disability, fractures and death in older men. *J Am Ger Soc*, 57, 492-49

[64] Searle SD, Mitnitski A, Gahbauer EA, Gill TM, Rockwood K.(2008): A standard procedure for creating a frailty index. *BMC Geriatr*, 30, 8-24.

[65] Xue QL, Bandeen-Roche K, Varadhan R et al l: Initial Manifestations of frailty criteria and the development of frailty phenotype in the Women Health and Aging Study II. *J Gerontol Med Sci* 2008, 63, 984-990

[66] Anonimous): Assessing Care of Vulnerable Elders-3 Quality Indicators. *J Am Ger Soc,* 2007, 55, supplement 2, s464-487

[67] Gabutti G: Vaccine against Papilloma Virus: a review of clinical studies. *J prev Med Hyg*, 2009, 50, 79-89

[68] Martino S, Costantino J, McNabb M, et al: The role of selective estrogen receptor modulators in the prevention of breast cancer: comparison of the clinical trials. *Oncologist*, 2004, 9, 116-125

[69] Thompson IM: Chemoprevention of prostate cancer: agents and study design. *J Urol,* 2007, 178, s9-s13.

[70] Wirth LJ, Haddad RI, Posner MR.: Progress and perspectives in chemoprevention of head and neck cancer. *Expert Rev Anticancer Ther.* 2003 Jun;3(3):339-55

[71] Andriole GL, Bostwick DG, Brawley OW, et al: Effec of dutasteride on the risk of prostate cancer *N Engl J Med.* 2010 Apr 1;362(13):1192-202.

[72] Zilli M, Iacobelli S.: Chemoprophylaxis in gastro-intestinal tumors. *Eur Rev Med Pharmacol Sci.* 2010 Apr;14(4):285-91

[73] Smith DL Jr, Elam CF Jr, Mattison JA, et al: Metformin supplementation and life span in Fischer 344 rats. *J Gerontol A Biol Sci Med Sci.* 2010 May;65(5):468-74

[74] Anisimov VN, Egormin PA, Piskunova TS, et al: Metformin extends life span of HER-2/neu transgenic mice and in combination with melatonin inhibits growth of transplantable tumors in vivo. *Cell Cycle*. 2010 Jan 1;9(1):188-97. Epub 2010 Jan 22.

[75] Balducci L; Beche' C: Secondary prevention of cancer in the older person. In: Balducci L; Lyman GH; Ershler WB; Extermann M: *Comprehensive Geriatric Oncology*. Taylor and Francis, London, 2004 pp 365-376

[76] Grce M.: primary and secondary prevention of cervical cancer. *Expert Rev Mol Diagn*. 2009 Nov;9(8):851-7.

[77] Walter LC, Lewis CL, Barton MB.: Screeing for colorectal, breast, and cervical cancer in the elderly: a review of the evidence. *Am J Med*. 2005 Oct;118(10):1078-86

[78] Walter LC, Bertenthal D, Lindquist K et al: PSA screening in older men with limited life-expectancy. *JAMA*. 2006 Nov 15;296(19):2336-42.

[79] Terret C, Castel-Kremer E, Albrand G, et al: Effects of comorbidity on screening and early diagnosis of cancer in elderly people. *Lancet Oncol*. 2009 Jan;10(1):80-7.

[80] Ramesh HS; Jain S; Audisio RA: Implications of age in surgical oncology *Oncologist*, 2005, 11, 488-494

[81] Kristjansson SR, Nesbakken A, Jordhøy MS, et al Comprehensive geriatric assessment can predict complications in elderly patients after elective surgery for colorectal cancer: A prospective observational cohort study. *Crit Rev Oncol Hematol*. 2010 in press

[82] Zachariah B, Balducci L, Venkattaramanabalaji GV, et al: Radiotherapy for cancer patients aged 80 and older: a study of effectiveness and side effects. *Int J Radiat Oncol Biol Phys*. 1997 Dec 1;39(5):1125-9.

[83] Olmi P, Ausili-Cefaro G. Radiotherapy in the elderly: a multicentric prospective study on 2060 patients referred to 37 Italian radiation therapy centers. *Rays*. 1997 Jan-Mar;22(1 Suppl):53-6.

[84] Mitsuhashi N, Hayakawa K, Yamakawa M, et al: cancer in patients aged 90 and older: radiation therapy. *Radiology*. 1999 Jun;211(3):829-33.

[85] Langer CJ. : elderly patients with lung cancer: biases and evidence *Curr Treat Options Oncol*. 2002 Feb;3(1):85-102.

[86] Balducci L. : Treating elderly patients with hormone-sensitive breast cancer: what do the data show? *Cancer Treat Rev*. 2009 Feb;35(1):47-56.

[87] Lattouf JB, Saad F. Bone complications of androgen deprivation therapy: screening, prevention, and treatment. *Curr Opin Urol*. 2010 May;20(3):247-52.

[88] Hollis BW: Assessment of vitamin D status and definition of a normal circulating range of 25-hydroxyvitamin D. *Curr Opin Endocrinol Diabetes, obesity*, 2008, 15, 489-494

[89] Yealtey EA: Assessing the Vitamin D Status of the US population. *Am J Clin Nutr*, 2008, 88, 558S-564S

[90] Casey R; Gesztesj Z; Rochford J: Long term zoledronic acid during androgen blockade for prostate cancer. *Can J Urol*, 2010, 17, 5170-5177

[91] Rizzoli R, Yasothan U, Kirkpatrick P. : Denosumab. *Nat Rev Drug Discov*. 2010 Aug;9(8):591-2.

[92] Scherr DS; Pitts WR: the non-steroidal effect of dyethilstiblbestrol. The rational for androgen deprivation without estrogen deprivation in the treatment of prostate cancer. *J Urol*, 2003, 170, 1703-1708

[93] Keating NL, O'Malley AJ, Freedland SJ et al: Diabetes and cardiovascular disease during androgen deprivation therapy: observational study of veterans with prostate cancer. *J Natl Cancer Inst.* 2010 Jan 6;102(1):39-46.

[94] Carreca I, Balducci L. Cancer chemotherapy in the older cancer patient *Urol Oncol.* 2009 Nov-Dec;27(6):633-42.

[95] Lyman GH, Kuderer NM. A primer in prognostic and predictive models: development and validation of neutropenia risk models. *Support Cancer Ther.* 2005 Apr 1;2(3):168-75.

[96] Kuderer NM, Dale DC, Crawford J, et al: Impact of primary prophylaxis with granulocyte colony-stimulating factor on febrile neutropenia and mortality in adult cancer patients receiving chemotherapy: a systematic review. *J Clin Oncol.* 2007 Jul 20;25(21):3158-67.

[97] Balducci L ; Al Halawani H ; Charu V et al: Elderly cancer patients receiving chemotherapy benefit from first-cycle pegfilgrastim. *Oncologist.* 2007 Dec;12(12):1416-24.

[98] Bohlius J, Schmidlin K, Brillant C, et al: Erythropoietin or Darbepoetin for patients with cancer--meta-analysis based on individual patient data. *Cochrane Database Syst Rev.* 2009 Jul 8;(3):CD007303. Review.

[99] Sonis ST. Regimen-related gastrointestinal toxicities in cancer patients.*Curr Opin Support Palliat Care.* 2010 Mar;4(1):26-30.

[100] Minton O, Richardson A, Sharpe M, et al A systematic review and meta-analysis of the pharmacological treatment of cancer-related fatigue.*J Natl Cancer Inst.* 2008 Aug 20;100(16):1155-66.

[101] Dy SM, Lorenz KA, Naeim A et al: Evidence-based recommendations for cancer fatigue, anorexia, depression, and dyspnea. *J Clin Oncol.* 2008 Aug 10;26(23):3886-95

[102] Broder H, Gottlieb RA, Lepor NE. :chemotherapy and cardiotoxicity *Rev Cardiovasc Med.* 2008 Spring;9(2):75-8

[103] Balducci L.: Molecular Insights in cancer Treatment and Prevention. *Int J Biochem Cell Biol.* 2007;39(7-8):1329-36

[104] Gonsalves W, Ganti AK.: targeted anti-cancer agents in the elderly. *Crit Rev Oncol Hematol.* 2010 in press

[105] Urban D, Cherny N, Catane R.: The management of cancer pain in the elderly. *Crit Rev Oncol Hematol.* 2010 Feb;73(2):176-83.

[106] Jones RN; Fong TG; Metzger E et al: Aging, brain disease, and reserve: implications for delirium. *Am J Geriatr Psych,* 2010, 18, 117-127

[107] Deeken JF, Taylor KL, Mangan P, et al: Care for the caregivers: a review of self-report instruments developed to measure the burden, needs, and quality of life of informal *J Pain Symptom Manage.* 2003 Oct;26(4):922-53

[108] Dominguez LJ.: Medicine and the arts: l'incendio di Borgo. *Commentary Acad Med.* 2009 Sep;84(9):1260-1.

[109] Manton KG, Gu X, Lowrimore GR. Cohort changes in active life expectancy in the U.S. elderly population: experience from the 1982-2004 National Long-Term Care Survey. *J Gerontol B Psychol Sci Soc Sci.* 2008 Sep;63(5):S269-81.

In: Essentials and Updates in Urologic Oncology
Editor: Philippe E. Spiess

ISBN: 978-1-62081-494-9
© 2013 Nova Science Publishers, Inc.

Chapter XXXVIII

Assessment of the Older Adult with Cancer

Ari Vanderwalde[*] and Arti Hurria

City of Hope Comprehensive Cancer Center, Duarte, California, US

Abstract

Cancer is a disease associated with aging and this is particularly true for urologic malignancies. Treating an older adult with cancer requires a number of special considerations because the aging process is characterized by a decrease in physiologic reserve. This decrease in reserve affects most organ systems and may impact cancer treatment tolerance. Additionally, aging is associated with an increased number of competing co-morbid medical conditions which may impact treatment tolerance, as well as life expectancy. A Comprehensive Geriatric Assessment (CGA) can be utilized to weigh the risks and benefits of cancer therapy for the individual patient. A CGA includes an evaluation of functional status, co-morbid medical conditions, cognitive status, psychological state, nutritional status, social support, and a review of medications. Each of these domains can predict for morbidity and mortality in older adults, and can identify patients that might benefit from targeted interventions prior to cancer treatment. Consensus panels have recommended the administration of a CGA both before and during treatment of older patients with cancer. A version of the CGA is currently being incorporated in cooperative group trials. This chapter describes the utility of the CGA in the care of older adults with urologic malignancies, as well as various means of administering the CGA in oncology practice.

---

[*] Ari Vanderwalde, MD, MPH, Fellow, Department of Medical Oncology & Experimental Therapeutics, Department of Hematology and Hematopoietic Cell Transplantation, City of Hope Comprehensive Cancer Center, Phone: (626) 256-4673, Fax: (626) 301-8233, E-mail: avanderwalde@coh.org

Introduction

Urologic cancers are generally diseases of older adults. Of the more than 200,000 patients diagnosed yearly with prostate cancer, the median age is 67 years. Likewise, the median age of the more than 70,000 patients diagnosed with bladder cancer is 73 years, with 27.4% of all bladder cancers diagnosed between the ages of 65 and 74; 32.1% between 75 and 84; and 12.8% 85+ years of age.[1] Of the almost 60,000 kidney cancers, the median age is 64 years.[1] Both the prevalence and the average age of all of these cancers will be further increasing over the next few decades as the population continues to age.[2, 3]

It is known that aging is associated with a progressive decrease in physiologic reserve.[4, 5] The age-related physiological decline in organ systems may not be evident at times of rest, but becomes most apparent when the body is stressed.[6] This age-related decrease in reserve may affect tolerance to cancer treatment. The decreased reserve affects every individual at a unique pace, and as such it may be difficult to achieve an *a priori* determination of who will be able to withstand the stressors of cancer therapy based on chronological age alone. A geriatric assessment provides a comprehensive overview of the older adult's physiologic reserve by evaluating independent risk factors of morbidity and mortality, such as functional status, comorbidity, cognitive function, medication review, nutritional status, and psychological and social support

In this chapter, we will discuss the domains of the comprehensive geriatric assessment, the rationale behind the domains, tools to perform the assessment, and methods to calculate life expectancy. Finally, this chapter will review time-effective ways to perform these assessments and how to interpret the results.

The Treatment Gap

Despite the large number of older adults with cancer, older adults are less likely to be offered treatment for cancer than younger adults. In an analysis using the SEER registry, one group of investigators found that adults over the age of 70 with bladder cancer were less than half as likely to undergo a radical cystectomy than adults age 55-59 years.[7, 8]

Age influences treatment decisions in prostate cancer as well. In a survey of 244 British urologists, 64% reported that they would recommend radical prostatectomy for a 55 year old man, 24% for a 69 year old man, and 0% for a man age 75 or older. On the other hand, conservative management was recommended by only 8% of urologists for the 55 year old man, 13% for a 69 year old man, and 24% for a man age 75 or older. Of note, no further information on comorbidity or functional status was provided to the urologists, and the treatment recommendations were largely driven by age alone.[9, 10] A retrospective study of 260,000 patients treated from the national cancer database showed that only 6% of men over age 75 with prostate cancer underwent a radical prostatectomy between 1992 and 1994, as compared to 48% of those aged 50-64. This difference was maintained even when controlling for stage of disease.[11]

This treatment gap extends across malignancies and modalities of treatment. In a study of a breast cancer cohort deemed to be eligible for adjuvant chemotherapy based on consensus guidelines, there was a strong relationship between increasing age of the patient and decreasing likelyhood that the physician will recommend chemotherapy. This was the case even though there was no observed difference in patient preference.[12] In fact, many older adults, regardless of cancer type, would be equally motivated to try chemotherapy, despite knowing the risks. In a survey of patients age 70 to 95 both with and without cancer, two thirds of those with cancer said that they would be willing to receive "strong" chemotherapy despite increased likelihood of toxicity. In addition, two thirds of all patients, whether they had cancer or not, expressed theoretical willingness to receive "mild" chemotherapy.[13]

Reasons for these treatment differences between older and younger adults are multi-factorial. Possible etiologies include poorer access to care, poorer perceived or actual treatment tolerance,[14] other comorbidities (outweighing the risk of cancer or influencing treatment tolerance), and/or patient or physician preference.[8, 10, 12-16] Furthermore, there are less data on older adults from randomized clinical trials to guide treatment decisions.[16-18]

Life Expectancy

An integral part of the cancer treatment decision is to determine whether the patient will die *of* cancer, or simply *with* cancer. Furthermore, one needs to weigh whether the cancer is likely to cause significant disability for the patient in his/her lifetime.[19] While younger patients with cancer can usually anticipate that having a diagnosis of cancer will shorten their life expectancy without treatment, the same may not be true for older adults. The prevalence of comorbid conditions increases with age.[20, 21] Additionally, some cancers appear more indolent in older adults.[22-24] Competing comorbidities increase the risk that the older adult with cancer may die of another cause, while indolent cancer may make it more likely that the cancer will not influence the lifespan or even quality of life of the patient.

However, the life expectancy of an older adult is often longer than might be thought. Total life expectancy changes with age. While a child born in the United States has an average expected life-span of 78 years, a person aged 65 can expect to live, on average, to 84 years (an additional 19 years).[25] Life expectancy can be further influenced by gender, race, socioeconomic factors, and area or country of residence.[25] The variability in these estimates is large. Walter and Covinsky, using US life-table data, described life expectancy by upper, middle, and lower quartiles. For example, while the median additional life expectancy for a 70 year old woman is 15.7 years, 25% of 70 year-old women can expect to live an additional 21.3 years or more, while 25% of these women can only expect an additional 9.5 years or less.[26] Validated tools are available to predict the risk of mortality. Carey et al developed a functional morbidity index that takes into account age, gender, and self-reported functional status to stratify adults age 70 or older into varying risk groups for 2-year mortality.[27] Lee et al developed a similar tool for clinicians to determine 4-year mortality. This tool takes into account comorbid conditions as well as age, gender, and functional status.[28]

Estimation of life-expectancy, however, may have significant intra-observer variability. In patients with cancer, physicians may well over- or underestimate life expectancy based on a variety of factors. Additionally, life expectancy on its own only provides a small part of the equation that ultimately will determine whether or not to treat an older adult.

Additional considerations include whether the cancer will influence life expectancy,[1] the short- and long-term toxicities of cancer treatment, and quality-of-life with or without cancer treatment, [29, 30]

Comprehensive Geriatric Assessment

A Comprehensive Geriatric Assessment (CGA) has been used in the general geriatric population to assist in an evaluation of life expectancy, to identify vulnerable older adults, and to guide interventions to optimize care in this population.[31-33] Consensus guidelines recommend the routine use of the CGA for older adults with cancer; however the exact means of integrating a CGA into oncology practice is an area of active research.[34, 35] It has been postulated that the CGA might be used to guide treatment strategies in older adults with cancer,[33, 36, 37] and various cancer-specific geriatric assessments have been proposed, with one currently being tested in cooperative groups.[37, 38] The domains of a CGA are summarized below and in Table 2.[39]

Table 1. Life Expectancy Based on Years Already Lived, 2007

Age (years)	Life expectancy (total years)	Median years of life remaining
0	78	78
60	83	23
65	84	19
70	85	15
75	87	12
80	89	9
85	92	7
90	95	5
95	98	3
100	102	2

Adapted from Table 7 in Xu et al. National Vital Statistics Reports. Deaths: Final Data for 2007. National Vital Statistics System, Centers for Disease Control and Prevention, US Department of Health and Human Services 2010; 58(19).[25]

Table 2. Geriatric Assessment Domains and Measures[147]

Domain	Possible Measures	Predictive Value	Number of Items
Physical Function	Activities of Daily Living (ADLs)[51]	Predicts institutionalization and mortality in geriatric populations	6
	Instrumental Activities of Daily Living[52]	Predicts survival in selected small studies of older cancer patients	8
	Vulnerable Elders Survey[148]	Predicts mortality and functional decline in geriatric populations	13
	Get Up and Go Test[149]	Correlates with ability to transfer independently	1
	Short Physical Performance Battery	Predicts future disability and mortality in geriatric populations	5

Domain	Possible Measures	Predictive Value	Number of Items
Comorbidity	Charlson Comorbidity Index[63]	Analyzed 1-year risk for mortality. Age-adjusted index is available	19
	Lee Prognostic Index[28]	Analyzed 4-year risk for mortality (includes age, sex, comorbid medical conditions, and functional status)	12
	ACE-27[64]	Analyzes the impact of comorbidity in patients with cancer	27
Cognition	Mini-Mental State Examination[150]	All are screening tools for cognitive impairment and have been associated with dementia and increased morbidity and mortality in community-dwelling samples	11
	Blessed Orientation-Memory Concentration (OMC) Test[151]	Associated with impaired survival in cancer patients	6
	Short Portable Mental Status Questionnaire (SPMC)[152]	Associated with mortality in community-dwelling older populations	10
Nutrition	Self-reported weight loss	Associated with impaired survival in cancer patients	1
	Body Mass Index (BMI)	<18.5 kg/m^2 cutoff per World Health Organization (WHO)	1
	Mini-Nutritional Assessment (MNA)[127]	Predictive of mortality in hospitalized elders	18
Psychological State	Distress Thermometer[98]	High concordance between scores on the Distress Thermometer and the Hospital Anxiety and Depression Scale Cutoff score of 4 had the greatest sensitivity and specificity when compared with the Center for Epidemiological Studies Depression scale Patients with cancer who scored $\geq$ 4 on the Distress Thermometer were more likely to also report physical, emotional, practical, and family problems	1
Social support	MOS Social Support Survey: Emotional/Information and Tangible Subscales[153]	Tangible subscale measures access to material aid or behavioral assistance and emotional/information subscales measure the expression of positive affect and empathetic understanding; the offering of advice, information, guidance, or feedback	20
Geriatric syndromes Incontinence Osteoporosis Frailty Dementia Delirium Falls Pressure sores Neglect and abuse	No comprehensive tool exists, but questions to ask include frequency and severity of syndromes that are not assessed within other measures of the CGA		

From Klepin, Mohile, Hurria. J Natl Compr Canc Netw 2009;7:226 Table 2.[147] Reprinted with permission from *JNCCN- Journal of the National Comprehensive Cancer Network*.

Functional Status

A diagnosis of cancer is associated with an increased need for functional assistance. In a population study of 9745 Medicare beneficiaries, cancer was reported by 17% of the study cohort. Those older adults with cancer had poorer health and more functional limitations than those without cancer.[40] Another study of 363 patients age 65 or older with cancer also showed high prevalence of functional limitations, with difficulties in function reported by over half of patients.[41]

Measures of functional status assess an individual's ability to perform daily tasks. In oncology practice, the tools most often used to assess a patient's functional capacity are the Karnofsky[42] and ECOG[43] performance status (PS) scales. Patients are assigned a score which provides a broad overview of their functional status, and predicts overall survival and treatment tolerance among patients with cancer of any age. However, this assessment misses the granular details regarding daily functioning which may be important to consider in cancer treatment planning.[20, 44-50] In comparison, a geriatrician's assessment of functional status includes an evaluation of the patient's ability to complete Activities of Daily Living (ADLs) and Instrumental Activities of Daily Living (IADLs). ADLs are the activities that are necessary for basic self-care such as feeding, transferring, grooming, dressing and toileting.[51] IADLs include activities necessary to function independently in the home and neighborhood, such as housekeeping, preparing meals, shopping, and managing finances and medications.[52]

Assessments of ADLs and IADLs are more likely to identify functional deficits than performance status measures. In a cohort of 363 cancer patients with ECOG PS scores of <2 (representing a higher functional level), 9% were found to have limitations in ADLs, while 38% were found to have limitations in IADLs.[45] Cancer is associated with an increased need for assistance with ADLs and IADLs. In a study of older adults with metastatic breast cancer, 26% required assistance with ADLs and 73% required assistance with IADLs.[53] This need for assistance persists among older cancer survivors.[40, 54]

Limitations in functional status have been found to be predictive of life expectancy and overall survival in older patients with cancer.[55] In a study of 566 patients age 70 or older with advanced lung cancer receiving chemotherapy, mortality was influenced by the need for assistance with IADLs. Those with the most independence in IADLs prior to chemotherapy lived significantly longer than those who had the least independence.[56] Other studies have indicated that the need for functional assistance is associated with an increased risk of chemotherapy toxicity. In a study of 83 patients age 70 or older with ovarian cancer receiving carboplatin and cyclophosphamide, independent predictors of chemotherapy toxicity included needing assistance (living alone with assistance or requiring assistance in a medical institution), ECOG PS ≥2, and depression.[33] A survey of oncologists and primary care providers demonstrated that functional status, when combined with an assessment of comorbidity, plays an important role in determining whether an older adult with breast cancer is offered adjuvant therapy.[57]

Finally, from a practical standpoint it is imperative to understand a patient's functional capacity in order to determine whether the patient can comply with the cancer treatment plan and recognize toxicity. Before prescribing oral chemotherapy, for example, it is important to know whether the patient is able to manage his/her own medications, and if not, who will administer them. Furthermore, it is important to determine if the patient understands the signs and symptoms of toxicity as well as the indications and means to seek medical attention.

Comorbidity

With increasing age, there is an increase in both the number and severity of comorbid medical conditions.[58-60] Competing risks make it more likely that any individual additional diagnosis (such as cancer) will have less of an impact on life expectancy. The threshold for when to start treatment may therefore be shifted to only those treatments with high likelihood of efficacy and a low risk of toxicity. Conversely, though, cancer may outweigh the risk of other comorbidities, such as with very aggressive tumors. In one study of older adults with node positive breast cancer, standard adjuvant chemotherapy was associated with a significant improvement in both disease-free and overall survival within a short follow-up period (2.4 years). Within this period, only 2% of patients died from causes unrelated to their cancer or treatment.[61] There are a number of tools available to assess for comorbidity.[62-66] A summary of some of these tools and their predictive ability are described in Table 2.

Increased numbers of comorbidities are associated with decreased overall survival in older adults with cancer. In a study of 120 patients age 70 or older with advanced lung cancer, increased comorbidity was found to independently predict poorer overall survival.[67] In another study of patients with early breast cancer, those patients with three or more selected comorbid conditions were 20 times more likely to die of a cause other than their breast cancer and 4 times more likely to die of any cause.[68] An observational prospective study of over 17,000 patients with a variety of cancers found that regardless of cancer type or stage, more severe comorbidity was associated with worse overall survival.[64]

Specific comorbid conditions may independently affect survival of older adults with cancer. Yancik et al. performed a SEER registry database search for patients older than 55 years who were diagnosed with colon cancer. The authors found that some cancers were more life-threatening than others depending on the comorbid conditions. Liver disease conferred a 3 fold increased risk of mortality, while emphysema conferred a 1.7 fold risk. A history of cardiac arrest, congestive heart failure, or renal failure conferred a very high risk of early mortality. Type 1 diabetes, cardiac arrhythmia, valvular heart disease, or prior malignant disease also conferred a higher risk of mortality.[69] In a randomized controlled trial of adjuvant chemotherapy in adults with colon cancer, the presence of diabetes was independently associated with worse disease-free survival and overall survival.[70]

The presence of comorbid conditions can potentially limit a patient's ability to tolerate cancer treatment.[71] In the study (described above) of 120 older adults with advanced lung cancer, a higher level of comorbidity was associated with an increased likelihood of patients discontinuing treatment.[67]

Advanced age alone, however, should not be confounded with comorbidity. A study of 1,255 patients with non-small cell lung cancer found that while comorbidity was associated with an increased risk of mortality, age itself was not an independent predictor. However, adults age 65 and older *were* more likely to have more comorbidity than younger adults.[72] Likewise, in a study of patients with breast cancer, comorbidity predicted the likelihood of toxicity from treatment better than age alone.[70, 71]

In the assessment of comorbid conditions, special consideration should be given to a certain number of conditions called "Geriatric Syndromes." These include dementia, depression, delirium, incontinence, a history of falls, bone fractures, vertigo, and neglect and abuse.[19] Geriatric syndromes have been associated with a decreased life expectancy.[73]

Importantly, assessment of functional status cannot substitute for an evaluation of comorbid medical conditions. In a study of 203 older adults with cancer, there was no correlation between comorbidity and functional status as measured using either ECOG performance status or IADLs.[21]

Cognitive Function

Rates of cognitive dysfunction increase with age, and an assessment of cognitive status is an integral part of the geriatric assessment. From a practical standpoint, assessment of cognitive status is necessary to ensure adequate understanding of the diagnosis and treatment plan. An assessment of cognitive function is also necessary to ensure that the patient can correctly take oral cancer therapy or home-administered supportive care medications.

A diagnosis of dementia is an independent predictor of morbidity and mortality;[74-77] however the diagnosis may not be readily apparent. In a study of 1,764 patients admitted to a post-acute rehabilitation setting, 24.1% were evaluated as having dementia. However, only one third of this number (301/425) carried a diagnosis of dementia prior to admission.[78] This has been demonstrated in older adults with cancer as well. In a retrospective study of 119 patients admitted to an Acute Care for Elders Unit, 27% scored in the abnormal range on a standard cognitive assessment, but only 36% of these had previously documented dementia.[79]

The presence of dementia affects the probability that a patient will receive care leading to cancer diagnosis or cancer treatment. One group of investigators reviewed cases of colon cancer in the SEER registry, and found that those patients with colon cancer and dementia were significantly more likely to have their colon cancer only reported at the time of death or found on autopsy. Those with dementia were less likely to have a pathologic diagnosis obtained, were less likely to undergo surgical resection, and were less likely to receive adjuvant chemotherapy.[80] Another study demonstrated that patients with Alzheimer's disease and breast cancer were more likely to be diagnosed at later stages and less likely to receive adjuvant chemotherapy.[81] In a study of 669 patients with a variety of cancers, decreased mental status was significantly and independently associated with a decreased likelihood of undergoing definitive surgical resection.[82] Various measures of cognitive status are available and can identify factors that may require more detailed screening and treatment (see Table 2).[35, 83-85]

Like functional status, cognitive function can change during the course of a patient's disease and treatment. In breast cancer, a number of studies have assessed whether cancer therapy can influence cognitive status. Though results are somewhat conflicting, it appears that, at least in the short term, chemotherapy is likely to affect cognition in a subset of patients.[86-90] This finding has been confirmed in older adults with breast cancer as well.[91, 92] Factors such as surgery, radiation, hormonal therapy, cancer-related fatigue, anesthesia, and depression can further influence cognitive status in older adults undergoing treatment for cancer.[93, 94] A recent study demonstrated that age and is related to post-treatment decline in processing speed in women exposed to chemotherapy for breast cancer.[95] Whether or not cognitive impairment is likely to occur during cancer treatment is of critical import for patients. In a study of adults age 60 or over with limited life expectancy due to a variety of illnesses, 89% stated that they would not undergo therapy even if the outcome was increased survival if there were to be severe cognitive impairment as a result.[96]

Psychological State

More than one-third of older adults with cancer experience psychological distress as a result of their diagnosis or treatment.[97, 98] Distress can be measured using the Distress Thermometer, which was specifically developed for adults with cancer.[99, 100] The tool can be completed by patients and contains questions in five categories; physical, emotional, family, spiritual, and practical. In reviewing this assessment, a physician can be alerted to potential problems. This tool has shown good correlation with the more comprehensive Hospital Anxiety and Depression Scale.[101]

Depression is commonly associated with distress. Clinically significant depression is present in up to 25% of older adults with cancer and can be a challenging diagnosis to recognize.[97, 102] Mood disorders in older adults are associated with functional decline, and may be associated with cognitive decline and physical disorders.[102-104] Greater numbers of other comorbid conditions among older adults are associated with an increased risk of depression and anxiety.[103]

Depression interferes with treatment compliance, and may therefore affect overall survival in adults with cancer.[105] In patients with cancer, there is a particular risk of exhibiting harmful behaviors as a result of depression. In a study of 2,924 patients with cancer, 7.8% (229 of 2,924; 95% CI, 6.9% to 8.9%) reported having suicidal thoughts or thinking that they were "better off dead" within the previous two weeks. Risk factors included older age, emotional distress, and significant pain.[106] A retrospective analysis of adults age 65 or older showed that the only medical condition significantly associated with an increased risk of suicide was cancer (OR 2.3, 95% CI, 1.1-4.8).[107]A variety of measures are available to screen for depression in the older adult (see Table 2).[108, 109]

Social Support

Social isolation can greatly increase the negative physical and psychological impact of cancer. Loneliness and poor social support have been associated with both increased morbidity and mortality in older adults,[110, 111] as well as a decreased sense of well-being.[112] Lack of social support is common among older adults. One group of investigators interviewed 1,299 older adults in their homes. Thirty-four percent of adults were found to have a non-integrated social network, and 38% were lonely.[112]

The home caregiver is often a crucial resource for an older patient with cancer. However, in most developed countries there have been shifts in the structure and location of family networks, making it less likely for older adults to have close family available in a geographically reasonable area to help provide care.[113] Most often, the caregiver is either an elderly spouse, who may have barriers to giving care because of his or her own poor health, or an adult child who does not live with the patient and therefore is providing "distant caregiving."

Social support can impact an older adult's psychological state,[112] and can affect medication adherence. In one meta-analysis, medication adherence was found to be 1.7 times higher among patients with a stable family structure.[114]

The presence and adequacy of social support may play a role in whether a patient receives treatment, what type of treatment is received, and ultimately the prognosis of the patient. In a study utilizing the SEER database of 32,268 women age 65 or older with breast cancer, unmarried status was associated with increased likelihood of being diagnosed at a later stage and a decreased likelihood of receiving definitive therapy. Additionally, even after controlling for tumor stage and size at diagnosis, unmarried women were more likely than married women to die from the breast cancer.[115]

The CGA includes identification of the patient's social network, identification of the primary caregiver, if any, and a determination of whether or not the patient is socially isolated. If a physician identifies that a patient has poor social support, it can be an opportunity for intervention to aid in the identification and education of potential caregivers.

Nutritional Status

Malnutrition is a common and serious condition in older adults. Low body mass index (BMI) and involuntary weight loss are both associated with an increased risk of mortality in community-dwelling older adults.[116, 117] In a large study of 7,527 patients age 70 or older, a BMI in the lowest 10% of the population was associated with a significantly increased risk of mortality.[118] In a study of 4,714 patients age 65 or older, weight loss of 5% or more was associated with an increased risk of mortality.[119]

Unintentional weight loss is associated with poorer overall survival among patients with cancer. In a study of 3,047 enrollees from 12 protocols administered by the Eastern Cooperative Oncology Group (ECOG), weight loss before starting chemotherapy was an independent predictor of survival. Additionally, weight loss was associated with poorer performance status.[120] Weight loss before initiating treatment has been associated with a poorer quality of life,[121, 122] poorer tolerance of chemotherapy,[120, 121] and decreased median survival.[120, 121] In patients with cancer, weight loss may be partly attributable to the underlying illness, a decreased appetite, and inadequate intake of calories.[35] Concerns regarding weight loss may cause significant distress.[123] Furthermore, social issues may compound under-eating.[124]

A nutritional evaluation should identify whether reversible factors are present that are causing weight loss, such as fatigue, lack of social support, mucositis, nausea, or medication side effects. Interventions by the treating team can range from counseling to enteral and parenteral nutrition. One commonly used measure of nutritional status in the CGA is the Mini-Nutritional Assessment (MNA). This assessment is composed of simple assessments and short questions that can identify older adults at risk for malnutrition at a point where the deleterious effects of malnutrition can be prevented.[125-127] While the long version takes approximately 15 minutes to administer, a validated short version that has good diagnostic accuracy has been developed that can be completed in about 4 minutes.[125, 128]

Review of Medication List

Older adults often take several medications (either prescribed or over the counter) placing them at risk for polypharmacy and drug interactions. [129] Furthermore, older adults often receive care across the multiple physicians and specialists, further increasing the potential for medication duplication or interactions.[130]

Additionally, there are age-related changes in physiology that effect the pharmacokinetics and pharmacodynamics of many drugs.[131] With aging, the percentage of body fat increases, changing the volume of distribution of many pharmaceutical agents.[132] Absorption of oral drugs can be affected by mucosal atrophy, decreased secretion of digestive enzymes, decreased intestinal motility, and decreased blood flow to the GI tract, which are all effects of aging.[133] Hepatic mass and hepatic blood flow decrease with age as well, which may effect metabolism and clearance of drugs.[134] Renal function declines in older adults, which may impact drug excretion.[14]

Therefore, a thorough review of an older adult's medications is an essential part of the CGA. Initial assessment of an older adult's medication list can allow for exploration of otherwise unidentified medical conditions, determination of medications that are duplicated, and identification of disorders that are not adequately treated. Furthermore, review of the medication list can identify potentially inappropriate medications with a high risk of side effects or drug interactions.[135] For example, patients taking inhibitors or inducers of the cytochrome P-450 system may need special tailoring of a treatment plan to prevent interactions that could influence the effect of the anti-cancer drug. Regular review of a medication list during therapy can allow the provider to discontinue any unnecessary medications, assess for drug-drug interactions, and assess adherence to a treatment plan.[132, 136]

Incorporating a CGA in Oncology Practice

The CGA has been shown to reveal multiple reversible conditions that could interfere and impact cancer treatment [21, 45]; however, there is no consensus on the optimal tools to use as part of the CGA. While the National Comprehensive Cancer Network (NCCN) and the International Society of Geriatric Oncology (SIOG) recommend the use of a CGA in all older adults with cancer,[34, 35] a number of methods have been studied to allow for a time-sensitive means of completing and reviewing the CGA. Additionally, various investigators are attempting to identify specific elements of the CGA that are most predictive of the outcomes of interest, including life expectancy, ability to tolerate chemotherapy, and surgical outcomes. Some of these time-saving methods and tools will be described below.

Provider-administered CGA: A full assessment by the healthcare provider as a part of the clinical interview has been evaluated in 30 older adults with cancer using the MACE (Multidimensional Assessment Protocol for Cancer). The mean time for administering this assessment was 27 minutes, and the tool included measurements of physical function, tumor characteristics, socioeconomic status, cognitive status, and psychological state.[37] While this tool is comprehensive, and was shorter than might be expected, a 27 minute assessment by the provider may remain prohibitive in a busy medical practice, especially if the assessment is readministered at sequential timepoints throughout treatment.

Self-administered CGA: Investigators from the Cancer in the Elderly Committee of the Cancer and Leukemia Group B have developed a CGA that is predominantly self-administered. Well-validated instruments that evaluate comorbidity, functional status, nutritional status, psychological state, and social support are all completed by the patient. The patient also lists the medications he or she is taking (both prescribed and over-the-counter). Healthcare providers perform a measure of cognition, a rating of the Karnofsky performance status, and a performance-based measure of functional status known as the Timed Up and Go. Pilot data have demonstrated that more than three quarters of participants are able to complete the self-administered portion on their own, and the mean time to completion is 27 minutes.[38] This type of assessment shows promise in being time saving for providers without sacrificing the detail of a CGA.

Mailed CGA: In theory, a full CGA could be mailed to patients prior to physician visits, and patients could fill out the assessment themselves or with the aid of their caregivers. Such a CGA was evaluated among a population of US Armed Services veterans with cancer at the North Carolina Veteran's Administration Hospital. While not all patients were older adults, the mean age was 67. Seventy-six percent of patients both completed the assessment and kept their appointment. The CGA captured important information, including functional status, polypharmacy, and comorbidity.[137] Disadvantages of this approach, however, include the lack of a cognitive screen. Furthermore, a proportion of patients did not complete the questionnaires.

Predicting Surgical Outcomes in Older Adults with Cancer

It is recognized that age alone is not the most important factor in the determination of surgical risk.[138, 139] The Preoperative Assessment of Cancer in the Elderly (PACE)[139-143] incorporates elements of the CGA, a brief fatigue inventory, performance status measures, and the American Society of Anesthesiologists grade.[141] In a prospective international study, 460 consecutive older adults with cancer underwent PACE prior to surgery. Poor performance status, dependence in IADLs, and moderate to severe fatigue were found to be independently associated with an extended hospital stay in the post-operative period.[142]Another recent trial demonstrated that measures of frailty, disability, and comorbidity are good predictors of 6-month post-operative mortality or institutionalization after major surgery in older adults.[144]

Predicting Chemotherapy Toxicity in Older Adults with Cancer: Investigators have sought to determine whether items in a CGA, in combination with those captured in daily clinical practice, can identify patients at risk for chemotherapy toxicity. A multi-institutional prospective study of 500 patients with cancer identified the following factors predictive of chemotherapy toxicity: 1) age $\geq$ 73, 2) cancer type (GI or GU), 3) receipt of poly-chemo-therapy, 4) receipt of standard dosing of chemotherapy, 5) creatinine clearance <34 ml/min (Jelliffe formula using ideal weight), 6) hemoglobin (male: <11 g/dL, female: <10 g/dL), 7) the need for assistance with taking medications, 8) $\geq$1 fall in the last 6 months, 9) hearing impairment, 10) limited in walking one block, and 11) decreased social activities due to physical or emotional health.[145] The Chemotherapy Risk Assessment Scale for High-Age Patients (CRASH) study evaluated 562 patients with cancer and found that albumin, IADLs, LDH, and diastolic blood pressure were predictive of hematologic toxicity, and hemoglobin, creatinine clearance, albumin, self-rated health, comorbidity, ECOG performance status, mini-mental status exam, and mini-nutritional assessment were predictive of non-hematologic toxicity.[146]

Conclusion

Cancer in older adults is understudied, and practice determinations are often extrapolated from studies of younger adults. Aging is associated with a decrease in physiologic reserve placing older adults at risk for treatment toxicity. However, as chronological age by itself cannot predict outcomes or tolerance to therapy, tools to determine "physiologic age" are necessary. The CGA identifies independent predictors or morbidity and mortality in older adults through an evaluation of functional status, comorbidity, cognition, psychological state, social support, nutrition, and concurrent medications. The CGA has been utilized to identify older adults with cancer at risk for chemotherapy toxicity and surgical complications. Research is underway to identify comprehensive yet time efficient means of incorporated the CGA into oncology practice.

References

[1]   Altekruse S, Kosary C, Krapcho M, Neyman N, Aminou R, Waldron W, et al. SEER Cancer Statistics Review, 1975-2007, National Cancer Institute. Bethesda, MD, *http://seer.cancer.gov/csr/1975_2007/ </csr/1975_2007/>*, based on November 2009 SEER data submission, posted to the SEER web site, 2010.

[2]   Yancik R, Ries LG. Cancer in the aged. An epidemiologic perspective on treatment issues. *Cancer*. 1991 Dec 1;68(11 Suppl):2502-10.

[3]   Yancik R. Population aging and cancer: a cross-national concern. *Cancer J*. 2005 Nov-Dec;11(6):437-41.

[4]   Sawhney R, Sehl M, Naeim A. Physiologic aspects of aging: impact on cancer management and decision making, part I. *Cancer J*. 2005 Nov-Dec;11(6):449-60.

[5]   Sehl M, Sawhney R, Naeim A. Physiologic aspects of aging: impact on cancer management and decision making, part II. *Cancer J*. 2005 Nov-Dec;11(6):461-73.

[6]   Duthie E. *Comprehensive Geriatric Oncology*: Taylor and Francis 2004.

[7]   Prout GR, Jr., Wesley MN, Yancik R, Ries LA, Havlik RJ, Edwards BK. Age and comorbidity impact surgical therapy in older bladder carcinoma patients: a population-based study. *Cancer*. 2005 Oct 15;104(8):1638-47.

[8]   Shariat SF, Sfakianos JP, Droller MJ, Karakiewicz PI, Meryn S, Bochner BH. The effect of age and gender on bladder cancer: a critical review of the literature. *BJU Int*. 2009 Feb;105(3):300-8.

[9]   Donovan JL, Frankel SJ, Faulkner A, Selley S, Gillatt D, Hamdy FC. Dilemmas in treating early prostate cancer: the evidence and a questionnaire survey of consultant urologists in the United Kingdom. *BMJ*. 1999 Jan 30;318(7179):299-300.

[10] Hall WH, Jani AB, Ryu JK, Narayan S, Vijayakumar S. The impact of age and comorbidity on survival outcomes and treatment patterns in prostate cancer. *Prostate Cancer Prostatic Dis.* 2005;8(1):22-30.

[11] Mettlin CJ, Murphy GP, Cunningham MP, Menck HR. The National Cancer Data Base report on race, age, and region variations in prostate cancer treatment. *Cancer.* 1997 Oct 1;80(7):1261-6.

[12] DeMichele A, Putt M, Zhang Y, Glick JH, Norman S. Older age predicts a decline in adjuvant chemotherapy recommendations for patients with breast carcinoma: evidence from a tertiary care cohort of chemotherapy-eligible patients. *Cancer.* 2003 May 1;97(9):2150-9.

[13] Extermann M, Albrand G, Chen H, Zanetta S, Schonwetter R, Zulian GB, et al. Are older French patients as willing as older American patients to undertake chemotherapy? *J Clin Oncol.* 2003 Sep 1;21(17):3214-9.

[14] Lichtman SM, Wildiers H, Chatelut E, Steer C, Budman D, Morrison VA, et al. International Society of Geriatric Oncology Chemotherapy Taskforce: evaluation of chemotherapy in older patients--an analysis of the medical literature. *J Clin Oncol.* 2007 May 10;25(14):1832-43.

[15] Droz JP, Aapro M, Balducci L. Overcoming challenges associated with chemotherapy treatment in the senior adult population. *Crit Rev Oncol Hematol.* 2008 Oct;68 Suppl 1(1):S1-8.

[16] Lane BR, Abouassaly R, Gao T, Weight CJ, Hernandez AV, Larson BT, et al. Active treatment of localized renal tumors may not impact overall survival in patients aged 75 years or older. *Cancer.* 2010 Jul 1;116(13):3119-26.

[17] Talarico L, Chen G, Pazdur R. Enrollment of Elderly Patients in Clinical Trials for Cancer Drug Registration: A 7-Year Experience by the US Food and Drug Administration. *J Clin Oncol.* 2004;22:4626-31.

[18] Chen H, Cantor A, Meyer JB, Corcoran M, Grendys E, Cavanaugh D, et al. Can older cancer patients tolerate chemotherapy? A prospective pilot study. *Cancer.* 2003 Feb 15;97(4):1107-14.

[19] Balducci L, Beghe C. Cancer in the Elderly: Biology, Prevention, and Treatment. In: Abeloff MD, Armitage JO, Niederhuber JE, Kastan MB, eds. *Abeloff's Clinical Oncology, 4th ed.* Philadelphia: Churchill Livingstone 2008:1039-49.

[20] Reuben D, Rubenstein L, Hirsch S, Hays R. Value of functional status as a predictor of mortality: results of a prospective study. *Am J Med.* 1992;93(6):663-9.

[21] Extermann M, Overcash J, Lyman GH, Parr J, Balducci L. Comorbidity and functional status are independent in older cancer patients. *Journal of Clinical Oncology.* 1998;16(4):1582-7.

[22] Balducci L. Geriatric oncology. *Crit Rev Oncol Hematol.* 2003 Jun;46(3):211-20.

[23] Balducci L, Beghe C. Cancer and age in the USA. *Crit Rev Oncol Hematol.* 2001 Feb;37(2):137-45.

[24] Audisio RA, Bozzetti F, Gennari R, Jaklitsch MT, Koperna T, Longo WE, et al. The surgical management of elderly cancer patients; recommendations of the SIOG surgical task force. *Eur J Cancer.* 2004 May;40(7):926-38.

[25] Xu J, Kochanek KD, Murphy SL, Tejada-Vera B. National Vital Statistics Reports. Deaths: Final Data for 2007. *US Department of Health and Human Services, Centers for Disease Control and Prevention, National Center for Health Statistics, National Vital Statistics System.* 2010 May;58(19).

[26] Walter LC, Covinsky KE. Cancer screening in elderly patients: a framework for individualized decision making. *JAMA.* 2001;285(21):2750-6.

[27] Carey EC, Walter LC, Lindquist K, Covinsky KE. Development and validation of a functional morbidity index to predict mortality in community-dwelling elders. *J Gen Intern Med.* 2004 Oct;19(10):1027-33.

[28] Lee SJ, Lindquist K, Segal MR, Covinsky KE. Development and Validation of a Prognostic Index for 4-Year Mortality in Older Adults. *JAMA.* 2006;295(7):801-8.

[29] Wedding U, Honecker F, Bockemeyer C, Pientka L, Hoffken K. Tolerance to chemotherapy in elderly patients with cancer. *Cancer Control.* 2007;14:44-56.

[30] Repetto L, Comandini D, Mammoliti S. Life expectancy, comorbidity, and quality of life: the treatment equation in the older cancer patients. *Crit Rev Oncol Hematol.* 2001;37:147-52.

[31] Rao AV, Seo PH, Cohen HJ. Geriatric Assessment and Comorbidity. *Semin Oncol.* 2004;31(2):149-59.

[32] Stuck AE, Siu AL, Wieland GD, Adams J, Rubenstein LZ. Comprehensive geriatric assessment: a meta-analysis of controlled trials. *Lancet.* 1993 Oct 23;342(8878):1032-6.

[33] Freyer G, Geay J, Touzet S, et al. Comprehensive geriatric assessment predicts tolerance to chemotherapy and survival in elderly patients with advanced ovarian carcinoma: a GINECO study. *Ann Oncol.* 2005;16(11):1795-800.

[34] Extermann M, Aapro M, Bernabei R, Cohen HJ, Droz JP, Lichtman S, et al. Use of comprehensive geriatric assessment in older cancer patients: recommendations from the task force on CGA of the International Society of Geriatric Oncology (SIOG). *Crit Rev Oncol Hematol.* 2005 Sep;55(3):241-52.

[35] Balducci L, Cohen HJ, Engstrom PF, Ettinger DS, Halter J, Gordon LI, et al. Senior adult oncology clinical practice guidelines in oncology. *J Natl Compr Canc Netw.* 2005 Jul;3(4):572-90.

[36] Bernabei R, Venturiero V, Tarsitani P, Gambassi G. The comprehensive geriatric assessment: when, where, how. *Crit Rev Oncol Hematol.* 2000 Jan;33(1):45-56.

[37] Monfardini S, Ferrucci L, Fratino L, Del Lungo I, Serraino D, Zagonel V. Validation of a multidimensional evaluation scale for use in elderly cancer patients. *Cancer.* 1996;77(2):395-401.

[38] Hurria A, Gupta S, Zauderer M, Zuckerman EL, Cohen HJ, Muss H, et al. Developing a cancer-specific geriatric assessment: a feasibility study. *Cancer.* 2005 Nov 1;104(9):1998-2005.

[39] Extermann M, Hurria A. Comprehensive geriatric assessment for older patients with cancer. *J Clin Oncol.* 2007;25:1824-31.

[40] Stafford RS, Cyr PL. The impact of cancer on the physical function of the elderly and their utilization of health care. *Cancer.* 1997;80(10):1973-80.

[41] Serraino D, Fratino L, Zagonel V. Prevalence of functional disability among elderly patients with cancer. *Crit Rev Oncol Hematol.* 2001 Sep;39(3):269-73.

[42] Karnofsky D, Burchenal J. The clinical evaluation of chemotherapeutic agents in cancer. In: Macleod C, ed. *Evaluation of chemotherapeutic agents.* New York: Columbia University Press 1948:191-205.

[43] Oken MM, Creech RH, Tormey DC, Horton J, Davis TE, McFadden ET, et al. Toxicity and response criteria of the Eastern Cooperative Oncology Group. *Am J Clin Oncol.* 1982 Dec;5(6):649-55.

[44] Hutchins LF, Unger JM, Crowley JJ, Coltman CA, Albain KS. Underrepresentation of Patients 65 Years of Age or Older in Cancer-Treatment Trials. *N Engl J Med.* 1999;341:2061-7.

[45] Repetto L, Fratino L, Audisio RA, Venturino A, Gianni W, Vercelli M, et al. Comprehensive Geriatric Assessment Adds Information to Eastern Cooperative Oncology Group Performance Status in Elderly Cancer Patients: An Italian Group for Geriatric Oncology Study. *J Clin Oncol.* 2002 January 15, 2002;20(2):494-502.

[46] Mor V, Wilcox V, Rakowski W, Hiris J. Functional transitions among the elderly: patterns, predictors, and related hospital use. *Am J Public Health.* 1994 August 1, 1994;84(8):1274-80.

[47] Barberger-Gateau P, Fabrigoule C, Helmer C, Rouch I, Dartigues J. Functional impairment in instrumental activities of daily living: an early clinical sign of dementia? *J Am Geriatr Soc.* 1999;47(4):456-62.

[48] Ponzetto M, Maero B, Maina P, Rosato R, Ciccone G, Merletti F, et al. Risk factors for early and late mortality in hospitalized older patients: the continuing importance of functional status. *J Gerontol A Biol Sci Med Sci.* 2003;58(11):1049-54.

[49] Inouye SK, Peduzzi PN, Robison JT, Hughes JS, Horwitz RI, Concato J. Importance of Functional Measures in Predicting Mortality Among Older Hospitalized Patients. *JAMA.* 1998 April 15, 1998;279(15):1187-93.

[50] Sleiman I, Rozzini R, Barbisoni P, Morandi A, Ricci A, Giordano A, et al. Functional Trajectories During Hospitalization: A Prognostic Sign for Elderly Patients. *J Gerontol A Biol Sci Med Sci.* 2009 June 2009;64A(6):659-63.

[51] Katz S, Ford A, Moskowitz R, Jackson B, Jaffe M. A standardized measure of biological and psychosocial function. *JAMA.* 1963;185:914-9.

[52] Fillenbaum GG. Screening the elderly. A brief instrumental activities of daily living measure. *J Am Geriatr Soc.* 1985 Oct;33(10):698-706.

[53] Del Mastro L, Perrone F, Repetto L, Manzione L, Zagonel V, Fratino L, et al. Weekly paclitaxel as first-line chemotherapy in elderly advanced breast cancer patients: a phase II study of the Gruppo Italiano di Oncologia Geriatrica (GIOGer). *Ann Oncol.* 2005 February 2005;16(2):253-8.

[54] Keating NL, Nørredam M, Landrum MB, Huskamp HA, Meara E. Physical and Mental Health Status of Older Long-Term Cancer Survivors. *J Am Geriatr Soc.* 2005;53(12):2145-52.

[55] Wedding U, Röhrig B, Klippstein A, Fricke H-J, Sayer H, Höffken K. Impairment in functional status and survival in patients with acute myeloid leukaemia. *Journal of Cancer Research and Clinical Oncology.* 2006;132(10):665-71.

[56] Maione P, Perrone F, Gallo C, Manzione L, Piantedosi F, Barbera S, et al. Pretreatment Quality of Life and Functional Status Assessment Significantly Predict Survival of Elderly Patients With Advanced Non--Small-Cell Lung Cancer Receiving Chemotherapy: A Prognostic Analysis of the Multicenter Italian Lung Cancer in the Elderly Study. *J Clin Oncol.* 2005 October 1, 2005;23(28):6865-72.

[57] Hurria A, Wong FL, Villaluna D, Bhatia S, Chung CT, Mortimer J, et al. Role of Age and Health in Treatment Recommendations for Older Adults With Breast Cancer: The Perspective of Oncologists and Primary Care Providers. *J Clin Oncol.* 2008 November 20, 2008;26(33):5386-92.

[58] Yancik R. Cancer burden in the aged: an epidemiologic and demographic overview. *Cancer.* 1997 Oct 1;80(7):1273-83.

[59] Asmis TR, Powell E, Karapetis CS, Jonker DJ, Tu D, Jeffery M, et al. Comorbidity, age and overall survival in cetuximab-treated patients with advanced colorectal cancer (ACRC)--results from NCIC CTG CO.17: a phase III trial of cetuximab versus best supportive care. *Ann Oncol.* 2010 Jul 5:Jul 5 (e-pub ahead of print).

[60] Extermann M, Aapro M. Assessment of the older cancer patient. *Hematol Oncol Clin North Am.* 2000;14:63-77.

[61] Muss HB, Berry DA, Cirrincione CT, Theodoulou M, Mauer AM, Kornblith AB, et al. Adjuvant Chemotherapy in Older Women with Early-Stage Breast Cancer. *N Engl J Med.* 2009 May 14, 2009;360(20):2055-65.

[62] Extermann M. Measuring comorbidity in older cancer patients. *Eur J Cancer.* 2000 Mar;36(4):453-71.

[63] Charlson M, Pompei P, Ales K, MacKenzie C. A new method of classifying prognostic comorbidity in longitudinal studies: development and validation. *J Chronic Dis.* 1987;40(5):373-83.

[64] Piccirillo JF, Tierney RM, Costas I, Grove L, Spitznagel EL, Jr. Prognostic Importance of Comorbidity in a Hospital-Based Cancer Registry. *JAMA.* 2004 May 26, 2004;291(20):2441-7.

[65] Charlson M, Szatrowski TP, Peterson J, Gold J. Validation of a combined comorbidity index. *J Clin Epidemiol.* 1994 Nov;47(11):1245-51.

[66] Miller MD, Paradis CF, Houck PR, Mazumdar S, Stack JA, Rifai AH, et al. Rating chronic medical illness burden in geropsychiatric practice and research: application of the Cumulative Illness Rating Scale. *Psychiatry Res.* 1992 Mar;41(3):237-48.

[67] Frasci G, Lorusso V, Panza N, Comella P, Nicolella G, Bianco A, et al. Gemcitabine Plus Vinorelbine Versus Vinorelbine Alone in Elderly Patients With Advanced Non-Small-Cell Lung Cancer. *J Clin Oncol.* 2000;18(13):2529-36.

[68] Satariano WA, Ragland DR. The Effect of Comorbidity on 3-Year Survival of Women with Primary Breast Cancer. *Ann Int Med.* 1994;120(2):104-10.

[69] Yancik R, Wesley MN, Ries LA, Havlik RJ, Long S, Edwards BK, et al. Comorbidity and age as predictors of risk for early mortality of male and female colon carcinoma patients: a population-based study. *Cancer.* 1998 Jun 1;82(11):2123-34.

[70] Meyerhardt JA, Catalano PJ, Haller DG, Mayer RJ, Macdonald JS, Benson AB, III, et al. Impact of Diabetes Mellitus on Outcomes in Patients With Colon Cancer. *Journal of Clinical Oncology.* 2003;21(3):433-40.

[71] Zauderer M, Patil S, Hurria A. Feasibility and toxicity of dose-dense adjuvant chemotherapy in older women with breast cancer. *Breast Cancer Research and Treatment.* 2009;117(1):205-10.

[72] Asmis TR, Ding K, Seymour L, Shepherd FA, Leighl NB, Winton TL, et al. Age and comorbidity as independent prognostic factors in the treatment of non small-cell lung cancer: a review of National Cancer Institute of Canada Clinical Trials Group trials. *J Clin Oncol.* 2008 Jan 1;26(1):54-9.

[73] Naeim A, Reuben D. Geriatric syndromes and assessment in older cancer patients. *Oncology* (Williston Park). 2001 Dec;15(12):1567-77, 80; discussion 81, 86, 91.

[74] Eagles JM, Beattie JA, Restall DB, Rawlinson F, Hagen S, Ashcroft GW. Relation between cognitive impairment and early death in the elderly. *BMJ: British Medical Journal.* 1990;300(6719):239-40.

[75] Landi F, Onder G, Cattel C, Gambassi G, Lattanzio F, Cesari M, et al. Functional Status and Clinical Correlates in Cognitively Impaired Community-Living Older People. *J Geriatr Psychiatry Neurol.* 2001;14(1):21-7.

[76] Wolfson C, Wolfson DB, Asgharian M, M'Lan CE, Ostbye T, Rockwood K, et al. A Reevaluation of the Duration of Survival after the Onset of Dementia. *The New England Journal of Medicine.* 2001;344(15):1111-6.

[77] Feil D, Marmon T, Unutzer J. Congitive impairment, chronic medical illness, and risk of mortality in an elderly cohort. *Am J Geriatr Psychiatry.* 2003;11(5):551-60.

[78] Ferretti M, Seematter-Bagnoud L, Martin E, Bula CJ. New diagnoses of dementia among older patients admitted to postacute care. *J Am Med Dir Assoc.* 2010 Jun;11(5):371-6.

[79] Flood KL, Carroll MB, Le CV, Ball L, Esker DA, Carr DB. Geriatric Syndromes in Elderly Patients Admitted to an Oncology-Acute Care for Elders Unit. *J Clin Oncol.* 2006 May 20, 2006;24(15):2298-303.

[80] Gupta SK, Lamont EB. Patterns of Presentation, Diagnosis, and Treatment in Older Patients with Colon Cancer and Comorbid Dementia. *J Am Geriatr Soc.* 2004;52(10):1681-7.

[81] Gorin SS, Heck JE, Albert S, Hershman D. Treatment for breast cancer in patients with Alzheimer's disease. *J Am Geriatr Soc.* 2005 Nov;53(11):1897-904.

[82] Goodwin JS, Hunt WC, Samet JM. Determinants of cancer therapy in elderly patients. *Cancer.* 1993;72(2):594-601.

[83] Davis PB, Morris JC, Grant E. Brief screening tests versus clinical staging in senile dementia of the Alzheimer type. *J Am Geriatr Soc.* 1990 Feb;38(2):129-35.

[84] Burch EA, Jr., Andrews SR. Comparison of two cognitive rating scales in medically ill patients. *Int J Psychiatry Med.* 1987;17(2):193-200.

[85] Crum RM, Anthony JC, Bassett SS, Folstein MF. Population-based norms for the Mini-Mental State Examination by age and educational level. *JAMA.* 1993 May 12;269(18):2386-91.

[86] Wefel JS, Lenzi R, Theriault RL, Davis RN, Meyers CA. The cognitive sequelae of standard-dose adjuvant chemotherapy in women with breast carcinoma: results of a prospective, randomized, longitudinal trial. *Cancer.* 2004 Jun 1;100(11):2292-9.

[87] Schagen SB, van Dam FS, Muller MJ, Boogerd W, Lindeboom J, Bruning PF. Cognitive deficits after postoperative adjuvant chemotherapy for breast carcinoma. *Cancer.* 1999;85(3):640-50.

[88] van Dam FS, Schagen SB, Muller MJ, Boogerd W, v.d. Wall E, Droogleever Fortuyn ME, et al. Impairment of cognitive function in women receiving adjuvant treatment for high-risk breast cancer: high-dose versus standard-dose chemotherapy. *J Natl Cancer Inst.* 1998;90(3):210-8.

[89] Brezden CB, Phillips KA, Abdolell M, Bunston T, Tannock IF. Cognitive function in breast cancer patients receiving adjuvant chemotherapy. *J Clin Oncol.* 2000 Jul;18(14):2695-701.

[90] Castellon SA, Ganz PA, Bower JE, Petersen L, Abraham L, Greendale GA. Neurocognitive performance in breast cancer survivors exposed to adjuvant chemotherapy and tamoxifen. *J Clin Exp Neuropsychol.* 2004 Oct;26(7):955-69.

[91] Hurria A, Rosen C, Hudis C, Zuckerman E, Panageas KS, Lachs MS, et al. Cognitive function of older patients receiving adjuvant chemotherapy for breast cancer: a pilot prospective longitudinal study. *J Am Geriatr Soc.* 2006 Jun;54(6):925-31.

[92] Hurria A, Goldfarb S, Rosen C, Holland J, Zuckerman E, Lachs MS, et al. Effect of adjuvant breast cancer chemotherapy on cognitive function from the older patient's perspective. *Breast Cancer Res Treat.* 2006 Aug;98(3):343-8.

[93] Hurria A, Somlo G, Ahles T. Renaming "chemobrain". *Cancer Invest.* 2007 Sep;25(6):373-7.

[94] Rogers LQ, Courneya KS, Robbins KT, Rao K, Malone J, Seiz A, et al. Factors associated with fatigue, sleep, and cognitive function among patients with head and neck cancer. *Head Neck.* 2008 Oct;30(10):1310-7.

[95] Ahles TA, Saykin AJ, McDonald BC, Li Y, Furstenberg CT, Hanscom BS, et al. Longitudinal Assessment of Cognitive Changes Associated With Adjuvant Treatment for Breast Cancer: Impact of Age and Cognitive Reserve. *J Clin Oncol.* 2010;28(29):4434-40.

[96] Fried TR, Bradley EH, Towle VR, Allore H. Understanding the treatment preferences of seriously ill patients. N Engl J Med. 2002 Apr 4;346(14):1061-6.

[97] Kua J. The prevalence of psychological and psychiatric sequelae of cancer in the elderly - how much do we know? Ann Acad Med Singapore. 2005 Apr;34(3):250-6.

[98] Hurria A, Li D, Hansen K, Patil S, Gupta R, Nelson C, et al. Distress in older patients with cancer. *J Clin Oncol.* 2009 Sep 10;27(26):4346-51.

[99] Hoffman BM, Zevon MA, D'Arrigo MC, Cecchini TB. Screening for distress in cancer patients: the NCCN rapid-screening measure. *Psychooncology.* 2004 Nov;13(11):792-9.

[100] Jacobsen PB, Donovan KA, Trask PC, Fleishman SB, Zabora J, Baker F, et al. Screening for psychologic distress in ambulatory cancer patients. *Cancer.* 2005 Apr 1;103(7):1494-502.

[101] Mitchell AJ. Pooled results from 38 analyses of the accuracy of distress thermometer and other ultra-short methods of detecting cancer-related mood disorders. *J Clin Oncol.* 2007 Oct 10;25(29):4670-81.

[102] Byrne GJ, Pachana NA. Anxiety and depression in the elderly: do we know any more? *Curr Opin Psychiatry.* 2010 Nov;23(6):504-9.

[103] Penninx BW, Guralnik JM, Ferrucci L, Simonsick EM, Deeg DJ, Wallace RB. Depressive symptoms and physical decline in community-dwelling older persons. *JAMA.* 1998 Jun 3;279(21):1720-6.

[104] Bruce ML, Seeman TE, Merrill SS, Blazer DG. The impact of depressive symptomatology on physical disability: MacArthur Studies of Successful Aging. *Am J Public Health.* 1994 Nov;84(11):1796-9.

[105] Kissane D. Beyond the psychotherapy and survival debate: the challenge of social disparity, depression and treatment adherence in psychosocial cancer care. *Psychooncology.* 2009 Jan;18(1):1-5.

[106] Walker J, Waters RA, Murray G, Swanson H, Hibberd CJ, Rush RW, et al. Better off dead: suicidal thoughts in cancer patients. *J Clin Oncol.* 2008 Oct 10;26(29):4725-30.

[107] Miller M, Mogun H, Azrael D, Hempstead K, Solomon DH. Cancer and the risk of suicide in older Americans. *J Clin Oncol.* 2008 Oct 10;26(29):4720-4.

[108] Yesavage JA. Geriatric Depression Scale. *Psychopharmacol Bull.* 1988;24(4):709-11.

[109] Yesavage JA, Brink TL, Rose TL, Lum O, Huang V, Adey M, et al. Development and validation of a geriatric depression screening scale: a preliminary report. *J Psychiatr Res.* 1982;17(1):37-49.

[110] Tomaka J, Thompson S, Palacios R. The relation of social isolation, loneliness, and social support to disease outcomes among the elderly. *J Aging Health.* 2006 Jun;18 (3):359-84.

[111] Iwasaki M, Otani T, Sunaga R, Miyazaki H, Xiao L, Wang N, et al. Social networks and mortality based on the Komo-Ise cohort study in Japan. *Int J Epidemiol.* 2002 Dec;31(6):1208-18.

[112] Golden J, Conroy RM, Bruce I, Denihan A, Greene E, Kirby M, et al. Loneliness, social support networks, mood and wellbeing in community-dwelling elderly. *Int J Geriatr Psychiatry.* 2009 Jul;24(7):694-700.

[113] Weitzner MA, Haley WE, Chen H. The family caregiver of the older cancer patient. *Hematol Oncol Clin North Am.* 2000 Feb;14(1):269-81.

[114] DiMatteo MR. Social support and patient adherence to medical treatment: a meta-analysis. *Health Psychol.* 2004 Mar;23(2):207-18.

[115] Osborne C, Ostir GV, Du X, Peek MK, Goodwin JS. The influence of marital status on the stage at diagnosis, treatment, and survival of older women with breast cancer. *Breast Cancer Res Treat.* 2005 Sep;93(1):41-7.

[116] Wallace JI, Schwartz RS, LaCroix AZ, Uhlmann RF, Pearlman RA. Involuntary weight loss in older outpatients: incidence and clinical significance. *J Am Geriatr Soc.* 1995 Apr;43(4):329-37.

[117] Reynolds MW, Fredman L, Langenberg P, Magaziner J. Weight, weight change, mortality in a random sample of older community-dwelling women. *J Am Geriatr Soc.* 1999 Dec;47(12):1409-14.

[118] Grabowski DC, Ellis JE. High body mass index does not predict mortality in older people: analysis of the Longitudinal Study of Aging. *J Am Geriatr Soc.* 2001 Jul;49(7):968-79.

[119] Newman AB, Yanez D, Harris T, Duxbury A, Enright PL, Fried LP. Weight change in old age and its association with mortality. *J Am Geriatr Soc.* 2001 Oct;49(10):1309-18.

[120] Dewys WD, Begg C, Lavin PT, Band PR, Bennett JM, Bertino JR, et al. Prognostic effect of weight loss prior to chemotherapy in cancer patients. Eastern Cooperative Oncology Group. *Am J Med.* 1980 Oct;69(4):491-7.

[121] Andreyev HJ, Norman AR, Oates J, Cunningham D. Why do patients with weight loss have a worse outcome when undergoing chemotherapy for gastrointestinal malignancies? *Eur J Cancer.* 1998 Mar;34(4):503-9.

[122] Nourissat A, Vasson MP, Merrouche Y, Bouteloup C, Goutte M, Mille D, et al. Relationship between nutritional status and quality of life in patients with cancer. *Eur J Cancer.* 2008 Jun;44(9):1238-42.

[123] Locher JL, Robinson CO, Bailey FA, Carroll WR, Heimburger DC, Saif MW, et al. Disruptions in the organization of meal preparation and consumption among older cancer patients and their family caregivers. *Psychooncology.* 2010 Sep;19(9):967-74.

[124] Locher JL, Robinson CO, Bailey FA, Carroll WR, Heimburger DC, Magnuson JS, et al. The contribution of social factors to undereating in older adults with cancer. *J Support Oncol.* 2009 Sep-Oct;7(5):168-73.

[125] Vellas B, Villars H, Abellan G, Soto ME, Rolland Y, Guigoz Y, et al. Overview of the MNA--Its history and challenges. *J Nutr Health Aging.* 2006 Nov-Dec;10(6):456-63; discussion 63-5.

[126] Guigoz Y, Lauque S, Vellas BJ. Identifying the elderly at risk for malnutrition. The Mini Nutritional Assessment. *Clin Geriatr Med.* 2002 Nov;18(4):737-57.

[127] [Guigoz Y, Vellas B, Garry PJ. Assessing the nutritional status of the elderly: The Mini Nutritional Assessment as part of the geriatric evaluation. *Nutr Rev.* 1996 Jan;54(1 Pt 2):S59-65.

[128] Rubenstein LZ, Harker JO, Salva A, Guigoz Y, Vellas B. Screening for undernutrition in geriatric practice: developing the short-form mini-nutritional assessment (MNA-SF). *J Gerontol A Biol Sci Med Sci.* 2001 Jun;56(6):M366-72.

[129] Maggiore RJ, Gross CP, Hurria A. Polypharmacy in older adults with cancer. *Oncologist.* 2010;15(5):507-22.

[130] Clarfield AM, Bergman H, Kane R. Fragmentation of care for frail older people--an international problem. Experience from three countries: Israel, Canada, and the United States. *J Am Geriatr Soc.* 2001 Dec;49(12):1714-21.

[131] Yuen G. Altered pharmacokinetics in the elderly. *Clin Geratr Med.* 1990 May;6(2):257-67.

[132] Vestal RE. Aging and pharmacology. *Cancer.* 1997;80(7):1302-10.

[133] Baker S, Grochow L. Pharmacology of chemotherapy in the older person. *Clin Geriatr Med.* 1997 Feb;13(1):169-83.

[134] Sotaniemi E, Arranto A, Pelkonen O, Pasanen M. Age and cytochrome P450-linked drug metabolism in humans: an analysis of 226 subjects with equal histopathological conditions. *Clin Pharmacol Ther.* 1997 Mar;61(3):331-9.

[135] Fick DM, Cooper JW, Wade WE, Waller JL, Maclean JR, Beers MH. Updating the Beers criteria for potentially inappropriate medication use in older adults: results of a US consensus panel of experts. *Arch Intern Med.* 2003 Dec 8-22;163(22):2716-24.

[136] Lichtman SM, Villani G. Chemotherapy in the elderly: pharmacologic considerations. *Cancer Control.* 2000 Nov-Dec;7(6):548-56.

[137] Ingram SS, Seo PH, Martell RE, Clipp EC, Doyle ME, Montana GS, et al. Comprehensive assessment of the elderly cancer patient: the feasibility of self-report methodology. *J Clin Oncol.* 2002 Feb 1;20(3):770-5.

[138] Kemeny MM, Busch-Devereaux E, Merriam LT, O'Hea BJ. Cancer surgery in the elderly. *Hematol Oncol Clin North Am.* 2000 Feb;14(1):169-92.

[139] Ramesh HS, Pope D, Gennari R, Audisio RA. Optimising surgical management of elderly cancer patients. *World J Surg Oncol.* 2005 Mar 23;3(1):17.

[140] Audisio RA, Ramesh H, Longo WE, Zbar AP, Pope D. Preoperative assessment of surgical risk in oncogeriatric patients. *Oncologist.* 2005 Apr;10(4):262-8.

[141] Pope D, Ramesh H, Gennari R, Corsini G, Maffezzini M, Hoekstra HJ, et al. Preoperative assessment of cancer in the elderly (PACE): a comprehensive assessment of underlying characteristics of elderly cancer patients prior to elective surgery. *Surg Oncol.* 2006 Dec;15(4):189-97.

[142] Audisio RA, Pope D, Ramesh HS, Gennari R, van Leeuwen BL, West C, et al. Shall we operate? Preoperative assessment in elderly cancer patients (PACE) can help. A SIOG surgical task force prospective study. *Crit Rev Oncol Hematol.* 2008 Feb;65(2):156-63.

[143] Ramesh HS, Jain S, Audisio RA. Implications of aging in surgical oncology. *Cancer J.* 2005 Nov-Dec;11(6):488-94.

[144] Bremmer MA, Beekman AT, Deeg DJ, Penninx BW, Dik MG, Hack CE, et al. Inflammatory markers in late-life depression: results from a population-based study. *J Affect Disord.* 2008 Mar;106(3):249-55.

[145] Hurria A, Togawa K, Mohile SG, Owusu C, Klepin HD, Gross C, et al. Predicting chemotherapy toxicity in older adults with cancer: a prospective 500 patient multicenter study. *J Clin Oncol.* 2010;28:15s (suppl; abstr 9001).

[146] Extermann M, Boler I, Reich R, Lyman GH, Brown RH, DeFelice J, et al. The chemotherapy risk assessment sclae for high-age patients (CRASH) score: design and validation. *J Clin Oncol.* 2010;28:15s (suppl;abstr 9000).

[147] Klepin H, Mohile S, Hurria A. Geriatric assessment in older patients with breast cancer. *J Natl Compr Canc Netw.* 2009 Feb;7(2):226-36.

[148] Saliba D, Elliott M, Rubenstein LZ, Solomon DH, Young RT, Kamberg CJ, et al. The Vulnerable Elders Survey: a tool for identifying vulnerable older people in the community. *J Am Geriatr Soc.* 2001 Dec;49(12):1691-9.

[149] Podsiadlo D, Richardson S. The timed "Up and Go": a test of basic functional mobility for frail elderly persons. *J Am Geriatr Soc.* 1991 Feb;39(2):142-8.

[150] Folstein MF, Folstein SE, McHugh PR. "Mini-mental state". A practical method for grading the cognitive state of patients for the clinician. *J Psychiatr Res.* 1975 Nov;12(3):189-98.

[151] Katzman R, Brown T, Fuld P, Peck A, Schechter R, Schimmel H. Validation of a short Orientation-Memory-Concentration Test of cognitive impairment. *Am J Psychiatry.* 1983 Jun;140(6):734-9.

[152] Pfeiffer E. A short portable mental status questionnaire for the assessment of organic brain deficit in elderly patients. *J Am Geriatr Soc.* 1975 Oct;23(10):433-41.

[153] Sherbourne CD, Stewart AL. The MOS social support survey. *Soc Sci Med.* 1991;32(6):705-14.

Index

C

D

E

F

G

H

I

S

T

U

V